2011
YEAR BOOK OF
PLASTIC AND
AESTHETIC SURGERY™

The 2011 Year Book Series

Year Book of Anesthesiology and Pain Management™: Drs Chestnut, Abram, Black, Gravlee, Lien, Mathru and Roizen

Year Book of Cardiology®: Drs Gersh, Cheitlin, Elliott, Gold, Graham, and Suri

Year Book of Critical Care Medicine®: Drs Dellinger, Parrillo, Balk, Dorman, Dries, and Zanotti-Cavazzoni

Year Book of Dermatology and Dermatologic Surgery™: Dr Del Rosso

Year Book of Diagnostic Radiology®: Drs Osborn, Abbara, Birdwell, Elster, Manaster, Oestreich, Offiah, Rosado de Christenson, and Walker

Year Book of Emergency Medicine®: Drs Hamilton, Bruno, Handly, Mullin, Quintana, and Ramoska

Year Book of Endocrinology®: Drs Schott, Apovian, Clarke, Eugster, Ludlam, Meikle, Ovalle, Schinner, Schteingart, and Toth

Year Book of Gastroenterology™: Drs Talley, Ambikaipaker, Bollipo, DeVault, Harnois, Pearson, Picco, Rombeau, Scolapio, and Smith

Year Book of Hand and Upper Limb Surgery®: Drs Yao and Steinmann

Year Book of Medicine®: Drs Barker, Berney, Garrick, Gersh, Khardori, LeRoith, Talley, and Thigpen

Year Book of Neonatal and Perinatal Medicine®: Drs Fanaroff, Benitz, Donn, Neu, and Papile

Year Book of Neurology and Neurosurgery®: Drs Klimo and Rabinstein

Year Book of Obstetrics, Gynecology, and Women's Health®: Drs Dungan and Shulman

Year Book of Oncology®: Drs Thigpen, Arceci, Bauer, Byhardt, Gordon, and Lawton

Year Book of Ophthalmology®: Drs Rapuano, Cohen, Flanders, Hammersmith, Milman, Myers, Nelson, Penne, Pyfer, Sergott, Shields, and Vander

Year Book of Orthopedics®: Drs Morrey, Beauchamp, Huddleston, Swiontkowski, and Trigg

Year Book of Otolaryngology-Head and Neck Surgery®: Drs Sindwani, Balough, Franco, Gapany, and Mitchell

Year Book of Pathology and Laboratory Medicine®: Drs Raab, Parwani, Bejarano, and Bissell

Year Book of Pediatrics®: Dr Stockman

Year Book of Plastic and Aesthetic Surgery™: Drs Miller, Gosain, Gurtner, Gutowski, Ruberg, Salisbury, and Smith

Year Book of Psychiatry and Applied Mental Health®: Drs Talbott, Ballenger, Buckley, Frances, Krupnick, and Mack

Year Book of Pulmonary Disease®: Drs Barker, Jones, Maurer, Raza, Tanoue, and Willsie

Year Book of Sports Medicine®: Drs Shephard, Cantu, Feldman, Jankowski, Khan, Lebrun, Nieman, Pierrynowski, and Rowland

Year Book of Surgery®: Drs Copeland, Behrns, Daly, Eberlein, Fahey, Huber, Jones, Mozingo, and Pruett

Year Book of Urology®: Drs Andriole and Coplen

Year Book of Vascular Surgery®: Drs Moneta, Gillespie, Starnes, and Watkins

2011

The Year Book of PLASTIC AND AESTHETIC SURGERY™

Editor-in-Chief
Stephen H. Miller, MD, MPH
Voluntary Clinical Professor of Surgery and Family Medicine, University of California at San Diego, San Diego, California

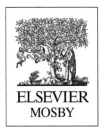

ELSEVIER
MOSBY

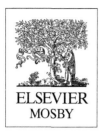

ELSEVIER
MOSBY

Vice President, Continuity: Kimberly Murphy
Senior Clinics Editor: Barbara Cohen-Kligerman
Production Manager, Electronic Year Books: Donna M. Skelton
Electronic Article Manager: Emily Ogle
Illustrations and Permissions Coordinator: Dawn Vohsen

Composition by TnQ Books and Journals Pvt Ltd, India

Editorial Office:
Elsevier
1600 John F. Kennedy Blvd.
Suite 1800
Philadelphia, PA 19103-2899

International Standard Serial Number: 1535-1513
International Standard Book Number: 978-0-323-08174-0

Printed and bound by CPI Group (UK) Ltd, Croydon, CR0 4YY

Transferred to Digital Print 2011

Editorial Board

Table of Contents

Journals Represented

Journals represented in this YEAR BOOK are listed below.

Acta Oto-Laryngologica
Aesthetic Plastic Surgery
Aesthetic Surgery Journal
American Journal of Orthodontics and Dentofacial Orthopedics
American Journal of Surgery
American Surgeon
Annals of Plastic Surgery
Annals of Surgery
Annals of Surgical Oncology
Archives of Facial Plastic Surgery
Archives of Surgery
Arthroscopy
Breast Journal
British Journal of Dermatology
British Journal of Oral & Maxillofacial Surgery
British Journal of Radiology
British Journal of Surgery
Burns
Cancer
Dermatologic Surgery
Dermatology
European Journal of Cancer
European Journal of Plastic Surgery
Fertility and Sterility
Foot & Ankle International
Injury
International Journal of Cancer
International Journal of Oral and Maxillofacial Surgery
Journal of Burn Care & Research
Journal of Clinical Microbiology
Journal of Computer Assisted Tomography
Journal of the European Academy of Dermatology and Venereology
Journal of Hand Surgery
Journal of Neurosurgery
Journal of Oral and Maxillofacial Surgery
Journal of Plastic, Reconstructive & Aesthetic Surgery
Journal of Reconstructive Microsurgery
Journal of the American Academy of Dermatology
Journal of the American College of Surgeons
Lancet
Medicine
Microsurgery
New England Journal of Medicine
Oral Surgery Oral Medicine Oral Pathology Oral Radiology and Endodontics
Otolaryngology-Head and Neck Surgery
Otology & Neurotology
Pediatrics

Plastic and Reconstructive Surgery
Surgery
The Cleft Palate-Craniofacial Journal
World Journal of Surgery
Wound Repair and Regeneration

STANDARD ABBREVIATIONS

The following terms are abbreviated in this edition: acquired immunodeficiency syndrome (AIDS), cardiopulmonary resuscitation (CPR), central nervous system (CNS), cerebrospinal fluid (CSF), computed tomography (CT), deoxyribonucleic acid (DNA), electrocardiography (ECG), health maintenance organization (HMO), human immunodeficiency virus (HIV), intensive care unit (ICU), intramuscular (IM), intravenous (IV), magnetic resonance (MR) imaging (MRI), ribonucleic acid (RNA), ultrasound (US), and ultraviolet (UV).

NOTE

The YEAR BOOK OF PLASTIC AND AESTHETIC SURGERY is a literature survey service providing abstracts of articles published in the professional literature. Every effort is made to assure the accuracy of the information presented in these pages. Neither the editors nor the publisher of the YEAR BOOK OF PLASTIC AND AESTHETIC SURGERY can be responsible for errors in the original materials. The editors' comments are their own opinions. Mention of specific products within this publication does not constitute endorsement.

To facilitate the use of the YEAR BOOK OF PLASTIC AND AESTHETIC SURGERY as a reference tool, all illustrations and tables included in this publication are now identified as they appear in the original article. This change is meant to help the reader recognize that any illustration or table appearing in the YEAR BOOK OF PLASTIC AND AESTHETIC SURGERY may be only one of many in the original article. For this reason, figure and table numbers will often appear to be out of sequence within the YEAR BOOK OF PLASTIC AND AESTHETIC SURGERY.

Introduction

As we present this hard copy edition of the 2011 Year Book of Plastic and Aesthetic Surgery, it seems worthwhile for this Editor, who has been with the Year Book for almost 20 years, to reflect on the current state of communication technology and how it has transformed the Year Book of Plastic and Aesthetic Surgery into a more timely, user-friendly, and interactive resource.

Several of the more important innovations have been (1) the opportunity to distribute selected articles for review to the appropriate associate editors within a very short time of their publication; (2) the ability to allow the associate editors to peruse a wide variety of literature from multiple journals, some of which are not usually associated with plastic surgery, to seek and incorporate articles into the Year Book of Plastic and Aesthetic Surgery that they believe may be of interest to our readership; and (3) the possibility to allow more than one associate editor to select the same article to review and critique, which gives readers the opportunity to benefit from the experience of more than one reviewer.

Another important innovation is eClips Consult (available at www.eclips.consult.com), which allows readers to access articles and commentaries online on an ongoing basis. An added feature of eClips Consult is that each reviewed article is assessed according to evidence-based medicine criteria and ranked according to its value and importance as perceived by the reviewer. Ultimately, in my opinion, one of the most important aspects of eClips Consult is the opportunity for the readers to participate and comment on the articles and reviews. This provides the authors of articles with insights from a wider audience than is currently possible and also expands the experience of readers to include the views of other readers.

I express my sincere appreciation to the following long-standing Associate Editors, Drs Robert L. Ruberg, Roger E. Salisbury, and David J. Smith, Jr, who continue to do a terrific job of combing through literature on a regular basis to find articles that they believe to be worthwhile and beneficial to our readership. I also express my appreciation to our new Associate Editors, Drs Arun Gosain, Geoffrey C. Gurtner, and Karol A. Gutowski, and to recognize their hard work and dedication in learning the ropes so quickly and in participating in bringing this 2011 Year Book to fruition. Thank you to Dr James Chao, Associate Professor of Surgery, University of California San Diego, for his contributions to this Year Book.

Thanks once again to Barbara Cohen-Kligerman, Senior Clinics Editor with Elsevier, for her patience with us and for her dedication to the many tasks required to publish the Year Book and facilitate posting of reviews on eClips.

I call the reader's attention to the expanded section on Skin, Soft Tissues, and Hair in Chapter 5, which now also includes fillers. The reader should also pay attention to the articles on "Benchmarking Outcomes in Plastic Surgery: National Complication Rates for Abdominoplasty and Breast Augmentation" in Chapter 5, and to "Assessing the Plastic Surgery Workforce: A Template for the Future of Plastic Surgery" and "Reviewing the World's Experience with Facial Transplantation" in Chapter 9.

Stephen H. Miller, MD, MPH

1 Congenital

Auricular Deformities

Auricular Reconstruction for Microtia: Personal 6-Year Experience Based on 350 Microtia Ear Reconstructions in China

Zhang Q, Zhang R, Xu F, et al (Shanghai JiaoTong Univ, People's Republic of China)
Plast Reconstr Surg 123:849-858, 2009

Background.—Favorable results in auricular reconstruction are difficult to achieve. The authors report 350 patients with different types of microtia who underwent total ear reconstruction. The youngest was aged 5.5 years and the oldest was aged 50 years.

Methods.—The authors performed auricular reconstruction using autologous costal cartilage with the combination of the Brent and Nagata

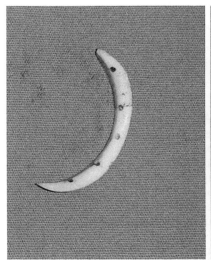 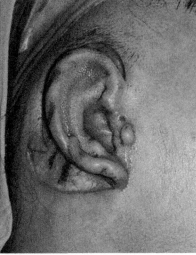

FIGURE 5.—(*Left*) Bone cement with a special semilunar shape and small pores. It is 2 mm wider at the north and south poles. (*Right*) Immediate view of an ideal long axis after fixation. (Reprinted from Zhang Q, Zhang R, Xu F, et al. Auricular reconstruction for microtia: personal 6-year experience based on 350 microtia ear reconstructions in China. *Plast Reconstr Surg.* 2009;123:849-858, with permission from the American Society of Plastic Surgeons.)

TABLE 2.—Age at Surgery

Age	No. of Patients (%)
5.5 years	3 (0.8)
6–7 years	34 (9.7)
8–10 years	45 (12.9)
11–15 years	112 (32.0)
16–20 years	87 (24.9)
21–40 years	65 (18.6)
41–50 years	4 (1.1)

TABLE 3.—Classification

Type	No. of Patients (%)
Lobule	278 (79.4)
Concha	72 (20.6)
Total	350 (100)

TABLE 5.—Complications at the Reconstructed Ear Side

Complications	Stage	Reasons	No. of Patients (%)
Broken helix	I	Calcified cartilage	1 (0.3)
Partial skin necrosis	I	Pedicle impairment	1 (0.3)
Blunted convolution	I	Failure of negative suction and body weight gain in a short period	5 (1.4)
Infection			
Extrusion of the cartilage	I	Block-corner like structure	1 (0.3)
No extrusion of the cartilage	I	Diabetes	1 (0.3)
Extrusion of the cartilage on the back of the framework	II	Strong tie-over dressing	3 (0.9)
Hypertrophic scars	II	Unclear	21 (6.0)

methods, with some modifications. At the first stage, an individualized framework fabrication based on different degrees of strength and thickness of the rib cartilages was performed. One piece of cartilage was added vertically under the reconstructed tragus to enhance conchal depth to provide a more prominent appearance. At the second stage, the elevated reconstructed ear was supported by bone cement with a special shape that was 2 mm wider at the end of two poles, giving the reconstructed ear more projection on the upper and lower poles. This external ear morphology occurs quite often in China.

Results.—In this series, the follow-up time in 322 patients ranged from 8 months to 6 years. Two hundred eighty-eight patients were satisfied with the results, including good shape, accurate size, right orientation, and duplication of more than 10 well-detailed structures. Surgery-related complications such as broken helix, skin necrosis, infection, blunted convolution, and extrusion of cartilage occurred in 13 cases and hypertrophic scars occurred in 21 patients.

Conclusions.—The authors' techniques produce acceptable results and fewer complications. This 6-year experience confirms the reliability, versatility, and reproducibility of this type of combined technique in auricular reconstruction, especially for Asian patients (Fig 5, Tables 2, 3 and 5).

▶ This article reviews microtia reconstruction in 350 patients operated on during a 6-year period. The patients ranged from age 5.5 to 50 years (see Table 2), with the most common age group being 11 to 15 years (32% of patients). Classification of microtia was approximately 80% lobule type and approximately 20% concha type (see Table 3), with 44% of patients having hemifacial microsomia. The interesting contribution of the article is the technique for microtia repair, which the authors state is a combination of the techniques developed by Dr Brent and Dr Nagata. The authors describe this technique in detail. The reconstructive technique that varies the most from that of the preceding authors is the use of bone cement for second stage elevation of the cartilage framework (see Fig 5). This varies from the techniques both of Nagata, who reharvests rib cartilage for second stage elevation, and of Brent. Coverage of bone cement is achieved using a retroauricular fascial flap, again departing from Nagata's technique that utilizes a temporoparietal fascia flap for coverage of the second stage cartilage elevation. The authors present several of their results, which appear to be of very high quality. Complications are minimal in the authors' hands, with hypertrophic scar being the most common complication observed, occurring in 6% of the cases (see Table 5). The authors point out that hypertrophic scars may be more common in the Oriental population, which is why a series in the United States may have a lower incidence of this problem. While the authors present a very effective technique in their patient population, some unanswered questions that remain are as follows: How do they handle patients who present with a low hairline? Is the flap depilated, or do the authors advocate the use of laser or electrolysis in these patients? If so, do they do so before or after construction of the cartilage framework? Handled? Is there ever a need for a temporoparietal fascia flap either at the first or second stage? Although the authors advocate the use of the retroauricular fascial flap at the second stage, is this flap ever found to be insufficient for adequate coverage? One questions whether the authors are augmenting the cartilage framework to the extent that Nagata does, which may be why the authors did not have difficulty obtaining adequate coverage with retroauricular fascia alone.

A. Gosain, MD

Auricular Reconstruction for Microtia: Personal 6-Year Experience Based on 350 Microtia Ear Reconstructions in China
Zhang Q, Zhang R, Xu F, et al (Shanghai JiaoTong Univ, People's Republic of China)
Plast Reconstr Surg 123:849-858, 2009

Background.—Favorable results in auricular reconstruction are difficult to achieve. The authors report 350 patients with different types of microtia who underwent total ear reconstruction. The youngest was aged 5.5 years and the oldest was aged 50 years.

Methods.—The authors performed auricular reconstruction using autologous costal cartilage with the combination of the Brent and Nagata methods, with some modifications. At the first stage, an individualized framework fabrication based on different degrees of strength and thickness of the rib cartilages was performed. One piece of cartilage was added vertically under the reconstructed tragus to enhance conchal depth to provide a more prominent appearance. At the second stage, the elevated reconstructed ear was supported by bone cement with a special shape that was 2 mm wider at the end of two poles, giving the reconstructed ear more projection on the upper and lower poles. This external ear morphology occurs quite often in China.

Results.—In this series, the follow-up time in 322 patients ranged from 8 months to 6 years. Two hundred eighty-eight patients were satisfied with the results, including good shape, accurate size, right orientation, and duplication of more than 10 well-detailed structures. Surgery-related complications such as broken helix, skin necrosis, infection, blunted convolution, and extrusion of cartilage occurred in 13 cases and hypertrophic scars occurred in 21 patients.

Conclusions.—The authors' techniques produce acceptable results and fewer complications. This 6-year experience confirms the reliability, versatility, and reproducibility of this type of combined technique in auricular reconstruction, especially for Asian patients (Figs 4-6).

▶ This is a large personal series detailing microtia reconstruction in an Asian population. Modifying the techniques of Brent[1] and Nagata[2] to suit their patient population has resulted in some very good aesthetic reconstructions (Figs 4-6). Particularly noteworthy are their discussions of individualizing the reconstructive technique, vis a vis sculpting or building the cartilage components depending on the thickness and strength of the patient's costal cartilage, adding cartilage to emphasize the conchal depth and using bone cement to elevate the ear from the side of the head (Figs 4,5). In several patients the helical rim-lobule junction is smooth and continuous, but in other patients it is not (Fig 6).

S. H. Miller, MD, MPH

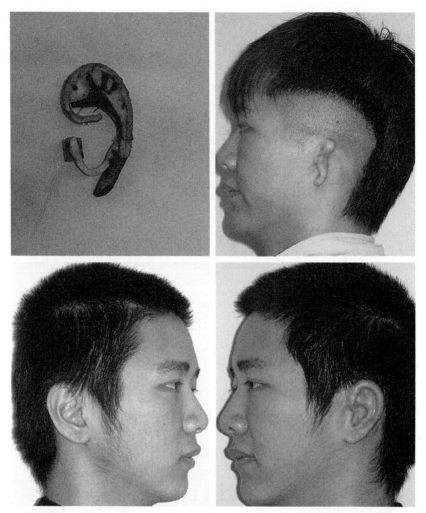

FIGURE 4.—A 19-year-old man with congenital microtia on the left side. (*Above, left*) One piece of cartilage is added vertically under the tragus (*red arrow*). (*Above, right*) Preoperative view. (*Below, left*) Normal side. (*Below, right*) Two-year postoperative view. For interpretation of the references to color in this figure legend, the reader is referred to web version of this article. (Reprinted from Zhang Q, Zhang R, Xu F, et al. Auricular reconstruction for microtia: personal 6-year experience based on 350 microtia ear reconstructions in china. *Plast Reconstr Surg.* 2009;123:849-858.)

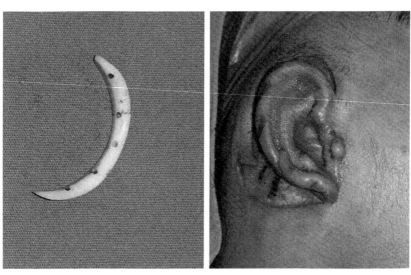

FIGURE 5.—(*Left*) Bone cement with a special semilunar shape and small pores. It is 2 mm wider at the north and south poles. (*Right*) Immediate view of an ideal long axis after fixation. (Reprinted from Zhang Q, Zhang R, Xu F, et al. Auricular reconstruction for microtia: personal 6-year experience based on 350 microtia ear reconstructions in china. *Plast Reconstr Surg.* 2009;123:849-858.)

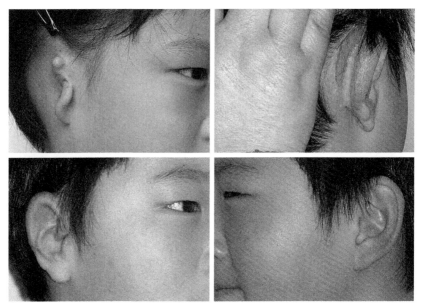

FIGURE 6.—An 8-year-old boy with congenital microtia on the right side. (*Above, left*) Preoperative view. (*Above, right*) The repaired auricular cephalic sulcus. (*Below, left*) Two-year postoperative view. (*Below, right*) Normal side. (Reprinted from Zhang Q, Zhang R, Xu F, et al. Auricular reconstruction for microtia: personal 6-year experience based on 350 microtia ear reconstructions in china. *Plast Reconstr Surg.* 2009;123:849-858.)

References

1. Brent B. Technical advances in ear reconstruction with autologous rib cartilage grafts: personal experience with 1200 cases. *Plast Reconst Surg.* 1999;104: 319-338.
2. Nagata S. Modification of the stages of total reconstruction of the auricle;part IV. *Plast Reconst Surg.* 1994;93:254-268.

A New Method for the Second-Stage Auricular Projection of the Nagata Method: Ultra-Delicate Split-Thickness Skin Graft in Continuity with Full-Thickness Skin

Chen Z-C, Goh RCW, Chen PK-T, et al (Chang-Gung Memorial Hosp, Taoyuan, Taiwan; Chang-Gung Univ, Taoyuan, Taiwan; Nagata Microtia and Reconstructive Plastic Surgery Clinic, Saitama, Japan)
Plast Reconstr Surg 124:1477-1485, 2009

Background.—Staged auricular reconstruction remains mainstream among the various techniques of microtia reconstruction using autogenous costal cartilage. The initial stage involves fabrication and implantation of the cartilage framework, followed by projection of the reconstructed auricle in the second stage. During the projection stage, the line of incision is usually made close to the helical rim, from the superoanterior margin of the helical rim to the region of the lobule. Generally, a fascial flap is raised and covered over a cartilage block to project the auricle, and a skin graft is inset over the raw surface of the newly created postauricular sulcus.

Methods.—The authors developed a new refinement for the second-stage auricular projection, whereby the skin cover for the raw surface over the posterior aspect of the auricle and the postauricular sulcus is an ultra-delicate split-thickness skin graft raised in continuity with the full-thickness skin over the anterior aspect of the auricle.

Results.—Incorporation of this new technique has minimized the visibility of suture lines and improved the appearance of the superior otobasion. In addition, the dimension of the skin cover required can be designed with greater precision. Postoperative outcomes using this new technique for auricular projection have been more than satisfactory.

Conclusion.—More favorable results that carry less surgical stigma can now be achieved in auricular reconstruction using this new modification of Nagata's two-stage method (Figs 2 and 6).

▶ This article from Nagata and his colleagues represents the state of the art in microtia reconstruction. Although the technique is not modified significantly, it provides an important review of the 2-stage reconstructive technique for microtia. These stages consist of (1) creation and implantation of the ear cartilage framework and (2) projection of the reconstructed auricle. Upon projection of the reconstructed auricle, the exposed postauricular region is covered with a temporoparietal fascial flap. This article describes a modification for lining of the elevated ear framework and temporoparietal fascial flap. In Nagata's

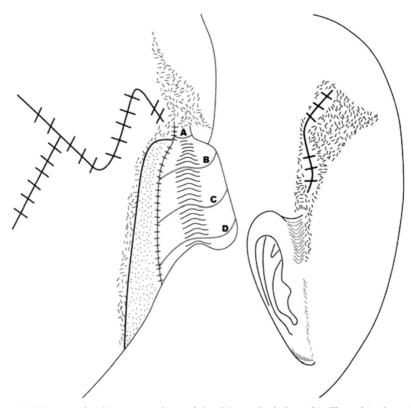

FIGURE 2.—(*Left*) Advancement and inset of ultra-delicate split-thickness skin. The graft is advanced caudally while the upper portion remains attached to the auricle. This posterior illustration reveals that the there is no incision along the outer margin of the helical rim as present in the original description of Nagata's second-stage auricular projection method. Overall, aesthetic appearance is enhanced as a result. (*Right*) The superior region of the reconstructed auricle is shown in this illustration. Note the absence of sharp angulations at the superior otobasion, which produces a more natural superior pole. (Reprinted from Chen Z-C, Goh RCW, Chen PK-T, et al. A new method for the second-stage auricular projection of the Nagata method: ultra-delicate split-thickness skin graft in continuity with full-thickness skin. *Plast Reconstr Surg.* 2009;124:1477-1485, with permission from the American Society of Plastic Surgeons.)

initial technique, a separate skin graft was harvested and inset over the temporoparietal fascial flap. In the present modification a single composite unit of ultra-delicate split-thickness skin is harvested in continuity with the native full-thickness skin over the reconstructed auricle (Fig 2). The split-thickness skin harvested from hair-bearing scalp with dimensions matching that of the contralateral postauricular surface. This composite unit of split-thickness skin and full-thickness skin is then advanced anterocaudally to cover the posterior surface of the auricle, as well as the postauricular sulcus, thereby avoiding a visible suture line in the superior half of the reconstructed auricle (Fig 6). While the modification described produces excellent results, it is not clear if there is a great advantage over simply harvesting a thin split-thickness skin graft from temporal scalp to resurface that area not covered by the full-thickness skin over the reconstructed auricle. The latter technique would be much less

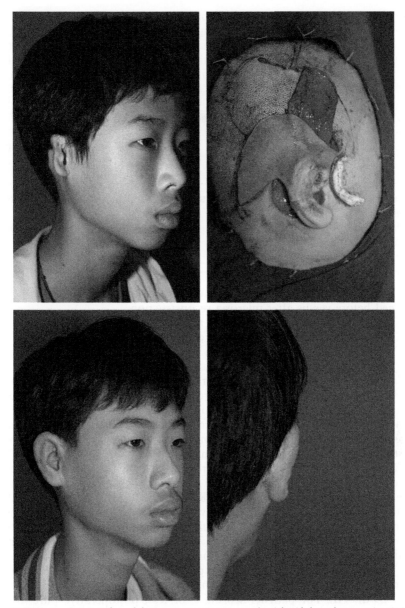

FIGURE 6.—Case 4. (*Above, left*) Preoperative appearance of a right-sided concha-type microtia in a 13-year-old boy. (*Above, right*) Intraoperative view shows the ultra-delicate split-thickness skin in continuity with the native full-thickness skin coverage. (*Below*) Postoperative views reveal a well-projected, natural-appearing auricle with no conspicuous scarring. (Reprinted from Chen Z-C, Goh RCW, Chen PK-T, et al. A new method for the second-stage auricular projection of the Nagata method: ultra-delicate split-thickness skin graft in continuity with full-thickness skin. *Plast Reconstr Surg.* 2009;124:1477-1485, with permission from the American Society of Plastic Surgeons.)

complex and not require the intricate planning shown in Fig 2. Maintaining continuity between the full-thickness and split-thickness skin is unlikely to provide vascularity to the split-thickness portion of the skin, and it appears that this unit functions as a graft rather than as a flap. The advantage of avoiding a visible suture line at the junction of full- and split-thickness skin is valid, but without showing photos of such a suture line long-term, it is difficult to judge whether the final outcome of the present technique is a significant advancement over that in which a separate split-thickness skin graft is harvested.

A. Gosain, MD

Atresia Repair Before Microtia Reconstruction: Comparison of Early With Standard Surgical Timing
Roberson JB Jr, Reinisch J, Colen TY, et al (California Ear Inst, Palo Alto/San Ramon; Cedar Sinai Med Ctr, CA)
Otol Neurotol 30:771-776, 2009

Objective.—To compare short-term results of atresia repair when performed before versus after microtia reconstruction.

Study Design.—Retrospective case review.

Setting.—Tertiary otologic referral center.

Patients.—Congenital aural atresia with or without microtia: 70 cases over 24 months.

Intervention.—Atresia repair before Medpor microtia reconstruction (ARM) versus atresia repair after microtia reconstruction with autogenous rib (ARR) versus atresia reconstruction without microtia (AR).

Main Outcome Measures.—Surgical outcomes, short-term postoperative audiometric results (at least 4 months after surgery but within the first postoperative year), complications.

Results.—Data from the 3 groups are as follows: ARM, 31 patients with median age 4.2 years (range, 2.5–9.3 yr); ARR, 28 patients with median age 12 years (range, 6.9–61); and AR, 11 patients with median age 5.9 years (range, 5.5–59 yr). Preoperative computed tomographic grading using the Jahrsdoerfer scale demonstrated an average score of 7.4 (range, 6–9) for the ARM group, 7.7 (range, 6–9) for the ARR group, and 8.5 (range, 8–9) for the AR group. For patients scoring 8 to 10 on the Jahrsdoerfer scale, postoperative pure-tone average 2 for each group were as follows: ARM, 28 dB hearing loss (HL); ARR, 32 dB HL; and AR, 29 dB HL. For patients scoring 7 or less, postoperative pure-tone average 2 were as follows: ARM, 42 dB HL; and ARR, 41 dB HL (AR, no patients). Surgical complications of infection and facial nerve injury were not seen in any group. Meatal stenosis was higher in the ARR group. One patient in the ARM group suffered a high-frequency sensorineural HL. No patient receiving Medpor microtia reconstruction suffered a complication due to the presence of the ear canal before microtia reconstruction.

TABLE 1.—Short-Term Complications of Atresia Repair in the 3 Study Groups

	ARM (31)	ARR (28)	AR (11)
Infection	0	0	0
Lateralized TM	1	1	1
Meatal stenosis	1	3	1
SNHL	1	0	0
Facial injury	0	0	0
TM perf	2	1	0

Conclusion.—Early results of ARM compare favorably with results achieved with atresia repair after microtia reconstruction with autogenous rib cartilage and with atresia repair without microtia repair. Hearing outcome and complications in this study are also comparable with previously reported expert results Because restoration of binaural hearing has been shown to be advantageous for auditory development and function, timing of atresia repair can be considered before microtia reconstruction on an individual case basis, provided preoperative computed tomographic evaluation shows an adequate chance of surgical success (Table 1).

▶ This article addresses an important question that is still a topic of debate: How should one coordinate auricular reconstruction for microtia and atresia repair, and is there any consequence on subsequent hearing by varying the sequence and timing of surgery? Seventy patients fell into 1 of the 3 protocols described (Atresia repair before Medpor microtia reconstruction [ARM], atresia repair after microtia reconstruction with autogenous rib [ARR], and atresia reconstruction without microtia [AR]). In 2 groups, atresia repair was performed without secondary delay due to microtia reconstruction, either because microtia reconstruction followed completion of atresia repair (ARM, $n = 31$) or because microtia reconstruction was not performed (AR, $n = 11$). Median age of atresia repair in these 2 groups was 4.2 years and 5.9 years, respectively, whereas median age of atresia repair in the ARR group was 12 years. However, the age range for atresia repair in the AR and ARR groups was significantly greater than in the ARM group, with the oldest patient in the ARM group being 9.3 years, the oldest patient in the AR group being 59 years, and the oldest patient in the ARR group was 61 years. The much more consistent age range for atresia repair in the ARM group suggests that these patients were placed on a protocol whereby atresia repair was completed before 10 years of age to allow these patients to undergo microtia reconstruction, whereas the latter 2 groups had no such protocol, and atresia repair may have been done as an afterthought in these patients. Despite this variability in protocol, the authors' findings that hearing loss postatresia repair was not significantly different between any of the groups is somewhat counterintuitive, as one would expect the ARM group to have the best hearing outcomes due to the younger age of repair. This finding suggests that with respect to hearing outcomes, age of atresia repair is not of consequence and should not be a factor in deciding the sequence of atresia repair and microtia reconstruction. The only other factors that the authors studied were complications of atresia repair in the 3 groups (Table 1). Of the 6 complications reviewed, the incidence of any given complication was too small to draw a valid conclusion. However, the authors comment that meatal stenosis was more common in the ARR group (3/28 patients) relative to the ARM group (1/31 patients) or the AR group (1/11 patients). This conclusion does not appear to be warranted, because the incidence of meatal stenosis was essentially the same in the ARR and the AR groups. Therefore, one cannot attribute the type of ear reconstruction or the sequence of ear reconstruction versus atresia repair on the likelihood of developing meatal stenosis, because patients who did not have any ear reconstruction were just as likely to develop this complication as those who had reconstruction with rib cartilage. In summary, it appears that the sequence of surgery—atresia repair and microtia reconstruction—remains the preference of the surgeon, because no convincing data are presented indicating that any of the approaches studied results in differences in the outcomes studied. This alone is useful information, because if a patient requests both microtia reconstruction and atresia repair, they should be informed that the sequence of surgical repairs can be individualized.

A. Gosain, MD

Combined Fascial Flap and Expanded Skin Flap for Enveloping Medpor Framework in Microtia Reconstruction
Yang S-L, Zheng J-H, Ding Z, et al (Shanghai Jiao Tong Univ, People's Republic of China)
Aesthetic Plast Surg 33:518-522, 2009

The Medpor implant is another choice for a new auricular framework besides autogenous costal cartilage. However, its relatively frequent exposure and less-matching skin coverage discourage surgeons from using it. In this article, we present a new two-flap method, a combination of the temporoparietal fascial flap and the expanded skin flap, for wrapping the Medpor implant in microtia reconstruction. A staged surgical procedure was performed, including soft tissue expansion in the mastoid region, soft tissue expander removal, expanded skin flap and temporoparietal fascial flap formation, Medpor framework implantation, and the combined two-flap envelopment. Conventional lobule transposition and tragus reconstruction were accomplished for selected patients. In this study, a total of 22 microtias were reconstructed consecutively using this method. Eighteen patients were followed since the first surgery. The postoperative follow-up time ranged from 3 to 12 months. The draped soft tissue covering was thin enough to show the reconstructed ear with excellent, subtle contour when edema gradually vanished 3-6 months postoperatively. The new ear had a stable shape, and its skin color and texture matched the normal surrounding skin very well. No exposure or extrusion of the framework was observed in the series. The Medpor implant enveloped by both a temporoparietal fascial flap and an expanded cutaneous flap appears to be a promising alternative for the auricular framework

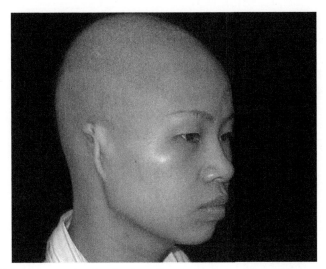

FIGURE 1.—A preoperative view showing unilateral microtia in a 26-year-old woman. (Reprinted from Yang S-L, Zheng J-H, Ding Z, et al. Combined fascial flap and expanded skin flap for enveloping medpor framework in microtia reconstruction. *Aesthetic Plast Surg.* 2009;33:518-522, with permission from Springer Science+Business Media.)

in microtia reconstruction. Because of the wrapping tissues, auricular construction using a Medpor implant can be a safe, steady, and easily acceptable choice for both microtia patients and their physicians (Figs 1, 3 and 5).

▶ Certainly autologous ear reconstruction in patients with microtia continues to be difficult, especially for the surgeon who attempts to do a case every now and then. One might make the point that these cases should be referred to those who have garnered and can demonstrate consistently good outcomes. Nonetheless, many have attempted to obviate the need for expertise in securing and carving autologous cartilage by using preformed implants. This study reports the use of a preformed Medpor implant covered/wrapped with a superiorly based temporoparietal fascial flap and a previously expanded mastoid skin flap in 22 reconstructions. The follow-up was between 3 and 12 months, but the authors describe good results and no evidence of exposure or extrusion of the implant within the limits of the time frame reported. However, almost 25% of the patients had downward shifting of the implant at 1 year and required further surgery for repositioning. In addition, most of the patients had some degree of baldness over the site of the temporoparietal fascial flap. This is obviously an early, albeit intriguing study, but requires a larger number of patients and longer follow-up as well as a solution to prevent late shift of the implant.

S. H. Miller, MD, MPH

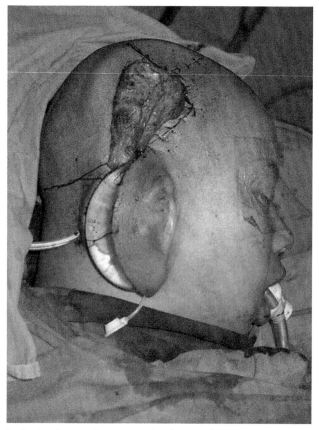

FIGURE 3.—During the second operation, after the expander was removed, an anteriorly based expanded skin flap was shaped and an ipsilateral temporoparietal fascia flap measuring 10 × 10 cm was harvested. (Reprinted from Yang S-L, Zheng J-H, Ding Z, et al. Combined fascial flap and expanded skin flap for enveloping medpor framework in microtia reconstruction. *Aesthetic Plast Surg.* 2009;33:518-522, with permission from Springer Science+Business Media.)

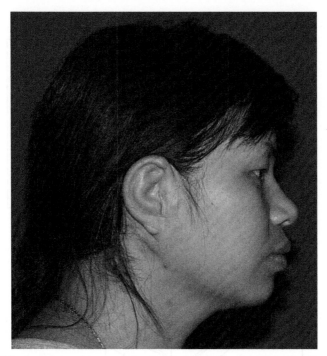

FIGURE 5.—Lateral view of the reconstructed ear 2 years after the second operation. (Reprinted from Yang S-L, Zheng J-H, Ding Z, et al. Combined fascial flap and expanded skin flap for enveloping medpor framework in microtia reconstruction. *Aesthetic Plast Surg.* 2009;33:518-522, with permission from Springer Science+Business Media.)

Cleft Lip and Palate

A quantitative radiological assessment of outcomes of autogenous bone graft combined with platelet-rich plasma in the alveolar cleft

Lee C, Nishihara K, Okawachi T, et al (Kagoshima Univ Graduate School of Med and Dental Sciences, Japan)

Int J Oral Maxillofac Surg 38:117-125, 2009

This longitudinal study evaluated the outcomes of secondary autogenous bone graft combined with platelet-rich plasma (PRP) in the alveolar cleft. Thirty-five alveolar clefts in 30 patients with grafted autogenous bone and PRP (PRP group), and 36 clefts in 30 patients with grafted autogenous bone alone (non-PRP group) were enrolled. PRP was extracted from autogenous blood using a plasma centrifuge system (SmartPReP SMP-1000). The density and resorption of grafted bone were evaluated at 1 week, and 1, 3, 6 and 12 months postoperatively. Bone density was quantitatively assessed as an aluminum-equivalence (Al-Eq) value. Moreover, relationships between bone resorption rate and prognostic factors

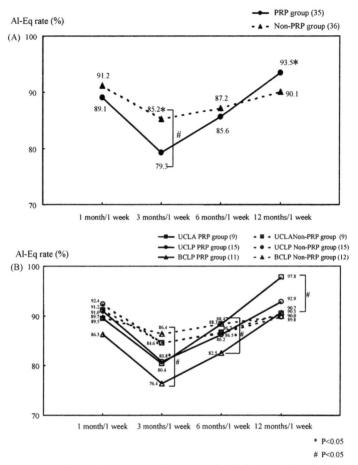

FIGURE 6.—(A) Radiographic assessment of Al-Eq rate of grafted bone and distributed by cleft type (B). *Significant change during the 1-year period (repeated measure ANOVA). #Significant change between PRP and non-PRP group (one-way ANOVA). (Reprinted from Int J Oral Maxillofac Surg, 38. Lee C, Nishihara K, Okawachi T, et al. A quantitative radiological assessment of outcomes of autogenous bone graft combined with platelet-rich plasma in the alveolar cleft. *Int J Oral Maxillofac Surg.* 2009;38:117-125. Copyright 2009 with permission from International Association of Oral and Maxillofacial Surgeons.)

were discussed. Al-Eq values decreased significantly until 3 months, and then increased up to 12 months in both groups. The Al-Eq rate in the PRP group was significantly smaller than that in the non-PRP group at 3 months. No significant differences were observed in the bone resorption rate between the groups. Regarding prognostic factors, continuous mechanical stress affected bone resorption with or without PRP. The authors suggest that PRP may enhance bone remodeling in the early phase, however, PRP seems to be insufficient as a countermeasure against bone resorption following secondary bone graft in the long term (Fig 6).

▶ This study evaluated 60 patients who underwent alveolar bone graft at approximately 9 years of age, obtaining autogenous bone from the iliac crest, without the addition of platelet rich plasma (PRP) in 30 patients and adding PRP in the remaining 30 patients. Bone density was measured as the aluminum-equivalence (Al-Eq) ratio. The Al-Eq rate in the PRP group was significantly smaller than that in the non-PRP group at 3 months, with no significant difference noted at 3 years (Fig 6). The authors conclude that PRP may enhance bone remodeling in the early phase; however, PRP seems to be insufficient as a countermeasure against bone resorption following secondary bone graft in the long-term. This study provides a careful analysis of outcomes relative to bone graft density and resorption over 1 year and provides an honest assessment of the outcomes. The study serves as a model for the evaluation of outcomes of a treatment strategy adhering to this rigorous assessment irrespective of the outcomes of the study.

A. Gosain, MD

The Natural History of Audiologic and Tympanometric Findings in Patients With an Unrepaired Cleft Palate
Zheng W, Smith JD, Shi B, et al (Sichuan Univ, the People's Republic of China; Oregon Health & Science Univ, Portland)
Cleft Palate Craniofac J 46:24-29, 2009

Objective.—To present the tympanometric findings In 552 patients (115 over 10 years of age) with unrepaired cleft palate (256 had audiologic findings) and to show the natural history and outcome of these cases.

Setting.—The cleft lip and palate clinic for the Division of Cleft Lip and Palate Surgery at the West China College of Stomatology, Sichuan University, Chengdu, People's Republic of China.

Design.—Pure-tone audiometric and tympanometric evaluations were performed on 552 patients with an unrepaired cleft palate. Results were analyzed by looking at the patient's age and cleft palate type.

Results.—This study demonstrated an age-related decrease in the frequency of hearing Impairment and abnormal tympanometry. The frequency of hearing impairment and abnormal tympanometry in patients with submucous cleft palate was significantly lower than in patients from the other four major cleft palate categories ($p = .001$, $p = .006$, respectively).

Conclusions.—The middle ear function and hearing levels of unrepaired cleft palate patients Improved with age, but at least 30% of the patients' ears demonstrated a hearing loss and abnormal tympanometry in each age group, including those over 19 years of age. In the crucial language-learning stage, the frequency of hearing impairment and abnormal

TABLE 3.—Hearing Level (dBHL) by Age in 508 Ears of Unrepaired Patients

		Ears in Each Hearing Loss Category, no. (%)					
Age (y)	No. of Ears	Normal	Very Mild	Mild	Moderate	Moderate to Severe	Severe to Profound
2.8 to 4	96	19 (20)	23 (24)	34 (36)	11 (11)	8 (8)	1 (1)
4	58	17 (29)	15 (26)	13 (22)	12 (21)	1 (2)	—
5	54	18 (33)	13 (24)	14 (26)	7 (13)	2 (4)	—
6 to 7	50	23 (46)	10 (20)	13 (26)	4 (8)	—	—
8 to 11	57	35 (61)	13 (23)	8 (14)	1 (2)	—	—
12 to 15	66	34 (52)	18 (27)	9 (14)	5 (7)	—	—
16 to 19	82	57 (70)	16 (20)	7 (8)	2 (2)	—	—
19 to 41	45	30 (67)	6 (13.5)	6 (13.5)	2 (4)	1 (2)	—
Total	508	233 (46)	114 (22.4)	104 (20.4)	44 (9)	12 (2)	1 (0.2)

TABLE 4.—Hearing Level (dBHL) by Cleft Type in 508 Ears of Unrepaired Patients

		Ears in Each Hearing Loss Category, no. (%)					
Cleft Type	No. of Ears	Normal	Very Slight	Slight	Moderate	Moderate to Severe	Severe to Profound
ICP*	229	100 (44)	61 (27)	51 (22)	14 (6)	3 (1)	—
RUCP±L	58	23 (40)	11 (19)	13 (22)	5 (8.5)	5 (8.5)	1 (2)
LUCP±L	115	52 (45)	24 (21)	21 (18)	15 (13)	3 (3)	—
BCP±L	66	30 (45)	14 (21)	12 (18)	9 (14)	1 (2)	—
SMCP	40	28 (70)	4 (10)	7 (17.5)	1 (2.5)	—	—
Total	508	233 (46)	114 (22.4)	104 (20.4)	44 (9)	12 (2)	1 (0.2)

*ICP = incomplete cleft palate; RUCP±L = right unilateral complete cleft palate with or without cleft lip; LUCP±L = left unilateral complete cleft palate with or without cleft lip; BCP±L = bilateral complete cleft palate with or without cleft lip; SMCP = submucous cleft palate.

tympanometry was as high as 60%. Considering these results, palate repair and surgical intervention, such as tube insertion, for otological problems should be considered at an early age (Tables 3 and 4).

▶ This study demonstrates the important relation between hearing impairment and unrepaired cleft palate in a large group of patients with unrepaired cleft palate (n = 552). Such a study could only take place in select areas of the world such as China because no centers in the United States would have this magnitude of unrepaired cleft palates over 4 years of age. Interestingly, hearing impairment decreased with age (Table 3) even though no intervention had taken place; impaired hearing was noted in 80% of the patients aged 2.8 to 4 years, compared with 33% of the patients aged 19 to 41 years. In overt cleft palate, the type of cleft did not have significant impact on hearing impairment. However, in submucous cleft palate, the incidence of hearing impairment was considerably less than in patients with overt cleft palate (Table 4). Since hearing impairment persisted in 30% or more of the patients in each age group, the authors conclude that palate repair and surgical intervention, such as tube insertion, for otological problems should be carried out at an early age. While the results of this study warrant attention, it is not clear that palate repair will decrease the audiologic outcomes because there was no cohort of repaired cleft palate patients for comparison. In addition, it is not clear whether cleft palate repair affects audiologic outcome or whether these benefits are from early tube insertion. Although few would disagree with the conclusion that children with cleft palate should have a palate repair, the outcomes of this repair on audiologic function remains speculative. To answer this question, one would need to compare audiologic findings in cleft palate patients who had palate repair without tube placement, tube placement alone, or no intervention. The study only addresses the latter group who had no intervention.

A. Gosain, MD

Craniofacial and Pharyngeal Cephalometric Morphology in Seven-Year-Old Boys With Unoperated Submucous Cleft Palate and Without a Cleft
Heliövaara A, Rautio J (Univ of Helsinki, Finland; Helsinki Univ Central Hosp, Finland)
Cleft Palate Craniofac J 46:314-318, 2009

Objective.—To evaluate cephalometrically the craniofacial and pharyngeal morphology in 7-year-old boys with unoperated submucous cleft palate and to compare the findings with the morphology of 7-year-old boys without clefts.

Setting and Patients.—Thirty-two boys with unoperated submucous cleft palate and 49 boys without a cleft were compared retrospectively from lateral cephalograms taken at the mean age of 7 years (range, 5.5 to 8.6 years).

Design.—A retrospective case-control study.

Outcome Measure.—Linear and angular measurements were obtained from lateral cephalograms. A Student's *t* test was used in the statistical analysis.

Results.—The maxilla of the boys with submucous cleft palate was shorter and slightly more retrusive in relation to the cranial base than that of boys without clefts. Also, the mandible of the boys with submucous cleft palate was smaller, with a steeper mandibular plane. The relationship between the jaws was similar in both groups; although, those without clefts showed higher values for soft tissue maxillary prominence. In the pharyngeal area, the boys with submucous cleft palate had larger nasopharyngeal depths, smaller hypopharyngeal depths, and shorter soft palates than the boys without a cleft.

Conclusions.—This small study suggests that the boys with unoperated submucous cleft palate have minor distinctive morphological features in the maxillary, mandibular, and pharyngeal areas (Fig 1, Table 1).

▶ This study compared 32 boys with unoperated submucous cleft palate (SMCP) with 49 boys without clefting in a retrospective case-control study. The data were collected from lateral cephalograms. Therefore, the study can only comment on AP projection of the facial structures and cannot comment

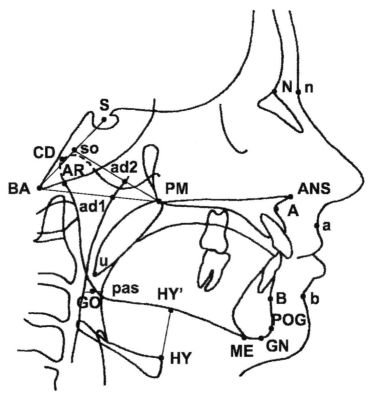

FIGURE 1.—Cephalometric landmarks (see Table 1 for abbreviations, full names, and definitions). (Reprinted from Heliövaara A, Rautio J. Craniofacial and pharyngeal cephalometric morphology in seven-year-old boys with unoperated submucous cleft palate and without a cleft. *Cleft Palate Craniofac J.* 2009;46:314-318.)

on other important parameters such as maxillary arch width. The cephalometric landmarks studied are summarized in Fig 1, and the results are summarized in Table 2. Findings were that the maxilla was slightly more retrusive relative to the cranial base in the patients with SMCP and that these patients also had a more retruded mandible with a steeper mandibular plane angle. Soft tissue findings were that the SMCP patients had increased nasopharyngeal depth and shorter soft palates than did the boys without clefts. Of note is that these findings are in boys who had not been operated on, suggesting that the differences were related to the cleft and not to surgical intervention as is often debated. This presents an interesting dilemma to the surgeon because we struggle to minimize final growth disturbance in children with clefts and try to choose operative procedures that are least likely to interfere with facial growth. We also try to maximize soft palate length postpalatoplasty. However, if the findings of this study are relevant, one would expect even more severe hypoplasia of the skeletal structures and a greater velopharyngeal gap in patients with complete cleft palate, making the dilemma as to how to design

TABLE 2.—The Mean (SD) and *p* Values of Cephalometric Variables Between Boys With Unoperated Submucous Cleft Palate (SMCP) and Controls Without a Cleft; Distances are Reported in Millimeters and Angles in Degrees

| | SMCP | | Controls | | SMCP/Controls |
	Mean	SD	Mean	SD	*p*
N-S-BA	130	3.4	131.7	4.5	.072
S-N-A	79.7	2.8	81.1	3.2	.05*
S-N-B	76.2	3.6	77.2	2.9	.164
A-N-B	3.5	2.3	3.9	1.9	.702
S-N-POG	75.8	3.9	77.1	2.9	.069
ANS-PM	45	2.5	46.8	2.1	.001**
N-ANS	42.4	3.1	42.7	2.6	.68
ANS-ME	56.7	4.1	57	3.4	.771
S-GO	59.3	4.9	62	4.1	.008*
NSL/ML	37.7	4.8	35.3	4	.017*
GN-CD	92.6	6	95.7	4.6	.012*
ME-GO	55.6	4.8	56.3	3.4	.967
AR-GO	33.6	3.6	37.4	3.2	.000***
S-n-a	91.4	3.8	93.4	3.6	.025*
S-n-b	82.9	3.9	81.4	3.4	.073
a-n-b	8.5	2.3	8	2	.054
BA-PM	38.6	2.6	41.1	2.7	.000***
ad1-PM	19.3	3.6	18.6	3.9	.367
ad1-BA	19.3	3.3	22.5	4.6	.001*
ad2-PM	16.4	3.5	14	3.7	.005*
ad2-so	18	3.3	22.4	4.3	.000***
pas	11.4	3.1	13.2	3.8	.026*
PM-u	25.5	2.8	28.1	2.7	.000***
HY-HY'	11.9	4.6	10.7	4.6	.241

*= *P* < 0.05.
**= *P* < 0.01.
***= *P* < 0.001.

the best operation to minimize growth disturbance even more complex. It may not be possible to extrapolate between patients with unoperated SMCP and those with complete cleft palate but getting a cohort of unoperated boys with complete cleft palate at age 7 years would be even more difficult. It would also be interesting if the authors had indicated the speech status of the boys with SMCP and correlated this with the cephalometric measurements, as one would expect the children with the greatest nasopharyngeal depth to be more prone to hypernasality. In summary, the study raises a host of questions that lay a groundwork for further investigation.

A. Gosain, MD

Cleft Surgery in Rural Bangladesh: Reflections and Experiences

Aziz SR, Rhee ST, Redai I (UMDNJ-New Jersey Med School, Newark; New York Presbyterian Hosp; Columbia Univ College of Physicians and Surgeons, NY)
J Oral Maxillofac Surg 67:1581-1588, 2009

Purpose.—The authors review their experiences during multiple cleft surgical missions to rural Bangladesh from 2006 to 2008. A significant number of patients who underwent primary palatoplasty or cheiloplasty were of adult age or size. Adult primary cleft lip and palate repair is often more challenging than repair at the standard age of fewer than 2 years. This patient population is rarely seen in the United States, but may be treated more often by American surgeons during surgical missions to the developing world. This report discusses the experiences of the authors' treatment of cleft lips and palates in rural Bangladesh.

Patients and Methods.—One hundred forty-six cleft-lip and cleft-palate patients were treated during 3 missions to rural Bangladesh, from 2006 to 2008. Thirty-three (23%) patients were of adult size, and aged 13 to 35 years. One hundred thirteen (77%) patients were aged 12 years or younger. Unilateral cleft lips were repaired with a Millard advancement-rotation technique. Bilateral cleft lips were repaired via the 1-stage procedure advocated by Mulliken and Salyer. Cleft palates were repaired using a 2-finger flap method.

Results.—Overall, 8 of 146 patients (5.5%) had nonlife-threatening complications (infection or wound dehiscence) requiring subsequent revision surgery. The adult-sized patients had clefts of significantly increased size secondary to patient growth, as well as maxillary expansion transversely and anteriorly. Adult cleft-lip repair required significant soft-tissue dissection to close the cleft adequately, and ensure symmetry to the upper lip and alar bases. However, this procedure sometimes resulted in placement of the lip cicatrix in an anatomically disadvantageous position. In addition, with the increased transverse dimension of the adult cleft palate, tension-free 3-layer closure was difficult. Again, aggressive dissection of the soft tissue was required: the nasal and muscular layers were closed without much tension, but oral closure was often under tension, requiring the assistance of dermal biomaterials to bolster the repair.

Conclusions.—Patients in the developing world often have limited access to specialized health care, and may not realize that cleft lips and palates can be repaired. As a result, there is an increased incidence of unrepaired clefts in adult-sized individuals in this part of the globe. The American surgeon may encounter these patients during surgical missions. The surgeon should be prepared to repair adult patients with clefts that are significantly enlarged in all 3 dimensions. Closure will require significant

TABLE 1.—Cleft Lip and Palate Patients Treated During Bangladesh Mission of 2006 to 2008

Age	<1 Year Old	1 to 12 Years Old	≥13 Years Old
UCCL	10	45	13
UICL	0	23	13
BCCL	3	4	2
BICL	0	5	1
CP	2	21	4
Total	15	98	33

Abbreviations: UCCL, unilateral complete cleft lip; UICL, unilateral incomplete cleft lip; BCCL, bilateral complete cleft lip; BICL, bilateral incomplete cleft lip; CP, cleft palate.

soft-tissue dissection as well as the use of biomaterials as needed to repair wide cleft palates (Table 1).

▶ This report brings light to a population in need of cleft repair, and the planning and execution of surgical missions performed over a 3-year period to provide care to these patients. The strengths of the article are reflected in the organization of the mission trips and the composition of the team, which consisted of 3 anesthesiologists, 2 to 3 attending surgeons, 2 nurses, and 1 or 2 surgical residents. The attending surgeon was either an oral surgeon or a plastic surgeon, and the surgical residents were from either specialty. The anesthesiologists point out that oral Ring-Adair-Elwyn (RAE) tubes used in the Caucasian cleft population were often too big for the smaller children in rural Bangladesh, and the tube often slipped into the right mainstem bronchus. It would be worthwhile to investigate if the tubes could be modified such that the length distal to the bend is shortened when dealing with a very small child, particularly since the cuff is normally not used in children under 1 year of age. The authors point out the composition of the patients they operated on (Table 1), in which 77% of patients were aged 12 years or younger (11% being less than 1 year old), and 23% of patients were aged 13 or over. The report raises questions that are not addressed. The authors state that adult patients with unrepaired cleft palate were found to have increased transverse dimension of the cleft palate. This is in contrast to the experience of surgeons who delay hard palate repair as they find that the transverse dimension of the cleft narrows when hard palate repair is delayed. Additional questions that remain unanswered are as follows: (1) What is the sequence of repair that the authors recommend in the adult patient with an unrepaired cleft lip and palate, given that the patient may only have one opportunity for surgery? Do the authors repair the lip and palate simultaneously, repair the lip first, or repair the palate first? If the repairs were done sequentially, how many of these patients then returned to complete the repairs? (2) Do the authors have any speech outcome data on the patients who had cleft palate repair as an adult? There remains controversy as to whether the refractory speech errors that these patients developed over their lifetime can be corrected following palate repair. (3) What postoperative regimens were in place to follow speech outcomes and to provide speech therapy for these patients? There is no question that cleft surgery on surgical missions is a challenge, and the authors provide a model for safe execution of this surgery, but questions as to how to optimize the outcomes of the surgery remain.

A. Gosain, MD

Revisional surgery following the superiorly based posterior pharyngeal wall flap. Historical perspectives and current considerations
Keuning KHDM, Meijer GJ, van der Bilt A, et al (Univ of Amsterdam, The Netherlands; Univ Med Ctr Utrecht, The Netherlands)
Int J Oral Maxillofac Surg 38:1137-1142, 2009

The aim of this study was to describe the surgical and functional complications following superiorly based posterior pharyngeal wall (SBPP) flap surgery. Records of 130 patients with velopharyngeal insufficiency (VPI) who had undergone SBPP flap surgery as a secondary procedure to reduce nasal resonance in speech were reviewed. Complications were defined as the incidence of revisional surgery required to obtain a more satisfactory result. 20 patients (15%) required revisional surgery. In 4 patients (3%) early revisional surgery was indicated to treat surgical complications (1 postoperative bleeding, 3 flap dehiscences). In 16 patients (12%) late revisional surgery was indicated to achieve a better functional result with regard to nasal resonance in speech. The low incidence of surgical complications indicates that SBPP flap surgery is a safe procedure. After SBPP flap surgery, a satisfactory functional result with respect to nasal resonance was obtained in 88% of patients. This result was improved after revisional surgery. The hypothesis that the patients of an experienced surgeon have fewer complications and better functional results than those of a less experienced one was tested. The individual skill of the surgeon rather than their experience led to a better functional result.

▶ This is an interesting commentary on a large series detailing the outcomes of 130 patients, based on the need for revisional surgery, following superiorly based posterior wall pharyngeal flaps to treat velopharyngeal incompetence. The results in general are quite good in almost 90% of the patients, but the major problem remains how to tailor the size of the flap and the relationship of the flap to the movement of the lateral pharyngeal walls. The authors' use of oral mucosa to cover the raw surface of the pharyngeal flap to prevent postoperative shrinkage is somewhat different than the approach I used, which was to use turn back flaps from the nasal side of the velum as described by Owsley and Blackfield.[1] Neither offers complete control of the outcome as the latter also depends on the degree of movement of the lateral pharyngeal walls. I too use the suction test described by Baker and Millard[2] to check on velopharyngeal competence at the conclusion of the operation. Intuitively, the greater the amount of experience of the surgeon, better the outcome. Although the authors state that the skill of the individual surgeon is more important for the outcome than the experience of that surgeon, no data are offered to prove this point.

S. H. Miller, MD, MPH

References

1. Owsley JQ Jr, Blackfield HM. The technique and complications of pharyngeal flap surgery; a continuing report. *Plast Reconstr Surg.* 1965;35:531-539.
2. Baker S, Millard DR. Intraoperative suction test as a predictor of velopharyngeal incompetence. *Cleft Palate Craniofac J.* 1993;30:452-453.

Nasoalveolar Molding Improves Long-Term Nasal Symmetry in Complete Unilateral Cleft Lip-Cleft Palate Patients
Barillas I, Dec W, Warren SM, et al (New York Univ Med Ctr)
Plast Reconstr Surg 123:1002-1006, 2009

Background.—Nasoalveolar molding was developed to improve dentoalveolar, septal, and lower lateral cartilage position before cleft lip repair. Previous studies have documented the long-term maintenance of columella length and nasal dome form and projection. The purpose of the present study was to determine the effect of presurgical nasoalveolar molding on long-term unilateral complete cleft nasal symmetry.

Methods.—A retrospective review of 25 consecutively presenting nonsyndromic complete unilateral cleft lip–cleft palate patients was conducted. Fifteen patients were treated with presurgical nasoalveolar molding for 3 months before surgical correction, and 10 patients were treated by surgical correction alone. The average age at the time of follow-up was 9 years. Four nasal anthropometric distances and two angular relationships were measured to assess nasal symmetry.

Results.—All six measurements demonstrated a greater degree of nasal symmetry in nasoalveolar molding patients compared with the patients treated with surgery alone. Five symmetry measurements were significantly more symmetric in the nasoalveolar molding patients and one measurement demonstrated a nonsignificant but greater degree of symmetry compared with the patients treated with surgery alone.

Conclusions.—The data demonstrate that the lower lateral and septal cartilages are more symmetric in the nasoalveolar molding patients compared with the surgery-alone patients. Furthermore, the improved symmetry observed in nasoalveolar molding–treated noses during the time of the primary surgery is maintained at 9 years of age (Figs 2 and 3, Table 1).

▶ This article is from the group at New York University (NYU) who pioneered nasoalveolar molding (NAM), and their findings represent the state of the art in this field. The authors studied 25 consecutive patients, in whom 15 had undergone NAM during the 3 months prior to cleft lip repair, and 10 had not had NAM prior to cleft lip repair. None of the patients had undergone secondary

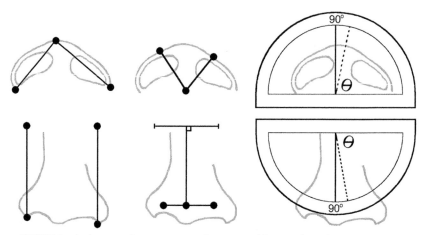

FIGURE 2.—Anthropometric measurements. Six anatomical linear and angular measurements were obtained to assess nasal symmetry. Three measurements were obtained from the basilar view: (*above, left*) nasal ala projection length, (*above, center*) nasal dome height, and (*above, right*) columellar deviation. Three measurements were obtained from the frontal view: (*below, left*) superoinferior alar groove position, (*below, center*) mediolateral nasal dome position, and (*below, right*) nasal bridge deviation. (Reprinted from Barillas I, Dec W, Warren SM, et al. Nasoalveolar molding improves long-term nasal symmetry in complete unilateral cleft lip-cleft palate patients. *Plast Reconstr Surg.* 2009;123:1002-1006, with permission from the American Society of Plastic Surgeons.)

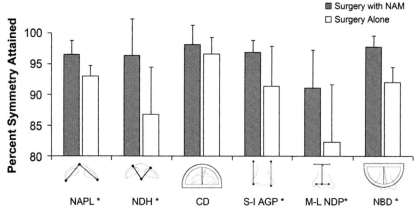

FIGURE 3.—Graph depicting nasal symmetry comparison measurements for the surgery with nasoalveolar molding group (*blue*) and surgery-alone control group (*white*). *Asterisk* indicates a statistically significant difference. Error bars = 1 SD. *NAPL*, nasal ala projection length; *NDH*, nasal dome height; *CD*, columellar deviation; *S-I AGP*, superoinferior alar groove position; *M-L NDP*, mediolateral nasal dome position; *NBD*, nasal bridge deviation. For interpretation of the references to color in this figure legend, the reader is referred to web version of this article. (Reprinted from Barillas I, Dec W, Warren SM, et al. Nasoalveolar molding improves long-term nasal symmetry in complete unilateral cleft lip-cleft palate patients. *Plast Reconstr Surg.* 2009;123:1002-1006, with permission from the American Society of Plastic Surgeons.)

nasal surgery following cleft lip repair. The patients were recalled an average of 9 years (range: 7-11 years) later, and nasal impressions were taken using a dental impression model. Anthropometric measures were taken from these

TABLE 1.—Nasal Symmetry Comparisons

	Surgery-Alone Control Group (%)	Surgery with NAM Group (%)
Nasal ala projection length*‡	93.0 ± 1.7	96.5 ± 2.3
Nostril dome height*‡	86.8 ± 7.5	96.4 ± 5.9
Columellar deviation†	96.6 ± 2.7	98.1 ± 3.2
Superoinferior alar groove position*‡	91.4 ± 6.5	96.9 ± 2.0
Mediolateral nasal dome position*‡	82.3 ± 9.3	91.1 ± 6.1
Nasal bridge deviation†‡	92.0 ± 2.4	97.9 ± 1.7

NAM, nasoalveolar molding.
*Linear measurement.
†Angular measurement.
‡Statistically significant difference.

nasal impressions, making 3 measures from the basilar view and 3 measures from the frontal view (Fig 2). There was a statistically significant increase in measures representative of nasal symmetry in 5 of the 6 measures from the group of patients who had undergone NAM (Table 1 and Fig 3). The only measure that was not significantly different was a measure of columellar deviation made on the basilar view. Objective measures of nasal aesthetics are very difficult to achieve, and the authors made a very thorough and meticulous study to recall these patients an average of 9 years following surgery and to obtain nasal impressions on all patients. The analysis presented is rigorous and may be used as a standard for subsequent studies of nasal symmetry, both in cleft and noncleft patients. The authors make valid conclusions on the efficacy of NAM in long-term maintenance of nasal aesthetics in cleft patients.

A. Gosain, MD

Cranio-Maxillo-Facial

Application-Specific Selection of Biomaterials for Pediatric Craniofacial Reconstruction: Developing a Rational Approach to Guide Clinical Use

Gosain AK, Chim H, Arneja JS (Case School of Medicine, Cleveland, OH; Children's Hosp of Michigan, Detroit; Wayne State Univ, Detroit, MI)
Plast Reconstr Surg 123:319-330, 2009

Background.—Biomaterials provide an invaluable alternative to autogenous bone graft for pediatric craniofacial reconstruction. However, there is no uniform agreement on the choice of biomaterial for different reconstructive needs.

Methods.—Patients who had reconstruction of the craniofacial skeleton with alloplastic materials from 1994 to 2006 by a single surgeon were reviewed. Biomaterials used consisted of three classes: cement pastes, biomaterials designed to be replaced by bone, and prefabricated polymers. The study included 25 patients with a mean age of 5.5 years and a mean follow-up of 3.3 years.

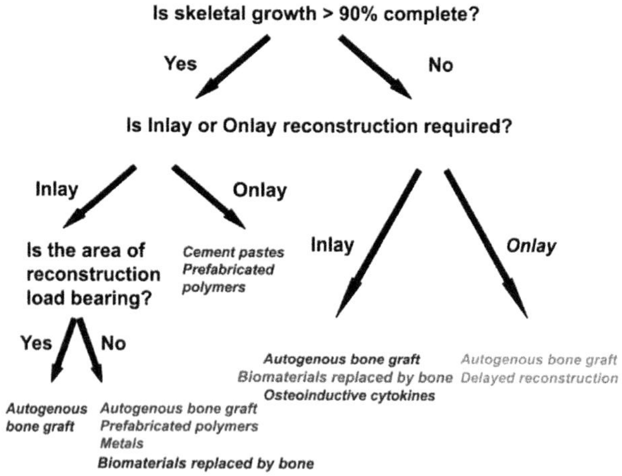

FIGURE 6.—Algorithm to guide the choice of biomaterials for use in craniofacial reconstruction. (Reprinted from Gosain AK, Chim H, Arneja JS. Application-specific selection of biomaterials for pediatric craniofacial reconstruction: developing a rational approach to guide clinical use. *Plast Reconstr Surg.* 2009;123:319-330, with permission from the American Society of Plastic Surgeons.)

Results.—Cement pastes used for onlay augmentation to the cranial skeleton in eight patients consisted of hydroxyapatite ($n = 5$) and calcium phosphate ($n = 3$). One patient had a postoperative infection that resolved with partial implant removal and antibiotics. Biomaterials designed to be replaced by bone consisted of bioactive glass ($n = 3$) and demineralized bone ($n = 8$), which were used for inlay reconstruction of full-thickness calvarial defects in 11 patients. Computed tomographic scanning showed adequate bone mineralization in nine patients; two of the three patients with calvarial defects greater than 5 cm in diameter demonstrated variable mineralization. Prefabricated porous polyethylene was used in six patients for either onlay malar augmentation ($n = 3$) or inlay calvarial reconstruction ($n = 3$). One patient had a peri-implant infection that resolved with aspiration, irrigation, and intravenous antibiotics.

Conclusions.—The authors developed an algorithm to guide use of biomaterials in craniofacial reconstruction based on whether (1) growth of the underlying craniofacial skeleton is nearly complete (>90 percent); (2) onlay or inlay reconstruction is to be performed; and (3) the reconstruction is performed in a load-bearing or non–load-bearing area (Fig 6).

▶ The selection of biomaterials in craniofacial reconstruction poses very difficult choices based on the available literature. Often, biomaterials are condemned, particularly in pediatric applications, based on a series of complications in which the biomaterial selected may not have had the appropriate properties for the specific reconstruction chosen. This article seeks to clarify some of the areas of confusion in the selection of biomaterials, separately evaluating a single author's experience with (1) cement pastes, (2) biomaterials designed to be replaced by bone (demineralized bone and bioactive glasses), and (3) prefabricated polymers such as porous polyethylene. The authors suggest that the clinician should ask the following questions when selecting a biomaterial for a specific application: (1) is the reconstruction to be performed for a loadbearing or nonload-bearing application? (2) is an onlay or inlay reconstruction to be performed? (3) is growth of the underlying facial skeleton (90%) nearly complete? Based on these parameters, the authors provide an algorithm for the selection of biomaterials in craniofacial reconstruction (Fig 6). Whereas these results are based on 1 author's experience and the series is limited (25 patients), it serves as a guide for future research for applications where biomaterial science has yet to develop the ideal constructs for craniofacial reconstruction.

A. Gosain, MD

A 3-dimensional method for analyzing the morphology of patients with maxillofacial deformities
Terajima M, Nakasima A, Aoki Y, et al (Kyushu Univ, Fukuoka, Japan; Shibaura Inst of Technology Univ, Saitama, Japan)
Am J Orthod Dentofacial Orthop 136:857-867, 2009

Introduction.—Traditionally, cephalograms have been used to evaluate a patient's maxillofacial skeleton and facial soft-tissue morphology. However, magnification and distortion of the cephalograms make detailed morphologic analysis difficult in patients with complex deformities. The purpose of this article was to introduce a new method for visualizing deformation and deviation of the maxillofacial skeleton and facial soft tissues.

Methods.—Standard 3-dimensional Japanese head models were sized to match the sella-to-nasion distance obtained from 2 patients' (1 man, 1 woman) maxillofacial skeletal images. Then, the scaled standard model was superimposed on each patient's 3-dimensional computed tomography image.

Results.—This system provided clear shape information independent of size and facilitated the visualization of shape variations in maxillofacial skeletal and facial soft-tissue morphology.

Conclusions.—This method will be useful for 3-dimensional morphologic analysis of patients with jaw deformities (Figs 5 and 6).

▶ This article addresses an important analytic point in craniofacial surgery: potential inadequacy of cephalometric data derived from plain radiographs, particularly in a craniofacial patient with facial asymmetries. The lateral cephalogram represents a superimposition of the right and left sides of the face, and therefore, asymmetry in anterior projection between the 2 sides is masked by the superimposition. In addition, magnification varies based on the depth of the

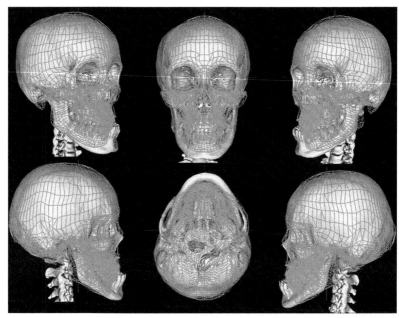

FIGURE 5.—Patient A: the superimposed images of the scaled female Japanese standard skeletal model (3D skeletal template) and the 3D CT images of the patient's preoperative maxillofacial skeleton. *Gray areas* represent the patient's image, and the *wire frame* represents the 3D skeletal template. (Reprinted from Terajima M, Nakasima A, Aoki Y, et al. A 3-dimensional method for analyzing the morphology of patients with maxillofacial deformities. *Am J Orthod Dentofacial Orthop.* 2009; 136:857-867, with permission from the American Association of Orthodontists.)

object being examined, with points closer to the X-ray film magnified less than those closer to the X-ray source. The authors have done a thorough analysis based on skull models of 2 subjects, creating virtual reality images of the skull models and superimposing these on images obtained by 3-dimensional (3D) CT scan. Superimposition of the skull (Fig 5) and mandible (Fig 6) of 1 patient demonstrates the discrepancy between the data sets. These analyses demonstrate the complexity of translating real skull landmarks onto recon-structed images. However, the data also point out that assumptions regarding the validity of 2-D images in placing any given skeletal landmark in a 3-D framework may be spurious. While this study is only a feasibility study, it brings key issues to light. The authors indicate that they plan to use this analytic method with cone beam CT (CBCT) data. This will be extremely valuable, as the CBCT is rapidly becoming a standard for facial analysis. Validation of the points represented by CBCT is therefore paramount in the evolution of this technique.

A. Gosain, MD

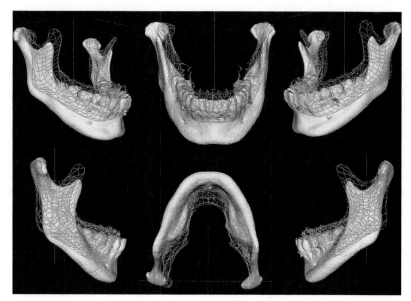

FIGURE 6.—Patient A: the superimposed images of the scaled female Japanese standard mandibular model (3D mandibular template) and the 3D CT images of the patient's preoperative mandible. *Gray areas* represent the patient's image, and the *wire frame* represents the 3D mandibular template. (Reprinted from Terajima M, Nakasima A, Aoki Y, et al. A 3-dimensional method for analyzing the morphology of patients with maxillofacial deformities. *Am J Orthod Dentofacial Orthop.* 2009;136:857-867, with permission from the American Association of Orthodontists.)

Vascular Malformations

Outcomes of Childhood Hemangiomas Treated with the Pulsed-Dye Laser with Dynamic Cooling: A Retrospective Chart Analysis

Rizzo C, Brightman L, Chapas AM, et al (New York Univ Skin; Laser and Skin Surgery Ctr of New York)
Dermatol Surg 35:1947-1954, 2009

Background.—Laser treatment of childhood hemangiomas remains controversial. Previous studies have used outdated technology, resulting in a potential overrepresentation of adverse outcomes.

Objective.—To evaluate outcomes of hemangiomas treated with the most current laser technology.

Methods.—A retrospective chart analysis of 90 patients with a median age of 3.0 months and a total of 105 hemangiomas were enrolled over a 2.5-year period. All were treated with the 595-nm long-pulse pulsed-dye laser (LP-PDL) with dynamic epidermal cooling at 2- to 8-week intervals depending on the stage of growth. Exclusion criteria were previous laser, surgical, or corticosteroid treatment. Three reviewers assessed outcomes.

Results.—Near-complete or complete clearance in color were achieved for 85 (81%) and in thickness for 67 (64%) hemangiomas. There was no scarring or atrophy. Ulceration occurred in one case and resolved during treatment. Hyperpigmentation and hypopigmentation occurred in 4% and 14% of hemangiomas, respectively.

Conclusion.—Early treatment of childhood hemangiomas with the 595-nm LP-PDL with dynamic cooling may reduce the proliferative phase and result in excellent rates of clearing and few adverse events.

▶ This is an interesting report of a retrospective study of the effects of 595-nm pulsed-dye laser with dynamic cooling on outcomes of childhood hemangiomas. The authors acknowledge that laser treatment of childhood hemangiomas remains controversial, due in large part to the use of "outdated" technology resulting in significant adverse outcomes reported by others. In this study, they report their use of current laser technology long-pulsed-dye laser treatment with dynamic epidermal cooling performed at 2- to 8-week intervals. They do seem to reduce the number of adverse events in their patients compared with those reported in other studies. They postulate that the particular laser used and dynamic cooling may reduce the proliferative phase, and thus promote reduction in the color and thickness of the hemangiomas they treated. However, little evidence is offered to conclusively prove their hypothesis as they themselves state that it is difficult to clearly identify whether the treatment produced a better outcome when these lesions spontaneously improve. Future efforts with regard to documenting the validity of using these or any treatment for involuting heamangiomas will hinge on being able to define markers of some type within the lesions that can determine those that will spontaneously disappear and over what time period the resolution will occur.

S. H. Miller, MD, MPH

Resection of Amblyogenic Periocular Hemangiomas: Indications and Outcomes

Arneja JS, Mulliken JB (British Columbia Children's Hosp, Canada; Children's Hosp Boston, MA)
Plast Reconstr Surg 125:274-281, 2010

Background.—Periocular hemangiomas can induce irreversible amblyopia by multiple mechanisms: visual deprivation, refractive error (astigmatism and/or anisometropia), or strabismus. There is a subset of complicated periocular hemangiomas most effectively managed by resection.

Methods.—The authors reviewed all patients from 1999 to 2008 with a periocular hemangioma that was either completely resected or debulked; whenever necessary, the levator apparatus was reinserted. Infants were included in the study if they had complete preoperative and postoperative ophthalmic assessments and there was more than a 6-month follow-up interval.

Results.—Thirty-three children were treated with a mean operative age of 6.2 months and a mean follow-up interval of 48.2 months. The majority of hemangiomas were well-localized and caused corneal deformation with astigmatism or blepharoptosis. Intralesional or oral corticosteroid administration was attempted in almost one-half of patients. Postoperatively, the degree of astigmatism was statistically improved: from 3.0 diopters to 1.11 diopters ($p < 0.001$). When resection was performed in infants younger than 3 months (19 patients), astigmatism was less severe preoperatively and the correction was slightly greater postoperatively (from 2.76 diopters to 0.80 diopters). Resection performed after 3 months (14 patients) of age also resulted in improvement of astigmatism (from 3.39 diopters to 1.38 diopters). Reinsertion of the levator expansion was required in 34 percent of patients.

Conclusions.—The authors advocate early resection of a well-localized periocular hemangioma to prevent potentially irreversible amblyopia caused by either corneal deformation or blepharoptosis. The longer a complicated periocular hemangioma is observed, the greater the astigmatism and the less amenable it will be to correction following tumor removal.

▶ This is a small, albeit important series detailing the surgical management of children with periocular hemangiomas. We agree with the authors that the primary danger for these children is the development of irreversible amblyopia and that early treatment, before age 3 months, is in most instances ideal to minimize astigmatism. Corticosteroids are still the mainstay for extensive and non-localized hemangiomas, but surgical excision is warranted when the lesions are localized and begin to cause visual deprivation.[1]

S. H. Miller, MD, MPH

Reference

1. Levi M, Schwartz S, Blei F, et al. Surgical treatment of capillary hemangiomas causing amblyopia. *J AAPOS.* 2007;11:230-234.

2 Neoplastic, Inflammatory and Degenerative Conditions

Benign and Malignant Tumors of the Skin

Does Shave Biopsy Accurately Predict the Final Breslow Depth of Primary Cutaneous Melanoma?
Moore P, Hundley J, Hundley J, et al (Wake Forest Univ School of Medicine, Winston-Salem, NC)
Am Surg 75:369-373, 2009

Shave biopsy (SB) is used for the diagnosis of suspicious skin lesions, including melanoma. Its accuracy for melanoma has not been confirmed. We examined our experience with SB to determine its ability to predict true Breslow depth (BD). We performed a retrospective review of the tumor registry for all patients diagnosed with melanoma by SB from 1995 to 2004. Site and depth of lesion, tumor stage, correlation of BD between SB and wide local excision (WLE), and changes in surgical management due to discordance were examined. Melanoma-in-situ was defined as a depth of 0 for this analysis. One hundred thirty-nine patients were diagnosed with melanoma by SB. Pathology after WLE were as follows: 54 (39%) patients had no residual disease, 67 (48%) had a BD equal to or less than the SB, and 18 (13%) had a thicker BD compared with the SB. For these 18 patients, the median BD by SB and WLE was 1.1 mm (range 0–6.5) and 3.5 mm (range 0.5–20.5), respectively ($P = 0.0017$). Upstaging of final BD from SB to WLE was significantly associated with increasing tumor depth and higher stage of melanoma ($P < 0.0001$). Only seven of the 139 patients (5%) required further surgery because of the increased depth of the WLE. SB underestimated the final BD of melanoma in 13 per cent of patients, but changed the management of few patients. SB is a valuable tool for practitioners in the diagnosis of

35

melanoma. Nevertheless, patients diagnosed with melanoma by SB should be counseled about the rare need for additional surgery.

▶ The advice offered by the authors based on this retrospective study is a bit disconcerting to me. First and foremost is the retrospective nature of the study, followed by the 13% under diagnosis of the Breslow depth to guide subsequent treatment, and then bringing into the equation that shave biopsies may be either "superficial or deep." The latter is particularly troublesome when the authors suggest that the expertise or resources to perform excisional biopsy may be too much for some practitioners, and that they may just observe or cauterize the lesions without a definitive diagnosis. Does that mean they would or should be able to distinguish between and perform "superficial or deep shave biopsies" more easily, or that their index of suspicion would not suggest that the patient should be sent to a physician with the expertise and resources to do an excisional biopsy?

S. H. Miller, MD, MPH

Does Shave Biopsy Accurately Predict the Final Breslow Depth of Primary Cutaneous Melanoma?
Moore P, Hundley J, Hundley J, et al (Wake Forest Univ School of Medicine, Winston-Salem, NC)
Am Surg 75:369-373, 2009

Shave biopsy (SB) is used for the diagnosis of suspicious skin lesions, including melanoma. Its accuracy for melanoma has not been confirmed. We examined our experience with SB to determine its ability to predict true Breslow depth (BD). We performed a retrospective review of the tumor registry for all patients diagnosed with melanoma by SB from 1995 to 2004. Site and depth of lesion, tumor stage, correlation of BD between SB and wide local excision (WLE), and changes in surgical management due to discordance were examined. Melanoma-in-situ was defined as a depth of 0 for this analysis. One hundred thirty-nine patients were diagnosed with melanoma by SB. Pathology after WLE were as follows: 54 (39%) patients had no residual disease, 67 (48%) had a BD equal to or less than the SB, and 18 (13%) had a thicker BD compared with the SB. For these 18 patients, the median BD by SB and WLE was 1.1 mm (range 0–6.5) and 3.5 mm (range 0.5–20.5), respectively ($P = 0.0017$). Upstaging of final BD from SB to WLE was significantly associated with increasing tumor depth and higher stage of melanoma ($P < 0.0001$). Only seven of the 139 patients (5%) required further surgery because of the increased depth of the WLE. SB underestimated the final BD of melanoma in 13 per cent of patients, but changed the management of few patients. SB is a valuable tool for practitioners in the diagnosis of melanoma. Nevertheless, patients diagnosed with melanoma by SB should be counseled about the rare need for additional surgery.

▶ This article was selected for its content, but not its conclusions. The authors noted that the most commonly used technique for diagnosis of melanoma is excisional biopsy (EB). However, a small number (reported at 10%) of practitioners use shave biopsy (SB) instead of EB. The authors set out to determine whether this was a reasonable alternative approach. After collecting and analyzing their data, they concluded that it was an acceptable approach, with limitations. The importance of the article is the demonstration of the limitations. In the series, 18 of the 139 patients had inadequate assessment of the thickness of the lesion using SB, and 7 (5%) required an additional operation because of this inadequate assessment. For surgeons who are facile in the performance of excisional biopsy, the shave should be considered as less than desirable. It is highly likely that the lesion will require complete excision, even if it is not proven to be melanoma. Why not do complete excision, initially? Or at least one or more punch biopsies (which were not discussed in the article)? So I applaud the collection of this valuable data, but disagree with the authors' conclusions.

R. L. Ruberg, MD

Staged Excision of Lentigo Maligna and Lentigo Maligna Melanoma: A 10-Year Experience

Bosbous MW, Dzwierzynski WW, Neuburg M (Med College of Wisconsin, Milwaukee)
Plast Reconstr Surg 124:1947-1955, 2009

Background.—The treatment of lentigo maligna and lentigo maligna melanoma presents a difficult problem for clinicians. Published guidelines recommend a 5-mm excision margin for lentigo maligna and a 1-cm margin for lentigo maligna melanoma, yet these are often inadequate. The authors' purpose is to report their 10-year experience using staged excision for the treatment of lentigo maligna and lentigo maligna melanoma of the head and neck.

Methods.—Staged excision was performed on 59 patients over a 10-year period. Data on patient demographics, lesion characteristics, and treatment were collected through an institutional review board–approved chart review.

Results.—Using staged excision, 62.7 percent of patients required a 10-mm or greater margin to achieve clearance of tumor. Two or more stages of excision were required in 50.9 percent of patients. Invasive melanoma (lentigo maligna melanoma) was identified in 10.2 percent of patients initially diagnosed with lentigo maligna. There was one (1.7 percent) documented recurrence during a median 2.25-year follow-up period (range, 0 to 10.17 years).

Conclusions.—Staged excision is an effective treatment for lentigo maligna and lentigo maligna melanoma. Previously published recommendations of 5-mm margins for wide local excision are inadequate for tumors located on the head and neck.

▶ This is an interesting variation of a technique originally described in 1997.[1] In essence, it is a permanent section technique, which uses some of the best concepts from Mohs' surgery and avoids some of the artifactual problems associated with the use of frozen sections in that technique. The authors clearly develop a case for the fact that national recommendations, currently extant in the United States for an adequate excision, require revision. One of the difficulties in determining the extent of the lesion during the planning of the primary excision is the fact that many times the margins of lentigo maligna are rather indefinite. Might the use of dermatoscopy help to better define the margins?[2] Finally, might there be a place for the use of imiquimod topical cream, an immune enhancing agent, as an adjunct to surgical excision similar to the use of bacillus Calmette-Guérin (BCG) in superficial bladder cancer?

S. H. Miller, MD, MPH

References

1. Johnson TM, Headington JT, Baker SR, Lowe L. Usefulness of the staged excision for lentigo maligna and lentigo maligna melanoma: the "square procedure". *J Am Acad Dermatol.* 1997;37:758-764.
2. Vestergaard ME, Macaskill P, Holt PE, Menzies SW. Dermatoscopy compared with naked eye examination for the diagnosis of primary melanoma: a meta-analysis of studies performed in a clinical setting. *Br J Dermatol.* 2008;59:669-676.

Staged Excision of Lentigo Maligna and Lentigo Maligna Melanoma: A 10-Year Experience

Bosbous MW, Dzwierzynski WW, Neuburg M (Med College of Wisconsin, Milwaukee)
Plast Reconstr Surg 124:1947-1955, 2009

Background.—The treatment of lentigo maligna and lentigo maligna melanoma presents a difficult problem for clinicians. Published guidelines recommend a 5-mm excision margin for lentigo maligna and a 1-cm margin for lentigo maligna melanoma, yet these are often inadequate. The authors' purpose is to report their 10-year experience using staged excision for the treatment of lentigo maligna and lentigo maligna melanoma of the head and neck.

Methods.—Staged excision was performed on 59 patients over a 10-year period. Data on patient demographics, lesion characteristics, and treatment were collected through an institutional review board–approved chart review.

Results.—Using staged excision, 62.7 percent of patients required a 10-mm or greater margin to achieve clearance of tumor. Two or more stages of excision were required in 50.9 percent of patients. Invasive melanoma (lentigo maligna melanoma) was identified in 10.2 percent of patients initially diagnosed with lentigo maligna. There was one (1.7 percent) documented recurrence during a median 2.25-year follow-up period (range, 0 to 10.17 years).

Conclusions.—Staged excision is an effective treatment for lentigo maligna and lentigo maligna melanoma. Previously published recommendations of 5-mm margins for wide local excision are inadequate for tumors located on the head and neck.

▶ The approach to lentigo maligna and lentigo maligna melanoma that is advocated by these authors would at first appear to be a step backward from modern treatment modalities. But the data that are presented in this series seem to entirely justify that step. Many surgeons (myself included) for years performed resection of lentigo maligna with a simple 5 mm margin. Others used Mohs' surgery with multiple excisions and frozen sections done in one "sitting." However, several recent articles have shown that 5 mm may be inadequate, and frozen sections may be unreliable for melanocytic lesions. The staged excision approach, carried out over several days, permits permanent sections and more complete verification of total removal of the lesions. As a result, the authors are able to report a much lower recurrence rate for their management of these sometimes challenging lesions.

R. L. Ruberg, MD

Incompletely excised skin cancer rates: a prospective study of 31 731 skin cancer excisions by the Western Australian Society of Plastic Surgeons
Dhepnorrarat RC, Lee MA, Mountain JA (Sir Charles Gairdner Hosp, Perth, Western Australia; Western Australian Audit of Surgical Mortality)
J Plast Reconstr Aesthet Surg 62:1281-1285, 2009

Background.—The incomplete excision of malignant skin lesions is an established measure of the standard of surgical care. It is one of the clinical indicators established by the Royal Australasian College of Surgeons and the Australian Council on Healthcare Standards.

Purpose of the Study.—The purpose of this study was to identify the rate of incomplete excisions of skin cancers by a group of plastic surgeons in Western Australia and to present the data in a way that enhances the audit process.

Methods.—Since 1996, 25 plastic surgeons in Western Australia have been collecting prospective data on incomplete clearances of skin cancer excisions in private practice. A standard data entry form is used and data were collected by clerical staff, independent of the surgeon, and submitted annually to the Western Australian Society of Plastic Surgeons.

A lesion was considered to be incompletely excised if tumour was found on histological examination to be present at the excision margin of a specimen.

Results.—From 1996 to 2002, 25 plastic surgeons performed 31 731 skin lesion excisions over a period of 6 years. Incomplete margins were found on histopathological examination of 1277 lesions (4.02%). Nineteen surgeons performed over 500 procedures.

Conclusion.—The 4.02% rate of incomplete lesion excisions compares favourably to the results of other series. Further development of the audit will yield valuable information on skin lesion management in Western Australia.

▶ This is an excellent prospective cooperative study to identify the percentages of incomplete excisions of various types of malignant skin lesions (basal cell carcinoma [BCC], squamous cell carcinoma [SCC], malignant melanoma [MM], and other types) by 25 plastic surgeons in Western Australia. It would have been very helpful to identify the numbers of surgeons in Western Australia who chose not to participate compared with those who did participate, and the reasons they made such a choice and whether they were different than those in the study group. The data was analyzed annually over the course of the study's duration. It was possible to identify those surgeons whose incomplete excision rate was above the norm during the course of the study, and presumably the data could be used as an outcome audit for quality improvement. It would have been useful to have some assurance that there was good interrater and intrarater reliability among the pathologists performing the histological examinations. The goals of the study need to be expanded to learn whether the low incomplete excision rate translates into an equally low recurrence rate and whether there are other demographic characteristics that impact patient outcome. Nonetheless, the authors are to be congratulated for organizing and participating in a study of this dimension.

S. H. Miller, MD, MPH

Facial Paralysis

Mini-Temporalis Transfer as an Adjunct Procedure for Smile Restoration
Terzis JK, Olivares FS (Eastern Virginia Med School, Norfolk)
Plast Reconstr Surg 123:533-542, 2009

Background.—The versatility of the temporalis muscle justifies its wide popularity in reconstructive craniomaxillofacial surgery. In late facial paralysis, results of neural reconstructive techniques such as cross-facial grafting or mini-hypoglossal-to-facial nerve transfer are partial at best. In this series, the authors have used a segmental temporalis transfer, the "mini-temporalis," to augment the function attained with neural microsurgery. The aim of this present study was to present the experience of the authors' center with the use of the mini-temporalis as an adjuvant to facial nerve microsurgery for smile restoration.

Methods.—Data were collected from 31 patients who underwent mini-temporalis transfer for smile restoration. In all patients, the mini-temporalis was used to augment the results of neural reconstructive techniques. Opting for the mini-temporalis related to a variety of reasons, after preoperative evaluation was weighed against the advantages and disadvantages of different reconstructive strategies on individual bases. Aesthetic and functional outcomes were evaluated by a panel of five independent observers using a five-category scale ranging from poor to excellent.

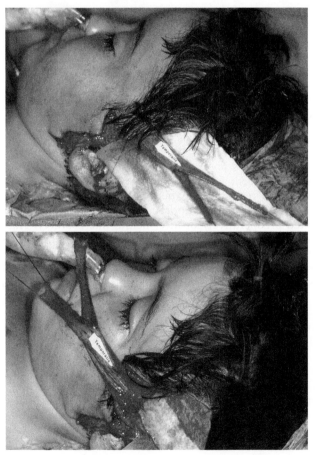

FIGURE 1.—Intraoperative photographs showing mini-temporalis transposition to the oral commissure. (*Above*) The middle section of the temporalis muscle is raised with the attached strip of deep temporal fascia and periosteum (divided in this case into two slips). Once transposed to the angle of the mouth, the elongated muscle reaches the modiolus and upper lip comfortably, where it will be anchored (*below*). (Reprinted from Terzis JK, Olivares FS. Mini-temporalis transfer as an adjunct procedure for smile restoration. *Plast Reconstr Surg* 2009;123:533-542.)

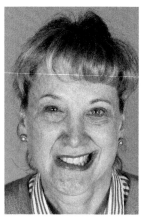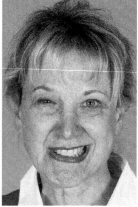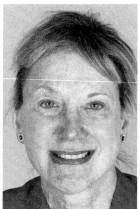

FIGURE 3.—Case 1. A 56-year-old woman presented with right-sided facial paralysis following the excision of an acoustic neuroma. She was first assessed at our center in October of 2001, 132 months after the insult. (*Left*) She had three cross-facial nerve grafts in January of 2003, and in December of 2003, she underwent secondary microcoaptations and mini-temporalis transposition to the oral commissure. (*Center* and *right*) Appearance at follow-up visits after neural microsurgery and temporalis transfer, respectively. The independent evaluators rated her smile as fair (2.4) preoperatively, moderate (3.2) after neural rehabilitation, and excellent (4.6) after mini-temporalis transfer. (Reprinted from Terzis JK, Olivares FS. Mini-temporalis transfer as an adjunct procedure for smile restoration. *Plast Reconstr Surg* 2009;123:533-542.)

Results.—All patients observed a follow-up longer than 3 months. Of 31 patients, 61.3 percent achieved excellent or good results and 29 percent achieved moderate results. All patients demonstrated an increase in the observers' scores after mini-temporalis transfer in comparison with the scores granted preoperatively or after neural microsurgery. Highly motivated patients committed to postoperative motor reeducation exhibited the best results.

Conclusion.—The clinical data presented support the use of mini-temporalis transposition in association with facial nerve microsurgery as a valuable alternative to free muscle transfer in selected cases (Figs 1 and 3).

▶ Mini-temporalis transfer is an excellent primary procedure in patients who are too old or infirm for free flap surgery or neural reconstruction. I frequently used it for both smile restoration and for eyelid closure in leprosy patients in Africa with very good results. The local periosteum and temporalis fascia were used to extend the muscle flaps to allow favorable insertion intraorally into the upper lip and modiolus. I am certain that given the opportunity to tailor the postoperative course and rehabilitation today results in better outcomes than were achieved in Africa in the 1970s. Virtually all patients were kept on a soft diet for 1 week and then dieted as tolerated. The only rehabilitation provided was to teach the patient how to use chewing gum and a mirror to practice using the muscle to achieve a smile.

S. H. Miller, MD, MPH

Thin-Profile Platinum Eyelid Weighting: A Superior Option in the Paralyzed Eye

Silver AL, Lindsay RW, Cheney ML, et al (Massachusetts Eye and Ear Infirmary and Harvard Med School, Boston)
Plast Reconstr Surg 123:1697-1703, 2009

Background.—A devastating sequela of facial paralysis is the inability to close the eye. The resulting loss of corneal protection can lead to exposure keratitis, corneal ulceration, and potentially permanent vision loss. Methods to address lagophthalmos historically have included tarsorrhaphy, lid weighting, levator palpebrae superioris lengthening, chemodenervation to yield protective ptosis, and the placement of magnetic eyelid springs. The gold eyelid weight, introduced nearly 50 years ago, continues to enjoy immense popularity, despite high complication rates and nearly uniform visibility under the skin. The authors hypothesized that a commercially available, thin platinum weight would combat the visibility of the thicker gold weights and herein compare complication rates and visibility rates with literature-reported data for gold weights.

Methods.—Beginning in 2004, 100 consecutive patients presenting to the authors' Facial Nerve Center with paralytic lagophthalmos requiring intervention were treated with thin-profile platinum eyelid weights. Ninety-six percent of cases were performed under local anesthesia in the office setting.

Results.—Median follow-up was 22 months. In 102 weights placed, there have been six complications (5.9 percent): three extrusions, two capsule formations, and one case of astigmatism. All of the extrusions involved irradiated patients with parotid malignancies.

Conclusions.—The authors report the first large series of thin-profile platinum eyelid weight implantations for the treatment of lagophthalmos. This implant significantly reduces both capsule formation phenomena and extrusion compared with gold weights and should be considered as alternative to the more conventional gold implants.

▶ The old style thick gold eyelid weighting device was often, if not always, visible in my experience. Not infrequently, patients had shifting of the implant, and in some instances extrusion. According to the authors, the thin platinum implants have a lower complication rate (roughly 6%), but the mean follow-up time was 19 months, and in some patients was only 4 months. The authors postulate that the thin platinum implants were 11% smaller than the same sized thin gold implants, due to the increased density of platinum, and viewed that difference in size as well as the lack of patient allergic reactivity to platinum as favorable, but no data are presented to validate those statements. Costs for the different thin implants as compared with the old gold implants were not addressed.

S. H. Miller, MD, MPH

Masseteric-facial nerve coaptation – an alternative technique for facial nerve reinnervation

Coombs CJ, Ek EW, Wu T, et al (Royal Children's Hosp, Parkville, Melbourne, Victoria, Australia; et al)
J Plast Reconstr Aesthet Surg 62:1580-1588, 2009

Background.—Reinnervation of the facial musculature when there is loss of the proximal facial nerve poses a difficult clinical problem. Restoration of spontaneous mimetic motion is the aim and, to this end, the use of cross-facial nerve grafts has long been considered the reconstruction of choice. The nerve to masseter has been used very successfully for reinnervation of microvascular functioning muscle transfers for facial reanimation in established facial palsy but its use as a direct nerve transfer to the facial nerve to reinnervate 'viable' facial musculature has been scarce.

Methods.—Electron micrographic studies of axonal counts in the nerve to masseter and nerve to gracilis in a clinical series of seven patients undergoing surgery for facial nerve palsy were made. Based on these results, and previous success with the use of the nerve to masseter for reinnervation of free gracilis transfers, we report our experience with the transfer of the nerve to masseter for direct coaptation with the ipsilateral facial nerve to restore facial motion.

Results.—Our axonal counts of the nerve to masseter have, on average, 1542 ± 291.70 (SD) axons. Historical data have shown that the buccal branch of the facial nerve has 834 ± 285 (SD) where the distal end of a cross-facial nerve graft has 100 to 200 axons. Our clinical use of the nerve to masseter as a direct nerve transfer in three patients based on these data has resulted in significant improvement in facial symmetry in repose (at a minimum of 1 year follow up), restoration of facial motion with occasional spontaneous activity and minimal synkinesis without any donor morbidity.

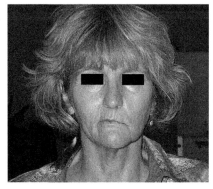 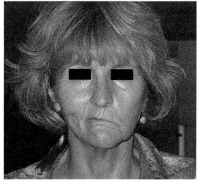

FIGURE 4.—Preoperative images of Case 2 in repose and smile – note facial cant, scleral show and left upper lip segment length. (Reprinted from Coombs CJ, Ek EW, Wu T, et al. Masseteric-facial nerve coaptation – an alternative technique for facial nerve reinnervation. *J Plast Reconstr Aesthet Surg.* 2009; 62:1580-1588, with permission from British Association of Plastic, Reconstructive and Aesthetic Surgeons.)

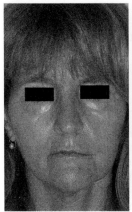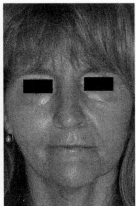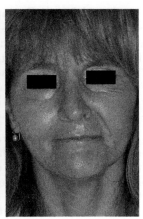

FIGURE 5.—Postoperative images at 11 months showing resolution of facial cant, scleral show and shortening of the left upper lip segment in repose, symmetrical small smile (middle image) and strength of reinnervated upper lip elevators. (Reprinted from Coombs CJ, Ek EW, Wu T, et al. Masseteric-facial nerve coaptation – an alternative technique for facial nerve reinnervation. *J Plast Reconstr Aesthet Surg.* 2009;62:1580-1588, with permission from British Association of Plastic, Reconstructive and Aesthetic Surgeons.)

Conclusions.—The advantages of this technique include the ease of dissection, constant and reliable anatomy, powerful reinnervation of the facial muscles without donor site morbidity and the potential for return of spontaneous facial movement (Figs 4 and 5).

▶ This is a small, but intriguing, report of 3 patients with unilateral facial nerve palsy who underwent a re-innervation of their distal facial nerves using the nerve to the ipsilateral masseter muscle. While the nerve to the masseter muscle has been used for re-innervation of functional gracilis muscle transfers to correct facial paralysis by the authors and others,[1] its use as a direct nerve transfer has been relatively infrequent. The major benefits cited include the fact that an intramuscular branch of the nerve to the masseter can be co-apted to the remaining facial nerve in a single-staged procedure, provides a large number of axons for neurotization, is readily available and easy to dissect, may produce spontaneous facial nerve function, and usually causes minimal donor site morbidity. The results obtained at a minimum follow-up of 1 year were quite good in 1 child and 2 middle-aged adults reported. Further studies are clearly warranted to evaluate the appropriate use of this procedure and the long-term results that can be achieved.

S. H. Miller, MD, MPH

Reference

1. Manketelow RM, Tomat LR, Zuker RM. Smile reconstruction with free muscle transfer innervated by the masseter motor nerve: effectiveness and cerebral adaption. *Plast Reconstr Surg.* 2006;118:885-899.

Head and Neck Reconstruction

Anatomical and Clinical Studies of the Supraclavicular Flap: Analysis of 103 Flaps Used to Reconstruct Neck Scar Contractures

Vinh VQ, Van Anh T, Ogawa R, et al (Vietnam Natl Inst of Burns, Hanoi, Vietnam; Nippon Med School Hosp, Tokyo, Japan)
Plast Reconstr Surg 123:1471-1480, 2009

Background.—The supraclavicular flap is an excellent flap that has been used widely, but its vascular reliability remains unclear. In this article, the authors report the results of their anatomical studies on 40 flaps from 20 preserved cadavers and their clinical studies of 103 supraclavicular flaps in 101 patients.

Methods.—In their anatomical study, the authors analyzed the important anatomical features that are useful for harvesting flaps. In their clinical study, the authors analyzed the cases in terms of flap reliability.

Results.—The supraclavicular artery branched from the transverse cervical artery in all 40 specimens (100 percent). Although it arose from the middle third of the clavicle in 90 percent of the specimens, it arose from the lateral third of the clavicle in four specimens (10 percent). Moreover, the transverse cervical artery originated from the subclavian artery in two of 40 specimens (5 percent) rather than from the thyrocervical trunk. The origins of the supraclavicular and transverse cervical arteries were on average 4.12 cm apart (range, 3 to 5.5 cm). In our clinical study, 101 of the 103 flaps (98.1 percent) were (vascular-pedicled) island flaps and five (4.9 percent) were transferred under a skin tunnel. We also performed a supercharged flap transfer using posterior circumflex humeral vessels. Of the 103 flaps, 97 survived completely (94.2 percent), but four and two exhibited superficial distal necrosis (3.9 percent) and total necrosis (1.9 percent), respectively.

Conclusions.—Supraclavicular flaps are reliable, but vascular anomalies exist. In the authors' experience, the posterior circumflex humeral artery could be used for supercharging the supraclavicular flap.

▶ The authors provide an excellent description of the anatomy of the vasculature of the supraclavicular flap, including its relationship to surface landmarks and the underlying structures based on cadaver dissections and clinical cases. Important in their dissections was the observation that the vascular leash could be lengthened significantly by including the transverse cervical artery. The latter observation also increases the diameter of the feeding artery should one wish to transfer it as a free flap. The incorporation of the transverse cervical artery is also useful, as it becomes the pivot point when the flap is rotated into its new position. In most instances (90%) the primary vasculature originated from within area of the middle third of the clavicle, but in 10% of their studies the primary vasculature originated in proximity to the lateral third of the clavicle. Surgeons who choose to use this flap must be aware, preoperatively, of these vascular anomalies. The flap can be increased in size by supercharging it. In most of the patients shown, the flaps were used for burn scars of the neck, limiting motion, and the results appeared to be quite functional and deemed to be cosmetically acceptable. However, the follow-up photos are all short-term (1 year), and virtually all scars appear to be keloidal. Donor sites were also reported as cosmetically acceptable, but no photographs of these sites were shown.

S. H. Miller, MD, MPH

A Horizontal V-Y Advancement Lower Eyelid Flap

Marchac D, de Lange A, Bine-bine H (Paris, France; Brussels, Belgium; Rabat, Morocco)

Plast Reconstr Surg 124:1133-1141, 2009

Background.—The authors were surprised to realize that the horizontal V-Y advancement flap of the lower eyelid is not even mentioned in the text-books about eyelid repair, and they wanted to report their very positive experience with this subcutaneous pedicled flap.

Methods.—Between 2000 and 2006, 21 patients were operated on, 13 women and eight men, aged 37 to 98 years, with a mean age of 67.5 years. The diagnosis was basal cell carcinoma in 20 cases and melanoma in one case. The size of the defect ranged from 10 to 30 mm, with a mean of 20 mm.

Results.—All flaps survived and the aesthetic quality of the repair was excellent in 17 of 21 cases. Postoperative recovery was usually very fast.

Conclusions.—The lower eyelid is covered with remarkably thin skin, and for the repair of defects, especially after removal of basal cell carci-nomas, it is preferable to avoid using tissues coming from another facial

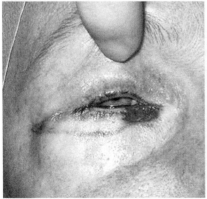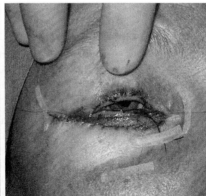

FIGURE 6.—Case 3. (*Left*) A 38-year-old woman after excision of a basal cell carcinoma in the lower eyelid. (*Right*) A long V-Y horizontal flap is moved medially, after the repair of a wedge resection. (Reprin-ted from Marchac D, de Lange A, Bine-bine H. A horizontal v-y advancement lower eyelid flap. *Plast Reconstr Surg.* 2009;124:1133-1141.)

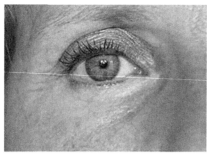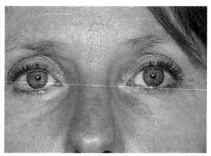

FIGURE 7.—Case 3. (*Left*) Close-up of the repaired eyelid 1 year postoperatively. (*Right*) Good symmetry has been obtained. (Reprinted from Marchac D, de Lange A, Bine-bine H. A horizontal v-y advancement lower eyelid flap. *Plast Reconstr Surg.* 2009;124:1133-1141.)

area (e.g., forehead, nose, or cheek), which has a different thickness and texture, or a full-thickness skin graft, which can leave a patch-like appearance. The ideal is to use the adjacent eyelid skin. For many years, the authors have used a horizontal large V-Y advancement flap on a muscular pedicle for the repair of lower eyelid defects, mostly after basocellular carcinoma excision, with very satisfactory results and often nearly invisible repairs (Figs 6 and 7).

▶ V-Y advancement flaps have proven value in reconstruction of facial defects, especially when the lines of the advancement are parallel to Langer's lines. In the authors' approach to defects of the lower eyelid, up to one third of the horizontal dimension of the lower eyelid can comfortably be repaired with the horizontal V-Y flap. The results reported are quite good, even in younger patients (Figs 6 and 7). Care must be taken to (1) make the flap sufficiently long, (2) make sure the width of the flap equals the width of the defect to be repaired, and (3) carefully maintain the subcutaneous pedicle.

S. H. Miller, MD, MPH

Palatomaxillary reconstruction with titanium mesh and radial forearm flap
Sun G, Yang X, Tang E, et al (Nanjing Univ, China)
Oral Surg Oral Med Oral Pathol Oral Radiol Endod 108:514-519, 2009

Objective.—The purpose of this study was to assess the treatment and prognosis of the palatomaxillary reconstruction with titanium mesh and the free radial forearm flap.
Study Design.—This is a retrospective study of 19 patients with palatomaxillary defects who underwent immediate reconstruction using titanium mesh and a radial forearm flap during the 4-year period from 2004 to 2008. Intraoperatively, the titanium mesh was fixed to the residual bones for the reconstruction of hard-tissue defect after the tumor

resection; then the free radial forearm flap was harvested to repair the soft-tissue defect, serving as the intraoral lining and titanium mesh covering.

Results.—Postoperative esthetic appearance and function were followed-up. All of the patients achieved a satisfactory facial appearance. The speech assessment was good, and the oronasal reflux did not occur in all patients. Only 3 patients had titanium mesh exposure during the follow-up period.

Conclusion.—The free radial forearm flap with folded titanium mesh is a reliable option for reconstruction of palatomaxillary defects. It is highly effective for swallowing and speech rehabilitation as well as esthetic reconstruction.

▶ Palatomaxillary reconstruction is often a daunting procedure. These authors confirm the earlier findings of Hashikawa et al[1] that use of titanium mesh plus a radial forearm flap can provide satisfactory functional and aesthetic reconstruction. As noted by the authors, care is required to make certain that technical errors (eg, inadequate amount of donor tissue being brought to the reconstructive site) do not occur, and to be aware that if high dose radiotherapy is necessary, there is an increased risk of exposure of the titanium. In spite of the fact that 3 of 19 patients required removal of the mesh, once exposed none developed oronasal incompetence or hypernasality.

S. H. Miller, MD, MPH

Reference

1. Hashikawa K, Tahara S, Ishida H, et al. Simple Reconstruction with titanium mesh and radial forearm flap after globe sparing total maxillectomy: a 5 year follow up study. *Plast Reconst Surg.* 2006;117:963-967.

Expanded Narrow Subcutaneous-Pedicled Island Forehead Flap for Reconstruction of the Forehead
Okazaki M, Ueda K, Sasaki K, et al (Tokyo Med and Dental Univ, Japan; Fukushima Med Univ, Japan; Horinouchi Hosp, Suginami-Ku, Japan; et al)
Ann Plast Surg 63:167-170, 2009

To reconstruct the subsequent defects after resection of a unilateral large forehead lesion, we devised a revised method, "expanded narrow subcutaneous-pedicled island forehead flap." After unilateral forehead skin was expanded by a tissue expander, the flap was designed on the upper half of the expanded forehead skin nourished by the subcutaneous adipomuscular pedicle, including the supratrochlear or supraorbital artery. The elevated flap was then transposed or rotated 180 degrees toward the defect. The donor site was closed with upward advancement of the lower half of the expanded skin. Four patients were treated with this method. The flaps survived completely without serious complications, and acceptable results were obtained in all patients. This method has the advantage of increased freedom of flap design and transfer, providing an effective use of unaffected skin, less scars left on the forehead, and less formation of the dog-ear compared with the conventional procedure.

▶ A nice variation on the use of forehead skin through expanding the proposed donor skin and basing the flap on a relatively narrow subcutaneous pedicle consisting of either the supratrochlear or supraorbital arteries (Figs 1 and 3 in the original article). The narrow pedicle allows the flap to be transposed or rotated 180°. Expansion of the forehead unquestionably promotes survival through delay of the flap. The limits of the flap were not defined as all survived, however, several of the photos do show elevation of the eyebrow on the side from which the flap was taken. I am sure that excessively large flaps will produce this elevation.

S. H. Miller, MD, MPH

New Method of Preparing a Pectoralis Major Myocutaneous Flap with a Skin Paddle that Includes the Third Intercostal Perforating Branch of the Internal Thoracic Artery

Rikimaru H, Kiyokawa K, Watanabe K, et al (Kurume Univ School of Medicine, Fukuoka, Japan)
Plast Reconstr Surg 123:1220-1228, 2009

Background.—Although the use of free flaps has become a major option for head and neck reconstruction, the pectoralis major myocutaneous flap still plays an important role because of its advantages and its convenience as a pedicle flap located adjacent to head and neck lesions. However, there remain two problems with the pectoralis major myocutaneous flap, namely, the difficulty in preparing a small, thin skin paddle with stable blood circulation for small defects and, particularly for female cases, sacrifice of the breast. The authors report a new method of preparing a pectoralis major myocutaneous flap to solve these problems.

Methods.—A skin paddle is designed just above the third intercostal perforating branch of the internal thoracic artery. The pectoralis major myocutaneous flap, including the muscular branch of the third intercostal perforating branch in its muscle, is elevated. The pectoralis major myocutaneous flap is moved to the reconstruction site through the subclavian route.

Results.—This method was used for 11 cases with small defects in the head and neck caused by lesions. Slight marginal necrosis was observed in one case, but the other skin paddles took completely. There was no infection or fistula formation, and almost satisfactory functional results were obtained in all cases. Deformity in donor sites that included a breast was also minimal.

Conclusions.—With this method, it was possible to prepare the pectoralis major myocutaneous flap using a small, thin skin paddle with stable

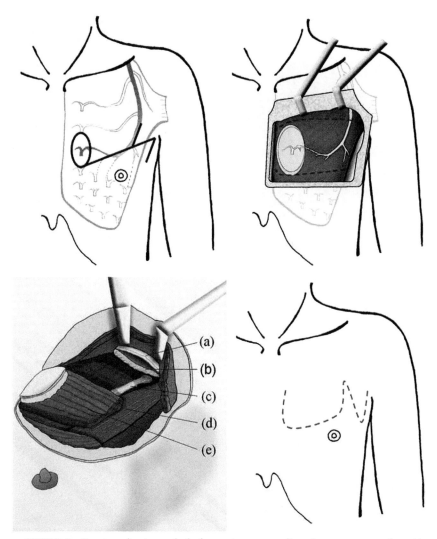

FIGURE 2.—Drawings showing method of preparing a pectoralis major myocutaneous flap with a skin paddle that includes the third intercostal perforating branch of the internal thoracic artery. (*Above, left*) Design of a skin paddle with an auxiliary incision line made toward the axilla. (*Above, right*) Upper and lower incision lines in the pectoralis major muscle (*blue broken lines*). (*Below, left*) Pectoralis major myocutaneous flap with pedicle made as a vascular pedicle only, and subclavian route. (*a*) Clavicle, (*b*) periosteum dissected beneath the clavicle, (*c*) loose areolar tissue enveloping thoracoacromial artery and vein, (*d*) pectoralis minor muscle, (*e*) pectoralis major myocutaneous flap. (*Below, right*) Method of donor-site closure. Performing a Z-plasty near the axilla and advancing the thoracic skin flap to cover the skin defect. This Z-plasty prevents scar contracture in the axilla after the operation. For interpretation of the references to color in this figure legend, the reader is referred to web version of this article. (Reprinted from Rikimaru H, Kiyokawa K, Watanabe K, et al. New method of preparing a pectoralis major myocutaneous flap with a skin paddle that includes the third intercostal perforating branch of the internal thoracic artery. *Plast Reconstr Surg.* 2009;123:1220-1228.)

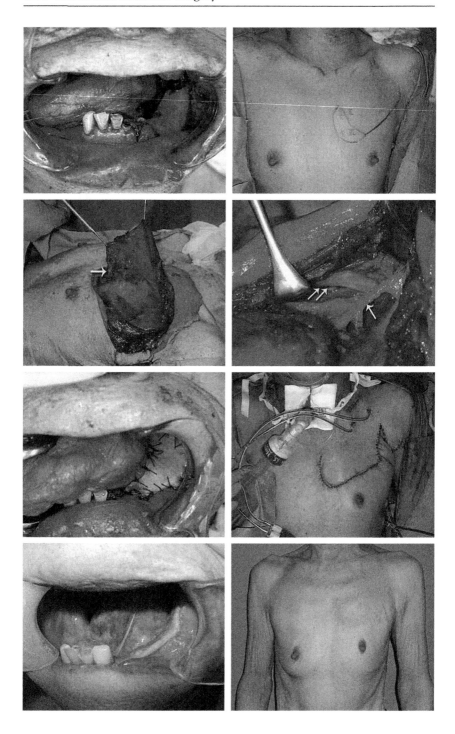

blood circulation. Breast deformation, particularly in female cases, was also kept to a minimum (Figs 2 and 3).

▶ This study looks at interesting findings that can increase the value of the pectoralis major myocutaneous flap for head and neck reconstruction. Especially useful has been the authors' elucidation of the blood supply to the thin skin of the anterior chest wall by inclusion of the third intercostal branch of the internal thoracic artery, as well as the pectoral branch of the thoracoacromial artery (Fig 2). While the modified flap seems relatively easy to prepare and better vascularized than the standard pectoralis major myocutaneous flap, it still appears to distort the female breast; however, this does not appear to be evident in the small-breasted Asian females shown in Fig 3 in this series.

S. H. Miller, MD, MPH

Pressure Ulcers

African Americans show increased risk for pressure ulcers: A retrospective analysis of acute care hospitals in America
Fogerty M, Guy J, Barbul A, et al (Vanderbilt Univ School of Medicine, Nashville, TN; Johns Hopkins Univ, Baltimore, MD)
Wound Rep Reg 17:678-684, 2009

In an earlier study, we reported a significantly increased risk of pressure ulcer hospital discharge diagnoses in African Americans, higher age groups, and those with certain medical conditions. The objectives of the present study were to: (a) investigate the demographics associated with a higher odds ratio (OR) in African Americans and (b) determine whether African Americans have different rates of medical risk factors. The 2003 Nationwide Inpatient Sample database was queried. Patients with pressure ulcers were identified by discharge diagnoses using ICD-9 codes 707.0–707.09. Discharge diagnosis was examined using the agency for healthcare research and quality clinical classifications software (CCS). The present study used identified CCS discharge diagnoses present in at least 5% of all patients,

---

FIGURE 3.—Case 1. (*Above, left*) Defect after tumor resection. Resection was performed using the pull-through method for carcinoma of the lower gingiva. (*Above, right*) Design of the skin paddle and auxiliary incision line. In this case, the skin paddle included both the third and second intercostal perforating branches of the internal thoracic artery. (*Second row, left*) Findings on dissection of the pectoralis major myocutaneous flap from the chest wall. The third intercostal perforating branch of the internal thoracic artery (yellow arrow) is tied off with an atraumatic ligature at the chest wall side. (*Second row, right*) Findings of the vascular pedicle with loose areolar tissue of which several branches were cut (*single yellow arrow*), and the subclavian root between the clavicle and its periosteum (*double yellow arrows*). (*Third row, left*) Immediate postoperative reconstruction site. (*Third row, right*) Donor site; a Z-plasty is performed near the axilla and the thoracic skin flap is advanced to cover the skin defect. (*Below, left*) Oral findings 6 months after the operation. The flap had taken completely. (*Below, right*) Donor-site findings 6 months after the operation. Almost no breast deformation can be observed. For interpretation of the references to color in this figure legend, the reader is referred to web version of this article. (Reprinted from Rikimaru H, Kiyokawa K, Watanabe K, et al. New method of preparing a pectoralis major myocutaneous flap with a skin paddle that includes the third intercostal perforating branch of the internal thoracic artery. *Plast Reconstr Surg.* 2009;123:1220-1228.)

with an OR > 2. African Americans exhibited a higher incidence of an OR > 2 for 28 identified CCS risk factors for pressure ulcers. The pressure ulcer diagnoses tended to occur at younger ages in African Americans. No significant differences were noted in African Americans with pressure ulcers when a subanalysis was conducted by zip code income quartile, region of the country, or teaching status of the hospital. Hospitalized African Americans exhibit an age-dependent, higher prevalence of pressure ulcers compared with Caucasians. Socioeconomic factors tracked within the Nationwide Inpatient Sample do not provide an explanation for this phenomenon.

▶ The results reported in this retrospective analysis of pressure ulcers are based on administrative data contained in the 2003 Nationwide Inpatient Sample database. The results are compelling, documenting that African Americans appear to have a higher incidence of risk factors for pressure ulcers to occur in hospital than do whites, and at an earlier age. However, while it is based on a large amount of data, the latter is administrative and retrospective, and a significant number of states reporting data do not classify patients according to race. Nonetheless, of the many socioeconomic factors studied, there does not appear to be a correlation between them and the higher incidence of pressure ulcers. It seems very clear that this is an important public health issue that requires careful prospective study to determine whether the findings are due to errors in data collection or interpretation, and more importantly why the incidence appears to be higher in African Americans.

S. H. Miller, MD, MPH

Treatment of large ischial ulcers communicating with the hip joint with proximal femoral resection and reconstruction with a combined vastus lateralis, vastus intermedius and rectus femoris musculocutaneous flap
Acartürk TO (Çukurova Univ School of Medicine, Turkey)
J Plast Reconstr Aesthet Surg 62:1497-1502, 2009

Pressure ulcers which communicate with the hip joint are very difficult to treat. Often, the hip joint is infected with osteomyelitis of the proximal femur resulting in bouts of sepsis and flap failure. These patients require proximal femoral resection and wide debridement in order to eradicate the infection, which in turn results in large and deep cavities. Reconstruction requires either a muscle flap or even a total thigh flap if the defect is very large and the pelvis is involved.

In a series of six ischial or ischio-trochanteric pressure sores communicating with the hip joint, following multiple serial debridements, the vastus lateralis, vastus intermedius and rectus femoris muscles were raised as a single musculocutaneous flap ('three muscle flap'), based on the descending branch of the lateral femoral circumflex artery, and transposed into the defect. All patients were paraplegics and had signs of sepsis during admission. Two patients had prior failed reconstructions within 3 months of admission and the others had not been operated on before. The external skin defect of the ulcers ranged from 7×5 cm to 30×12 cm. After 12 months follow up there was no recurrence of pressure sores or sepsis.

The 'three muscle flap' offers the advantage of providing large bulk to fill deep cavities, while preserving the rest of the thigh. The flap elevation is fast and safe and the vascular pedicle is reliable. This technique is not for simple pressure sores, but should be reserved for large pressure sores complicated with large cavities created after resection of the proximal femur.

▶ This article describes an aggressive approach to a challenging problem. The major value of this surgical technique is that it combines 3 muscles into a single flap. When faced with a large pressure sore after debridement of the acetabulum and a proximal femoral resection, I have usually tried to find the largest muscle or musculocutaneous flap available and transferred this tissue into the defect. If there was not enough tissue to obliterate the defect and cover all of the exposed bone, I would add a second and perhaps even a third flap. The author starts with the appropriate assumption that defects of this type very frequently require a great deal of tissue for coverage. Instead of progressively adding more tissue, the author immediately dissects all 3 muscles as a single unit. This approach preserves the blood supply, offers excellent dead space obliteration, and— perhaps most important—saves the time needed to dissect 3 different flaps. For appropriate defects, this approach makes very good sense. The results, as reported by the author, seem to be durable and long standing.

R. L. Ruberg, MD

Treatment of Ischial Pressure Sores Using a Modified Gracilis Myofasciocutaneous Flap

Lin H, Hou C, Chen A, et al (The Second Military Med Univ, Shanghai, People's Republic of China)
J Reconstr Microsurg 26:153-158, 2010

Despite the availability of a variety of flap reconstruction options, ischial pressure sores continue to be the most difficult pressure sores to treat. This article describes a successful surgical procedure for the coverage of ischial ulcers using a modified gracilis myofasciocutaneous flap. From August 2000 to April 2004, 12 patients with ischial sores were enrolled in the study. All patients underwent early aggressive surgical debridement followed by surgical reconstruction with a modified gracilis myofasciocutaneous flap. The follow-up period ranged from 13 to 86 months, with a mean of 44 months. Overall, 91.7% of the flaps (11 of 12) survived primarily. Partial flap necrosis occurred in one patient. Primary wound healing occurred without complications at both the donor and recipient sites in all cases. In one patient, grade II ischial pressure sores recurred 13 months after the operation. There was no recurrence in other 11 patients. A modified gracilis myofasciocutaneous flap provides a good cover for ischial pressure sores. Because it is easy to use and has favorable results, it can be used in the primary treatment for large and deep ischial pressure sores.

▶ The abstract describes the use of a modified gracilis flap for coverage of ischial pressure sores. Only a total of 12 patients were enrolled in the study. The follow-up median time of 44 months speaks to the longevity of the flap integrity. The study reports a survival rate of 92% with only 1 flap with partial necrosis. My experience with this flap has not been as positive. Orienting the skin portion longitudinally helps. The gracilis is not a particularly robust muscle to begin with and with the atrophy of paraplegia, orientation is ever more difficult. This flap should be kept in mind, but my overall algorithm won't change based on this experience.

D. J. Smith, Jr, MD

Increased fluid intake does not augment capacity to lay down new collagen in nursing home residents at risk for pressure ulcers: A randomized, controlled clinical trial
Stotts NA, Hopf HW, Kayser-Jones J, et al (Univ of California San Francisco; Univ of Utah, Salt Lake City; et al)
Wound Repair Regen 17:780-788, 2009

Prevention of pressure ulcers is fundamental to safe care of nursing home residents yet the role of hydration in pressure ulcer prevention has not been systematically examined. This randomized clinical trial was undertaken to determine whether administration of supplemental fluid to nursing home residents at risk for pressure ulcers would enhance collagen deposition, increase estimated total body water, augment subcutaneous tissue oxygenation, and was safe. After a baseline period, 64 subjects were randomized to receive the fluid volume prescribed or additional fluid (prescribed plus 10 mL/kg) for 5 days. Participants' potential to heal as measured with hydroxyproline was low at baseline and did not increase significantly during treatment when additional fluid was systematically provided. Fluid intake increased significantly during treatment. Estimates of total body water and subcutaneous oxygen did not increase, indicating hydration was not improved. Supplemental fluid did not result in overhydration as measured by clinical parameters. Further work is needed to examine the relationship between fluid intake and hydration in nursing home residents as well as the role of hydration in pressure ulcer prevention.

▶ Preventing pressure sores in the elderly is a significant unmet medical need. It is known that 1 in 4 patients who are admitted to a nursing home will eventually develop a pressure sore—a staggering burden for the health care system. This study examines one approach to pressure sore prevention, namely, increasing the hydration status of the elderly patients. The authors' previous work led them to believe that increasing the hydration status would increase collagen deposition, perfusion, and tissue oxygenation. These surrogate endpoints were used rather than skin breakdown itself. The study itself was well designed and randomized and examined endpoints by invasively implanting wound chambers and oxygen catheters. Unfortunately, the overall results of the study were negative and demonstrated that supplemental hydration did not have the expected effect on collagen deposition of tissue oxygenation. Interestingly, tissue oxygenation actually decreased with hydration, perhaps illustrating some of the age-related changes in oxygen sensing that have been described by others.[1] Hopefully, focusing on these defects in oxygen sensing and tissue PO_2 may lead to more robust treatments to prevent pressure ulceration in this vulnerable population.

G. C. Gurtner, MD

Reference

1. Chang EI, Loh SA, Ceradini DJ, et al. Age decreases endothelial progenitor cell recruitment through decreases in hypoxia-inducible factor 1alpha stabilization during ischemia. *Circulation.* 2007;116:2818-2829.

A 25-Year Experience with Hemicorporectomy for Terminal Pelvic Osteomyelitis

Janis JE, Ahmad J, Lemmon JA, et al (Univ of Texas Southwestern Med Ctr, Dallas; Univ of Colorado, Denver)
Plast Reconstr Surg 124:1165-1176, 2009

Background.—Hemicorporectomy involves amputation of the pelvis and lower extremities by disarticulation through the lumbar spine with concomitant transection of the aorta, inferior vena cava, and spinal cord. In addition, conduits are constructed for diversion of both the urinary and fecal streams. Of 57 cases reported in the literature, limited experience exists with hemicorporectomy for terminal pelvic osteomyelitis, with only 11 cases described. Furthermore, there is little information available regarding perioperative mortality and long-term survival. This article describes the largest reported series of hemicorporectomies performed for terminal pelvic osteomyelitis.

Methods.—A retrospective review of the medical records for nine patients who underwent hemicorporectomy at the authors' institution was conducted followed by interviews with all surviving patients.

Results.—At follow-up, four patients were alive and five patients were dead. For all patients, the average survival after hemicorporectomy was 11.0 years (range, 1.7 to 22.0 years). There was no perioperative mortality within 30 days of surgery. None of the surviving patients suffered from recurrent decubitus ulcers.

Conclusions.—Including this clinical series, a total of 66 hemicorporectomies have now been reported in the literature. Twenty cases were performed for terminal pelvic osteomyelitis with no mortality within

30 days of surgery, and 53.3 percent of patients were alive and well at long-term follow-up. Given the low perioperative mortality along with the ability of patients to achieve long-term survival following this operation, hemicorporectomy should be offered to appropriate patients suffering from terminal pelvic osteomyelitis.

▶ Hemicorporectomy is a radical approach to a devastating problem. Most surgeons who deal regularly with pressure ulcers and chronic osteomyelitis (me included) have at times considered this operation but then made every effort to avoid it. Somehow, it just did not seem "right" to amputate and discard half of the body. Now these authors make a good case for performance of this operation in carefully selected circumstances. They are able to support their argument for the procedure with several important observations based on their extensive literature review and personal experience at their own institutions: (1) survival (both short-term and long-term) is actually quite good; (2) patient satisfaction seems to be remarkably good; and (3) attention to specific surgical details can substantially reduce the operative risk. In fact, based on their observations, they even recommend abandoning the classic approach, which regards hemicorporectomy as a "last resort" procedure, and moving toward earlier performance of the operation to minimize the adverse effects of previous, unsuccessful, less-aggressive surgical procedures. The bottom line is what is best for the patient, and sometimes surgeons must make a decision that a seemingly radical approach may actually be the most conservative in terms of ultimate survival and patient satisfaction. This appears to be one of those situations.

R. L. Ruberg, MD

Trunk and Perineal Reconstruction

Surgical Management of the Symptomatic Unstable Sternum with Pectoralis Major Muscle Flaps

Cabbabe EB, Cabbabe SW (Univ of Alabama at Birmingham)
Plast Reconstr Surg 123:1495-1498, 2009

Background.—Sternal nonunion after median sternotomy is an uncommon but potentially disabling complication. The management of nonunion varies based on the discretion of the cardiovascular surgeon.

Methods.—An analysis of all patients with symptomatic sternal nonunion who underwent wire removal, subtotal sternal débridement, and muscle flap reconstruction from 1993 to 2008 was conducted. A retrospective review was performed to evaluate preoperative and postoperative symptoms, pain scores, procedures, length of hospital stay, operating time, complications, morbidity, and mortality.

Results.—A total of 24 patients were identified. The male-to-female ratio was 11:1. Time from initial median sternotomy to consultation ranged from 5 to 48 months. All were referred when stability was not achieved by other means. None of the patients had clinical or laboratory evidence of sternal wound infection at presentation. The patients rated their preoperative pain severity at an average of 7.7 and a maximum of 10 on a scale of 1 to 10. All intraoperative cultures showed no growth. The operating time averaged 104 minutes. The average length of stay for these patients was 2.5 days. Follow-up ranged from 2 to 15 months, with an average of 4.2 months. All patients had clinically improved sternal stability.

Conclusions.—All patients experienced improvement of their preoperative symptoms, particularly pain, popping, and grinding. Average pain severity dropped from 7.7 preoperatively to 2.2, with a maximum of 4. Two patients developed seroma and required operative drainage. Both went on to complete healing. The mortality rate was 0 percent.

▶ This is a short but valuable report that addresses a relatively uncommon but potentially vexing problem. There are many reports that address various aspects of, and approaches to, the management of sternal wound infections or acute sternal wound dehiscence. This report focuses only on those patients who do not have sternal infection or open sternal wounds. These are patients who have healed the soft tissues of their sternotomy wound, but have symptoms (usually significant pain) related to nonunion and motion of the boney structures. One might assume that any effort to address this problem should include an effort to restabilize the sternum (eg, with modern plating techniques). But these authors have been highly successful using only muscle transposition into the boney defect. In light of the fact that restabilization of the sternum often is unsuccessful, this relatively simple and well-described technique may indeed provide the best long-term results and pain relief, even though it might not appear to be the most logical approach.

R. L. Ruberg, MD

A "Buttressed Mesh" Technique for Fascial Closure in Complex Abdominal Wall Reconstruction

Davison SP, Parikh PM, Jacobson JM, et al (Georgetown Univ, Washington, DC)

Ann Plast Surg 62:284-289, 2009

Today, plastic surgeons are increasingly faced with the problem of complex abdominal wall reconstruction. Obesity, bariatric surgery, and failed prior herniorrhaphy contribute to high rates of hernia recurrence in these difficult tertiary cases.

We reviewed 50 consecutive complex abdominal wall reconstructions to identify the roles of 3 technical variables in successful outcomes: use of mesh, use of a flap buttress to reinforce the fascial repair, and the use of concomitant body-contouring techniques. Six groups were identified based on the presence or absence of each of these variables. Incidence of hernia recurrence and incidence of complications were compared for each group. Patient satisfaction with reconstructive outcome was assessed at follow-up using a 5-point scale.

At a mean follow-up of 24 months, we observed an overall hernia recurrence rate of 4.0%, and an overall complication rate of 34%. Tension-free primary fascial repair and mesh repair of tension defects had equivalent recurrence rates (3.3% vs. 5%) and complication rates (40% vs. 25%). Repairs buttressed with flaps and repairs without buttressing had equivalent recurrence rates (3% vs. 6%) and complication rates (38% vs 28%). Repairs with and without body contouring techniques as part of the reconstructive plan had equivalent recurrence rates (7.7% vs. 0%) and complication rates (31.7% vs. 53%). Mean patient satisfaction was 4.8 of 5.

Reconstruction of complex and recurrent hernias can be successfully performed. When tension-free primary fascial closure is not possible, an inlay mesh with a soft-tissue buttress leads to a 10-fold reduction in hernia recurrence as compared to historical norms. Concomitant body contouring surgery does not impact recurrence or complication rates and may contribute to reconstructive success.

▶ The authors present 50 consecutive complex abdominal wall reconstructions and present 3 pearls to maximize success and minimize morbidity in this difficult population: (1) body contouring incisions to provide abdominal wall access and to optimize the quality of skin closure by resecting redundant and attenuated tissue; (2) liberal use of mesh in an intraperitoneal position when primary closure is not possible; and (3) vascularized soft tissue buttressing of the fascial closure to reinforce the repair and protect it from superficial wound breakdown.

The knowledge and understanding of where to place body contouring incisions helps with exposure as well as allowing one to develop good surgical planes in unoperated areas leading to easier dissections. This is supported by the fact that the authors reported no enterotomies in their surgical complications.

The liberal use of composite mesh is not a new idea of general surgeons who regularly repair hernias. The key is a wide intraperitoneal placement of mesh to decrease and distribute tension of the suture to a wider area. Knowledge about and the use of different types of mesh, including biologicals, should be evaluated by the surgeon for each patient.[1,2]

The use of vascularized tissues to buttress the repair clearly reinforces the well-known plastic surgery dogma of bringing in healthy vascularized tissue to heal wounds. This certainly protects the mesh from future infections and may improve incorporation of the mesh into host tissues.

These clinical pearls will clearly help us understand future directions of abdominal wall reconstruction.

J. Chao, MD

References

1. Mathes SJ, Steinwald PM, Foster RD, et al. Complex abdominal wall reconstruction: a comparison of flap and mesh closure. *Ann Surg.* 2000;232:586-596.
2. Grevious MA, Cohen M, Jean-Pierre F, et al. The use of prosthetics in abdominal wall reconstruction. *Clin Plas Surg.* 2005;33:181-197.

Surgical Outcomes of VRAM versus Thigh Flaps for Immediate Reconstruction of Pelvic and Perineal Cancer Resection Defects

Nelson RA, Butler CE (Univ of Texas M. D. Anderson Cancer Ctr, Houston)
Plast Reconstr Surg 123:175-183, 2009

Background.—Reconstruction following abdominoperineal resection or pelvic exenteration is commonly performed with regional flaps from the thigh or abdomen. This study compared the surgical outcomes and complications in cancer patients who underwent immediate reconstruction of these defects with vertical rectus abdominis myocutaneous (VRAM) versus thigh flaps.

Methods.—One hundred thirty-three patients who underwent abdominoperineal resection or pelvic exenteration for cancer resection and immediate VRAM ($n = 114$) or thigh flap ($n = 19$) reconstruction of the perineal/pelvic defect were studied. Patient, tumor, and treatment characteristics; surgical outcomes; and postoperative donor- and recipient-site complications were compared between the two groups. Multivariate logistic regression analysis was used to identify predictive/protective factors for complications.

Results.—The thigh flap group had a significantly greater incidence of major complications (42 percent versus 15 percent) than the VRAM flap group. They also had significantly higher rates of donor-site cellulitis (26 percent versus 6 percent) and recipient-site complications, including cellulitis (21 percent versus 4 percent), pelvic abscess (32 percent versus 6 percent), and major wound dehiscence (21 percent versus 5 percent). Abdominal wall complications were not increased in the VRAM group despite flap harvest from the abdominal wall. Obesity was an independent predictor of any donor-site complication (odds ratio, 3.3) and previous abdominal surgery was a predictor of any complication (odds ratio, 3.6), any recipient-site complication (odds ratio, 3.5), and any major complication (odds ratio, 3.6).

Conclusion.—Immediate VRAM flaps result in fewer major complications than thigh flaps without increased early abdominal wall morbidity when used to repair abdominoperineal resection and pelvic exenteration defects.

▶ The introduction of pedicle flap reconstruction of the perineum, particularly the use of the gracilis musculocutaneous flap, greatly enhanced the outcome of radical resections in this area 30 years ago. More recent advances, particularly the use of the vertical rectus abdominis myocutaneous (VRAM) flap, gave the surgeon multiple options for reconstruction. Is there one operation that is clearly better than the others? At least in the hands of these investigators, the VRAM is clearly better when evaluated by a variety of parameters, which seems logical because the transfer of a vigorously perfused muscle with a tightly adherent skin island should do the best job of coverage and closure of the perineum. My own experience with multiple cases using the gracilis musculocutaneous flap (a flap with less consistent blood supply and tenuous connection of the skin island) encouraged me to look for other options. The main limitation of this study is the very low number of thigh flaps, suggesting that perhaps the authors' lesser experience with this type of procedure contributed to their higher complication rate. I would still go with the VRAM now.

R. L. Ruberg, MD

Reconstruction of Pelvic Exenteration Defects with Anterolateral Thigh–Vastus Lateralis Muscle Flaps

Wong S, Garvey P, Skibber J, et al (Univ of Texas M.P. Anderson Cancer Ctr, Houston)
Plast Reconstr Surg 124:1177-1185, 2009

Background.—The rectus abdominis may be unavailable or insufficient to reconstruct large pelvic exenteration defects. The purpose of this study was to report the authors' experience with the pedicled anterolateral thigh–vastus lateralis muscle flap for such reconstructions.

Methods.—Eighteen patients with pelvic exenteration underwent reconstruction with this flap between 2003 and 2007. When the perineal defect could be closed primarily, the vastus lateralis muscle was tunneled over the

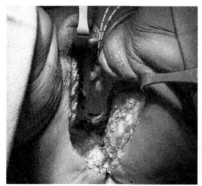 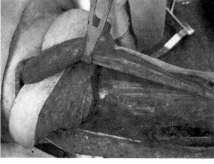

FIGURE 1.—A typical vaginal defect involving the posterior vaginal wall following a posterior pelvic exenteration (*left*). An anterolateral thigh flap with the vastus lateralis muscle was elevated from the right thigh and passed under the rectus femoris muscle to gain additional pedicle length (*right*). (Reprinted from Wong S, Garvey P, Skibber J, et al. Reconstruction of pelvic exenteration defects with anterolateral thigh-vastus lateralis muscle flaps. *Plast Reconstr Surg.* 2009;124:1177-1185, with permission from the American Society of Plastic Surgeons.)

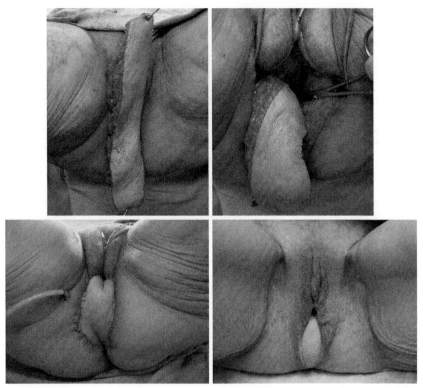

FIGURE 2.—The flap was brought to the perineal defect through a subcutaneous tunnel in the medial thigh (*above, left*). The proximal part of the flap skin was used for vaginal reconstruction (*above, right*) and the distal part was used to reconstruct the perineal defect (*below, left*). A photograph obtained 3 years after surgery showed a well-healed flap (*below, right*). (Reprinted from Wong S, Garvey P, Skibber J, et al. Reconstruction of pelvic exenteration defects with anterolateral thigh-vastus lateralis muscle flaps. *Plast Reconstr Surg.* 2009;124:1177-1185.)

inguinal ligament into the pelvis (inguinal route). For concomitant perineal-vaginal reconstruction, the anterolateral thigh–vastus lateralis muscle was tunneled over the medial thigh to the defect (perineal route).

Results.—All 18 patients (five men and 13 women) received preoperative chemoradiation. Nine patients received intraoperative pelvic brachytherapy. After pelvic exenteration, a colostomy was created in all patients, and a urostomy with ileal conduit was created in eight patients. The inguinal route was used in six patients and the perineal route was used in 10 patients. In the remaining two patients, the anterolateral thigh–vastus lateralis muscle from one thigh was delivered through the perineal route and the contralateral vastus lateralis flap was delivered through the inguinal route. Postoperative complications included five small perineal wound dehiscences that healed spontaneously, one flap failure caused by pedicle tension in an obese patient with a short thigh, an enterocutaneous fistula, and an ileal conduit leak that healed spontaneously. No hernias occurred.

Conclusions.—The pedicled anterolateral thigh–vastus lateralis flap is a good alternative for reconstruction of large pelvic exenteration defects when the rectus abdominis flap is unavailable. Obese patients with short thighs may not be good candidates for this procedure (Figs 1 and 2).

▶ Large perineal and pelvic wounds secondary to pelvic exenteration and chemoradiation therapy for cancers of this region are fraught with significant healing problems and considerable postoperative morbidity. If the rectus abdominus is not available or not large enough for reconstruction of defects secondary to pelvic exenteration, the anterolateral thigh vastus lateralis muscle flaps appear to be a good alternative for reconstruction. Although the authors report that 33% of their patients had small perineal wound healing problems, virtually all healed without further surgery. Three patients had significant complications and one flap failed due to compromise of the vascular pedicle in an obese patient. Seven of the 18 patients presented with primary tumors, and 11 patients presented with recurrent disease; the latter included 10 patients with colostomies and 3 of these with parastomal hernias. All patients had received radiation therapy before the surgical procedures reported. The small number of patients studied make generalizations difficult, but the admonition about trying to perform these operations on patients who are obese and have a short thigh is well worth noting, as is the indication for converting the flap from a pedicle flap to a free flap. The authors offer the opinion—which most of us experienced in operating in irradiated tissues agree with—that it is better to perform these reconstructions by bringing in healthy nonirradiated tissues preemptively than to perform them after these wounds have broken down postoperatively.

S. H. Miller, MD, MPH

Complex Torso Reconstruction with Human Acellular Dermal Matrix: Long-Term Clinical Follow-Up
Nemeth NL, Butler CE (Univ of Texas M. D. Anderson Cancer Ctr, Houston)
Plast Reconstr Surg 123:192-196, 2009

Although reports have demonstrated good early outcomes with human acellular dermal matrix even when used for complex, contaminated defects, no long-term outcomes have been reported. The authors reviewed the long-term outcomes of 13 patients who had complex torso reconstructions that included human acellular dermal matrix. All patients were at increased risk for mesh-related complications. Eight patients died as a result of progression of their oncologic disease at a mean of 258 days postoperatively. The mean follow-up for the remaining five patients was 43.7 months. Six patients had early complications (none were human acellular dermal matrix–related) and were reported on previously. Two patients had developed complications since the initial report. One patient developed a flap donor-site seroma remote from the reconstruction site, and another developed a recurrent ventral hernia. No patients have required additional surgery for human acellular dermal matrix–related complications. This follow-up report indicates that human acellular dermal matrix repair of large, complex torso defects can result in good long-term outcomes even when patients are at high risk for mesh-related complications.

▶ This is a long-term follow-up of an article that the senior author published in 2005.[1] They now present 3.5-year follow-up of these patients. Unfortunately, only 5 patients could be followed as 6 sucuumbed to their cancers. This small sample size limits significant statistical analysis in a highly specialized patient population. The authors present a nice description of the use of acellular dermal matrix and how it can become incorporated into host tissue. Histology shows cellular infiltration and neovascularization of the acellular dermal matrix. More studies documenting the long-term outcomes of patients who undergo reconstruction with acellular dermal matrix are clearly necessary.

J. Chao, MD

Reference

1. Butler CE, Languerin HN, Kronowitz SJ. Pelvic, abdominal and chest wall reconstruction with AlloDerm in patients at increased risk for mesh-related complications. *Plast Reconstr Surg.* 2005;116:1263-1275.

Extremity Reconstruction

Experimental Assessment of Autologous Lymph Node Transplantation as Treatment of Postsurgical Lymphedema

Tobbia D, Semple J, Baker A, et al (Univ of Toronto, Ontario, Canada)
Plast Reconstr Surg 124:777-786, 2009

Background.—The authors' objective was to test whether the transplantation of an autologous lymph node into a nodal excision site in sheep would restore lymphatic transport function and reduce the magnitude of postsurgical lymphedema.

Methods.—As a measure of lymph transport, iodine-125 human serum albumin was injected into prenodal vessels at 8 and 12 weeks after surgery, and plasma levels of the protein were used to calculate the transport rate of the tracer to blood (percent injected per hour). Edema was quantified from the circumferential measurement of the hind limbs.

Results.—The transplantation of avascular lymph nodes at 8 ($n = 6$) and 12 weeks ($n = 6$) produced lymphatic function levels of 12.3 ± 0.5 and 12.6 ± 0.8, respectively. These values were significantly less ($p < 0.001$) than those measured at similar times in the animals receiving sham surgical procedures (16.6 ± 0.7, $n = 6$; and 16.1 ± 0.7, $n = 6$, respectively). When vascularized transplants were performed, lymphatic function was similar to the sham controls and significantly greater ($p < 0.001$) than that of the avascular group (8 weeks, 15.8 ± 0.9, $n = 8$; 12 weeks, 15.7 ± 1.0, $n = 10$). Lymph transport correlated significantly with the health of the transplanted nodes (scaled with histologic analysis)

($p < 0.0001$). The vascularized node transplants ($n = 18$) were associated with the greatest clinical improvement, with the magnitude of edema in these limbs exhibiting significantly lower levels of edema ($p = 0.039$) than nontreated limbs ($n = 18$).

Conclusions.—The successful reimplantation of a lymph node into a nodal excision site has the potential to restore lymphatic function and facilitate edema resolution. This result has important conceptual implications in the treatment of postsurgical lymphedema.

▶ This is an interesting experimental study of the effects of autologous vascularized and nonvascularized transplantation of lymph nodes as treatment for postsurgical lymphedema in a sheep model. In all cases of experimental animals undergoing vascularized and nonvascularized transplants, the nodes were removed and replaced during the same operative procedure. Sham animals had incisions that were made and kept open for the same duration of time required to complete the experimental operations (3 hours). Lymphatic function and resolution of clinical edema occurred best after vascularized lymph node transplantation. The evidence presented is convincing in this animal model, but does this model really mirror the clinical situation? For example, what might occur if the lymph nodes were removed in one stage and lymph nodes from other sites in the animal were transplanted several weeks to months later, or if other modalities that might affect lymphatic function such as radiation therapy intervened before lymph node transplantation? Some of these questions were addressed in a clinical study of postmastectomy lymphedema patients reported in 2006. Good results occurred in some of the patients, primarily those with early lymphedema.

For further reading on this subject, I suggest an article by Becker et al.[1]

S. H. Miller, MD, MPH

Reference

1. Becker C, Assouad J, Riquet M, Hidden G. Postmastectomy lymphedema: long term results following microsurgical lymph node transplantation. *Ann Surg.* 2006;243:313-315.

3 Trauma

Head and Neck

The association between depression and anxiety disorders following facial trauma—A comparative study
Islam S, Ahmed M, Walton GM, et al (Univ Hosp Coventry & Warwickshire (UHCW), UK; et al)
Injury 41:92-96, 2010

Aim.—Although the surgical care provided for patients who have sustained a maxillofacial injury has advanced in recent years, psychological disorders may develop. Anxiety and depression may be a cause of significant morbidity in these patients. Such problems are often unrecognised and untreated.

Patients & Methods.—We undertook a comparative cross-sectional study in a cohort of adult patients to assess the association between traumatic facial injury and the presence of anxiety and depressive disorders. Study subjects were recruited during the period of June 2008 through August 2008. Fifty consecutive adult patients attending the maxillofacial outpatient clinic following facial trauma were asked to complete the Hospital Anxiety and Depression Scale (HADS). Data gathered from this group of patients were compared to 50 adult control subjects who were under follow-up following elective oral and maxillofacial surgery. We also looked at several demographic and other variables to assess its association with poor mental health outcomes.

Results.—Ten patients (20%) in the facial trauma group achieved high scores in both subscales suggesting a probable anxiety and depression state. The mean score for the depression subscale was significantly higher in the facial trauma group compared to the control group ($p = 0.006$). The mean score for anxiety was also higher but did not reach statistical significance ($p = 0.07$). Stratified analysis (Mantel–Haenszel) was used to control for possible confounding variables. The odds ratio for probable depression, for facial trauma patients compared with "control" patients, was 9.02, 95% CI = 2.45, 33.1, $p < 0.001$. Variables with significant associations ($p < 0.05$) with high depression scores in the facial trauma group were female sex, presence of a permanent facial scar, and a past psychiatric history. There was also significant correlation between patients' self-perception of facial disfigurement scores and scores obtained in both anxiety subscale ($r = 0.41$, $p = 0.003$) and depression subscale ($r = 0.46$, $p = 0.001$).

Conclusion.—Our results support the findings of previous studies and provide further evidence to clinicians for the critical identification and treatment of anxiety and depression in facial trauma victims.

▶ This is an interesting case-control study of known, but little appreciated, psychological disorders associated with maxillofacial injuries.[1] The authors documented that 20% of the 50 patients in their study group, postmaxillofacial injury, had significant, 9-fold difference in posttraumatic depression, and a 2-fold higher difference in posttraumatic anxiety than a control group of 50 patients undergoing elective oral and maxillofacial surgery. The study was conducted using the well-validated Hospital Hand Anxiety Depression Scale tool between 3.5 months in the traumatic group and 4.2 months in the control group.[2] While difficult to prove a causal relationship because of the cross-sectional nature of the study, the differences between the study and control groups, and the possibility that changes in the psychological outcomes might be time dependent, it nonetheless is suggestive enough to warrant awareness on the part of surgeons treating patients with maxillofacial trauma, especially when those patients are female, have associated permanent visible scarring, and a past psychiatric history.

S. H. Miller, MD, MPH

References

1. Bisson JL, Shepherd JP, Dhutia M. Psychological sequelae of facial trauma. *J Trauma.* 1997;43:495-500.
2. Herrmann C. International experiences with the Hospital Anxiety Depression Scale-a review of validation data and clinical results. *J Psychosom Res.* 1997;42: 17-41.

Facial Fractures in Children: Unique Patterns of Injury Observed by Computed Tomography
Chapman VM, Fenton LZ, Gao D, et al (The Children's Hosp, Denver; The Children's Hosp Res Inst, Denver, CO; et al)
J Comput Assist Tomogr 33:70-72, 2009

Objective.—To determine the patterns of facial fractures observed in pediatric patients after acute trauma.

Materials and Methods.—The computed tomography studies of 338 patients (63% male, 37% female; 7 months to 18 years of age) performed after acute nonpenetrating facial trauma were retrospectively reviewed to evaluate for facial fractures and associated orbital hematomas or contiguous skull fractures. Fracture patterns were characterized as orbital roof, orbital floor, medial orbital wall, nasal bone, naso-orbital-ethmoid, zygomatic complex, isolated zygomatic arch, Le Fort type (I, II, or III), maxillary sagittal, alveolar ridge, or mandibular. The frequency of the various fracture types was determined. The correlation between fracture type and orbital hematomas or contiguous skull fractures was assessed (Kendall tau rank correlation).

Results.—Computed tomography demonstrated facial fractures in 188 (54%) patients. The number and frequency of the fractures observed were as follows: orbital roof, 67 (36%); zygomatic complex, 38 (20%); naso-orbital-ethmoid, 30 (16%); orbital floor, 28 (15%); nasal bone, 25 (13%); mandibular, 24 (13%); medial orbital wall, 16 (9%); maxillary sagittal, 11 (6%); alveolar ridge, 8 (4%); isolated zygomatic arch, 3 (2%); Le Fort type I, 4 (2%); Le Fort type II, 4 (2%); and Le Fort type III, 0 (0%). Fifty children (27%) had multiple fractures. Orbital hematomas were seen in 28 patients (15%), and contiguous skull fractures were seen in 54 patients (29%). There was strong correlation between orbital hematomas and orbital roof fractures (0.62, $P < 0.0001$), orbital hematomas and naso-orbital-ethmoid fractures (0.18, $P = 0.001$), contiguous skull and orbital roof fractures (0.57, $P < 0.0001$), and contiguous skull and naso-orbital-ethmoid fractures (0.39, $P < 0.0001$).

Conclusions.—Fractures of the orbital roof are the most common facial fractures observed in pediatric patients after acute nonpenetrating trauma. Orbital roof and naso-orbital-ethmoid fractures are frequently associated with orbital hematomas and contiguous skull fractures.

▶ It is important to be cognizant of the fact that facial bone fractures in the pediatric population are less common than they are in adults. The most common anatomic locations for these fractures in children differ considerably from those seen in adult populations. The high incidence of orbital roof fractures, uncommon in adults, is due to the differences in the anatomy of the facial bones and sinuses of adults and children and the usual mechanisms of injury in each. It is important to be aware that orbital roof fractures may be associated with orbital hematomas and fractures of the adjacent skull, the latter if depressed will likely require neurosurgical intervention.

S. H. Miller, MD, MPH

Burns

Burn Hazards of the Deployed Environment in Wartime: Epidemiology of Noncombat Burns from Ongoing United States Military Operations
Kauvar DS, Wade CE, Baer DG (United States Army Inst of Surgical Res, Fort Sam Houston, TX)
J Am Coll Surg 209:453-460, 2009

Background.—Service in the deployed military environment carries risks for accidental (noncombat-related) burns. Examining these risks can assist in the development of military burn prevention measures. This study endeavored to examine noncombat burn epidemiology in the context of similar civilian data.

Study Design.—We performed a retrospective cohort study of consecutive casualties evacuated from operational military theaters in Iraq and Afghanistan to the sole tertiary military burn center in the US. Military data were compared with database samples of the US population from the American Burn Association and the Centers for Disease Control and Prevention.

Results.—The main causes of the 180 noncombat burns seen from March 2003 to June 2008 were waste burning, fuel mishaps, and unintentional ordinance detonations. Overall prevalence of noncombat burns was 19.5 burns/100,000 person-years lived. If causes specific to military operations are removed, military prevalence was 13.0/100,000. More than one-third of noncombat burns occurred in the first year of the study; a period of stability followed. A similar US population had an accidental burn prevalence of 7.1/100,000 from 2003 to 2007. Burn size, presence of inhalation injury, and burn center mortality were not different from those in a similar civilian cohort.

Conclusions.—Deployed service members have a greater risk of unintentional burns than a similar civilian cohort does. This is in part because of the specific dangers of military activities. More attention to deployed military burn prevention is needed, especially early in combat support operations.

▶ This burn prevention article is extremely interesting because it reveals that even in a well regimented and organized setting (ie, the United States military) there is an unacceptable incidence of burn injury from lack of education or foolish behavior. Recognizing the risks inherent in handling flammable military materials, there is still significant room for improvement in burn prevention education. For instance, the leading cause of burn injury was waste burning, which simply should not occur.

R. E. Salisbury, MD

Plastic surgery and burns disasters. What impact do major civilian disasters have upon medicine? Bradford City Football Club stadium fire, 1985, King's Cross Underground fire, 1987, Piper Alpha offshore oil rig disaster, 1988
Vaghela KR (Centre for the History of Science, Technology & Medicine, South Kensington, London, UK)
J Plast Reconstr Aesthet Surg 62:755-763, 2009

Major disasters involving multiple casualties are neither new nor infrequent. Such events have important implications for medicine and can provide crucial lessons for the future. However, while the medical aspects of war have received considerable attention, rather less is known about civilian disasters. To redress this imbalance, this article reviews three major British disasters of the 1980s where serious burns injury was a significant feature of the human casualty: the Bradford City Football Club fire of 1985, the King's Cross Underground fire of 1987 and the Piper Alpha oil rig disaster of 1988. Four related themes are used to examine in detail the ways in which these events impacted on medicine: plastics and reconstructive surgery, clinical psychology, disaster management and long-term structural change. Drawing on articles in specialist burns and psychiatric journals, together with the personal communications and recollections of surgeons and psychiatrists involved, it is revealed that while groundbreaking advances are a relative rarity in medicine, numerous small but significant lessons did emerge from these events, although often in subtle and highly specialised fields of medicine.

▶ This broad overview article is obviously very timely considering the political landscape in 2009. Of greatest interest are the author's comments on civilian casualties when compared with wartime disaster. While the military makes provisions for managing large numbers of casualties on a routine basis, the same cannot be said for civilian care. Unfortunately, the costs of preparation are extremely high. Holding drills, establishing training protocols, training personnel, and allotting funds for the unthinkable are beyond the budget of most tertiary care institutions.

The author's formulas for disaster management differ somewhat from that practiced in the United States. While understanding that the methodology will vary from region to region, we do not believe that it is feasible to bring all the specialists to 1 institution, but rather triage the patients out to level 2 trauma centers depending on the extent of injury, then not to inundate 1 or 2 institutions and bring civilian care to a standstill.

R. E. Salisbury, MD

Burns surgery handover study: Trainees' assessment of current practice in the British Isles

Al-Benna S, Al-Ajam Y, Alzoubaidi D (Ruhr Univ Bochum, Bochum, Germany; Royal Free Hosp, London, UK; Broomfield Hosp, Chelmsford, UK)
Burns 35:509-512, 2009

Introduction.—Effective handover of clinical information between working shifts is essential for patient safety. The aim of this study was to identify current practice and trainees' assessment of handover in the burns units of the British Isles.

Methods.—A telephone questionnaire was conducted to trainee burns surgeons (at junior and senior grades) currently working at all 30 burns surgery units in the British Isles. Information regarding timing, location, duration, participation and quality of handover was collated anonymously. Trainees commented on satisfaction with current practice and its perceived safety.

Results.—A 100% response from all 30 units was obtained. 23/30 units (76.7%) had junior to junior trainee handovers. 17/30 (56.7%) had senior to senior trainee handovers. 19/30 units (63.3%) reported that handover took place with more than one grade of doctor present (range 1–4 grades). 3/30 (10%) reported that handover was bleep-free. 3/30 (10%) had received formal training on good burns handover. 5/30 (16.7%) were working in a unit that operated a "burns surgeon of the week" pattern of emergency cover. Mean satisfaction level was 3.8 out of 5. Those working in "surgeon of the week" teams had significantly higher scores, 4.4 versus 3.68 ($p = 0.037$). Other healthcare professionals were present at only 4/30 (13.3%) handovers. Overall 26/30 (86.7%) of trainees judged their current handover practice "safe" (100% in 'surgeon of week' group and 84% in the remaining group, $p = 0.289$).

Conclusions.—Effective handover remains a keystone in safe and effective communication between doctors. The study highlights areas for improvement in handover practice, including greater involvement of an integrated multidisciplinary team. Those working under the "surgeon of the week" pattern are more satisfied.

▶ This article gives a clue to what medical care may look like after the current administration hammers out a new bill. Only 16% of the units had a surgeon-of-the-week pattern for emergency coverage, our equivalent of an attending of the week. Critical care management of the severely burned patient is a niche specialty that will not do well with the sign out and handover to those who are either unfamiliar or disinterested in good burn care. Twenty percent of the burn centers in the United States have closed within the last 10 years, and it remains to be seen what financial pressures will do to the next 5 years in burn care. If there is the lack of funding for materials and professionals that are predictive, the niche willl disappear and care will plummet.

R. E. Salisbury, MD

Fire-related deaths in India in 2001: a retrospective analysis of data
Sanghavi P, Bhalla K, Das V (Cambridge, MA; Harvard Univ, Cambridge, MA; Johns Hopkins Univ, Baltimore, MD)
Lancet 373:1282-1288, 2009

Background.—Hospital-based studies have suggested that fire-related deaths might be a neglected public-health issue in India. However, no national estimates of these deaths exist and the only numbers reported in published literature come from the Indian police. We combined multiple health datasets to assess the extent of the problem.

Methods.—We computed age–sex-specific fire-related mortality fractions nationally using a death registration system based on medically certified causes of death in urban areas and a verbal autopsy based sample survey for rural populations. We combined these data with all-cause mortality estimates based on the sample registration system and the population census. We adjusted for ill-defined injury categories that might contain misclassified fire-related deaths, and estimated the proportion of suicides due to self-immolation when deaths were reported by external causes.

Findings.—We estimated over 163 000 fire-related deaths in 2001 in India, which is about 2% of all deaths. This number was six times that reported by police. About 106 000 of these deaths occurred in women, mostly between 15 and 34 years of age. This age–sex pattern was consistent across multiple local studies, and the average ratio of fire-related deaths of young women to young men was 3:1.

Interpretation.—The high frequency of fire-related deaths in young women suggests that these deaths share common causes, including kitchen accidents, self-immolation, and different forms of domestic violence. Identification of populations at risk and description of structural determinants from existing data sources are urgently needed so that interventions can be rapidly implemented.

▶ These authors have highlighted a monstrous problem that requires attention and correction before India is considered a modern country. The issue of female abuse by burning is not a new one, and it has been mentioned at international surgical meetings repetitively in the past. The domestic violence of young women, especially because of an insufficient dowry, is ongoing and has not been addressed honestly and vigorously. The authors highlight all of the issues and deserve congratulations for their honesty and integrity, but the obvious solutions have yet to be addressed.

R. E. Salisbury, MD

Epidemiology of burn injuries presenting to North Carolina emergency departments in 2006–2007
DeKoning EP, Hakenewerth A, Platts-Mills TF, et al (Univ of North Carolina at Chapel Hill)
Burns 35:776-782, 2009

Approximately 600,000 burns present to Emergency Departments each year in the United States, yet there is little systematic or evidence-based training of Emergency Physicians in acute burn management. We retrospectively accessed the North Carolina Disease Event Tracking and Epidemiologic Collection Tool (NC DETECT) database to identify all thermal burns and electrical injuries with associated thermal burns presenting to 92% of North Carolina Emergency Departments over a 1-year period.

Results.—10,501 patients met inclusion criteria, 0.3% of all state-wide reported ED visits. Ninety-two percent of burn visits were managed exclusively by Emergency Physicians without acute intervention by burn specialists, including 87% of first degree, 82% of second degree, and 53% of third degree injuries. Only 4.3% were admitted; 4.3% were transferred to another institution. Fifty-five percent were male; 33% were aged 25–44 and 33% presented on weekends.

Conclusion.—This is the first state-wide study of burn injury and identifies Emergency Physicians as the major providers of acute burn care. Ninety-two percent of 10,501 burn visits, including the majority of severe injuries, were managed exclusively by Emergency Physicians. This supports a need for improved, evidence-based training of Emergency Physicians in the acute management of burns of all types.

▶ This nicely done epidemiology study shows the importance for evidence-based training of emergency physicians and the acute management of burns. In their study, most of the burn patients in the state of North Carolina were seen by emergency physicians. Unfortunately, there is little uniformity in burn education across the country. The results of this lack of education lead to wide disparity in the quality of care. Inaccurate estimation of burn size and the presence or absence of third degree burns or inhalation injury in particular results in inappropriate transfer, delayed transfer, and needless complications.

R. E. Salisbury, MD

A Case-Matched Controlled Study on High-Voltage Electrical Injuries vs Thermal Burns

Handschin AE, Vetter S, Jung FJ, et al (Univ Hosp of Zurich, Switzerland)
J Burn Care Res 30:400-407, 2009

The aim of this study was to provide an increased level of evidence on surgical management of high-tension electrical injuries compared with thermal burns using a case-controlled study design. Sixty-eight patients (64 males, 4 females, aged 33.7 ± 13 years) with high-tension electrical burns were matched for age, gender, and burnt extent with a cohort of patients sustaining thermal burns. Data were analyzed for cause of accident (occupational vs nonoccupational), concomitant injuries, extent of burn and burn depth, surgical management, complications, and hospital stay. High-tension electrical burn patients required an average of 5.2 ± 4 operations (range, 1–23 operations) compared with 3.3 ± 1.9 (range, 1–10 operations) after thermal burns ($P = .0019$). Amputation rates (19.7% vs 1.5%), escharotomy/fasciotomy rates (47% vs 21%), and total hospitalization days (44 d vs 32 d) were significantly higher in high-tension electrical injuries ($P < .05$). Creatinine kinase levels were significantly elevated during the first 2 days in patients with subsequent amputations. Free flap failure was observed during the first 4 weeks after the trauma, whereas no flap failure occurred at later stages. Local, pedicled, and distant flaps were used in 15% of the patients. The mortality in both groups was 13.2% vs 11%, respectively (nonsignificant). High-voltage electrical injury remains a complex surgical challenge. When performing free flap coverage, caution must be taken for a vulnerable phase lasting up to 4 weeks after the trauma. This phase is likely the result of a progressive intima lesion, potentially hazardous to microvascular reconstruction. The use of pedicle flaps may resemble an alternative to free flaps during this period.

▶ The authors discuss clinical care issues, which for the most part are already known but are certainly worth review. Of particular interest, however, is the timing of the performance of free flaps in high-voltage electrical injury patients. The high failure rate during the first 4 weeks after injury when compared with elective free flaps thereafter is certainly significant and noted by others. There are many ways to cover viable tissue that has been exposed following a high-voltage injury besides using a free flap, and the authors innumerate some of them. Often the desire to do an early free flap turns out to be misplaced enthusiasm. If there is no other way to salvage an extremity then the risk may be worth this effort, but otherwise it is obviously better to use an alternate form of tissue closure.

R. E. Salisbury, MD

Evaluation of the spontaneous breathing trial in burn intensive care patients
Smailes ST, Martin RV, McVicar AJ (Broomfield Hosp, Chelmsford, UK; Anglia Ruskin Univ, Chelmsford, UK)
Burns 35:665-671, 2009

Background.—The extubation failure rate in our burn patients is 30%.
Objective.—To evaluate the influence of the 30 min spontaneous breathing trial on extubation outcome in burn patients.
Methods.—A prospective, observational study in a burn intensive care unit. All adult patients requiring mechanical ventilation for >24 h and meeting the inclusion criteria underwent a 30 min spontaneous breathing trial (SBT). Extubation was undertaken after a successful SBT.
Results.—Of 49 planned extubations, 9 failed (18%), much lower than the 30% extubation failure rate identified prior to the implementation of the SBT. The duration of ventilation was significantly shorter ($p = 0.04$) in the patients who passed a SBT and those who failed extubation were significantly older ($p = 0.003$). The logistic regression analysis identified that age independently predicted extubation outcome. Patients who failed extubation, after a successful SBT, had a significantly longer duration of ventilation ($p = 0.0001$) and ITU length of stay ($p = 0.001$).
Conclusions.—The incidence of extubation failure was much lower and the duration of ventilation significantly shorter in patients who were extubated after a successful SBT. These findings support the use of the SBT in

burn patients. Age independently predicts extubation outcome in burn patients who have passed a SBT.

▶ This topic is extremely important as it concentrates on the most critically ill patients in burn centers. The authors have found that a spontaneous breathing trial of 30 minutes that was accomplished successfully markedly improved the ability to predict which patients could be extubated and do well. Certainly, they are correct in attempting to find objective criteria that will predict the ability for successful extubation. One wonders, however, why they settle on a 30-minute trial period? It has been our finding that many patients who have large burns and pulmonary compromise require a slow approach to extubation. Specifically, a 30-minute trial can be increased to 2 hours and then the patient placed back on the ventilator when he or she tires. The time off the ventilator can be slowly increased over a period of several days as the patient becomes more accustomed to breathing on his own with a simple T-piece. The authors don't mention any metabolic factors, but it has been our finding that when the patient is in positive nitrogen balance the success rate also improves. The success is multifactorial. Lastly, extubation should be performed early in the day when a full complement of nurses and physicians are present to allow for the possibility of a problem developing requiring reintubation.

R. E. Salisbury, MD

The Utility of Bronchoscopy After Inhalation Injury Complicated by Pneumonia in Burn Patients: Results From the National Burn Repository

Carr JA, Phillips BD, Bowling WM (Hurley Med Ctr, Flint, MI; American Burn Association, Chicago, IL)
J Burn Care Res 30:967-974, 2009

There are no guidelines to determine when bronchoscopy is appropriate in patients with inhalation injury complicated by pneumonia. We reviewed the National Burn Repository from 1998 to 2007 to determine if there is any difference in outcome in burn patients with inhalation injury and pneumonia who did and did not undergo bronchoscopy. Three hundred fifty-five patients with pneumonia did not undergo bronchoscopy, 173 patients underwent one bronchoscopy, and 96 patients underwent more than one bronchoscopy. Patients with a 30 to 59% surface area burn and pneumonia who underwent bronchoscopy had a decreased duration of mechanical ventilation compared with those who did not (21 days, 95% CI: 19–23 days vs 28 days, 95% CI: 25–31 days, P =.0001). When compared with patients who did not undergo bronchoscopy, patients having a single bronchoscopy had a significantly shorter length of intensive care unit stay and hospital stay (35 ± 3 vs 39 ± 2, P =.04, and 45 ± 3 vs 49 ± 2, P =.009). The hospital charges were on average much higher in those patients who did not undergo bronchoscopy, compared with those who did ($473,654 ± 44,944 vs $370,572 ± 36,602, P =.12). When compared with patients who did not undergo bronchoscopy, patients who did have one or more bronchoscopies showed a reduced risk of death by 18% (OR = 0.82, 95% CI: 0.53–1.27, P =.37). Patients with inhalation injury complicated by pneumonia seem to benefit from bronchoscopy. This benefit can be seen in a decreased duration of mechanical ventilation, decreased length of intensive care unit stay, and decreased overall hospital cost. In addition, there was a trend toward an improvement in mortality. The aggressive use of bronchoscopy after inhalation injury may be justified.

▶ This very nice article taps into the data from 82 Burn Centers in the United States. The findings are not surprising to those who care for critically ill patients demanding aggressive pulmonary care. The removal of foreign debris, accumulated secretions, and plugs that impair ventilation leads to not only improved results but also decreased hospital costs.

R. E. Salisbury, MD

Duration of Antibiotic Therapy for Ventilator-Associated Pneumonia in Burn Patients

Wahl WL, Taddonio MA, Arbabi S, et al (Univ of Michigan Health System, Ann Arbor; Univ of Washington/Harborview Med Ctr, Seattle)
J Burn Care Res 30:801-806, 2009

Shorter compared with longer courses of antibiotic therapy for ventilator-associated pneumonia (VAP) in mixed medical-surgical intensive care units (ICUs) have been reported to produce equivalent outcomes. There have been few studies on the duration of antibiotic therapy for VAP in the burn population. We hypothesized that a shorter duration of antibiotic therapy for VAP would produce similar outcomes in our burn ICU. All burn patients from July 2001 to December 2006 admitted to the burn ICU requiring mechanical ventilation were studied. VAP was diagnosed prospectively by our Infection Control Liaison using bronchoalveolar lavage for cultures. Patients were cohorted into two groups: before July 1, 2004, antibiotic therapy duration was directed by the discretion of the attending physician (preprotocol), and after, the goal was 8 days of appropriate therapy or longer based on physician discretion (postprotocol). There were 98 patients treated for VAP with similar rates of inhalation injury, %TBSA burn size, age, and need for mechanical ventilation between the groups. The incidence of recurrent VAP was the same: 17% for the preprotocol and 15% for the postprotocol periods. The overall duration of antibiotic therapy did not change from 11 ± 4 to 12 ± 6 days. For patients treated longer than the target of 8 days, 66% had positive respiratory cultures at 4 days after initiation of antibiotic therapy. For the majority of patients with aspiration-type organisms or nonvirulent strains, there were fewer antibiotic days overall at 10 ± 5 days (P < .05), with no episodes of recurrent VAP with the same bacteria. Despite a focused effort to decrease antibiotic usage for VAP in burn patients, the overall duration of therapy did not change. The majority of patients with virulent organisms such as methicillin-resistant *Staphylococcus aureus* or nonfermenting Gram-negative rods still had clinical signs of pneumonia and positive cultures, leading clinicians to continue antibiotics. In patients without virulent pathogens, a shorter antibiotic course was well-tolerated without recurrences.

▶ A shorter compared with a longer course of antibiotic therapy for ventilator-associated pneumonia in mixed medical/surgical intensive care units has been reported to produce equivalent outcomes. The authors attempted to use a shorter course of treatment in the burn ICU. Unfortunately, they found that despite intense effort to decrease the antibiotic usage, the duration of therapy did not change. The bulk of the patients with virulent organisms such as methicillin-resistant *Staphylococcus aureus* still had clinical signs of pneumonia and positive cultures forcing clinicians to continue antibiotics. These results are not surprising because patients with significant burn injuries, inhalation injury, and ventilator-associated pneumonia are immunosuppressed and do not clear organisms from their respiratory tree rapidly.

R. E. Salisbury, MD

Escharotomy and Decompressive Therapies in Burns
Orgill DP, Piccolo N (Brigham and Women's Hosp, Boston, MA; Pronto Socorro para Queimaduras, Goiânia, Brazil)
J Burn Care Res 30:759-768, 2009

Experienced clinicians treating burns recognize the need for escharotomy and decompressive therapies. The burning process causes the integument to become stiff, and the underlying tissues can swell during the fluid resuscitation process. We reviewed the literature that supports the current clinical practice of decompressive therapies following burn injury.

▶ This article is an updated review of the subject in Practice Guidelines. This review is extremely thorough and complete. The literature review is especially beneficial and is a must-read for anyone involved in the acute care of patients with severe burn injuries.

R. E. Salisbury, MD

Intraabdominal Hypertension and the Abdominal Compartment Syndrome in Burn Patients
Kirkpatrick AW, Ball CG, Nickerson D, et al (Univ of Calgary, Alberta, Canada; Emory Univ, Atlanta, GA; et al)
World J Surg 33:1142-1149, 2009

Severe burns represent a devastating injury that induces profound systemic inflammation requiring large volumes of resuscitative fluids. The consequent massive swelling and peritoneal ascites raises intraabdominal pressures (IAP) to supraphysiologic levels commensurate with intraabdominal hypertension (IAH) and with the abdominal compartment syndrome (ACS) if consistently associated with IAP > 20 mmHg and associated with new organ failure. Severe burn injuries are an example of the secondary ACS (2° ACS), wherein there has been no primary inciting intraperitoneal injury, yet severe IAH/ACS develops, setting the stage for progressive multiorgan dysfunction. These definitions along with practice management guidelines have recently been promulgated by the World Society of the Abdominal Compartment Syndrome (WSACS) in an effort to standardize terminology and communication regarding IAH/ACS in critical care. It is currently unknown whether these syndromes are iatrogenic consequences of excessive or poorly managed fluid resuscitation or unavoidable sequelae of the primary injury. It occurs frequently with burns of >60% body surface area, especially with associated inhalational injury, delayed resuscitation, and abdominal wall injuries. IAH/ACS is often a hyperacute phenomenon that occurs within the first hours of admission and thereafter with any complication requiring aggressive fluid resuscitation. Despite a number of noninvasive management strategies, interventions such as percutaneous peritoneal drainage and, ultimately, decompressive laparotomy are often required once the ACS is established. Whether novel resuscitation strategies can avoid or minimize IAH/ACS is unproven at present and requires further study. Truly understanding postburn ACS may require further insights into the basic mechanisms of injury and resuscitation.

▶ This article is a must-read for clinicians, as it nicely summarizes the history of intra-abdominal hypertension in burn patients, the pathophysiology, and the treatment. Unfortunately it is unknown whether intra-abdominal hypertension is a necessary sequelae of large severe burn injuries or the result of injudicious fluid administration. Are we simply more aware of the syndrome, or is it becoming more prevalent? It is the reviewer's suspicion that this problem is the result of excessive fluid administration because in the very large burn there is even increased capillary permeability in unburned tissues. It is the patient with large total body burn with or without inhalation injury who is most at risk and represents the greatest challenge for good fluid administration. Comorbidity factors, such as the aged with chronic systemic diseases or very small infants, must also be considered.

R. E. Salisbury, MD

Intensive insulin therapy confers a similar survival benefit in the burn intensive care unit to the surgical intensive care unit

Gibson BR, Galiatsatos P, Rabiee A, et al (Johns Hopkins Bayview Med Ctr, Baltimore, MD)
Surgery 146:922-930, 2009

Background.—In contrast to the benefits of intensive insulin therapy (IIT) in the surgical intensive care unit (SICU), its benefits in the burn ICU (BICU) remain unclear. Furthermore, IIT and tight glycemic control has received little attention in elderly ICU patients.

Methods.—We evaluated the normalization of blood glucose level with IIT in BICU and SICU patients. From October 2006 to July 2007, 970 patients were admitted to our BICU and our SICU. A total of 79 of these patients met criteria for initiation of IIT, 37 of who required IIT for at least 72 hours. Data were analyzed to determine if tight glycemic control (blood glucose ≤150 mg/dL by day 3) is associated with reduced morbidity and mortality.

Results.—Tight control was better achieved in SICU patients (45%) than in BICU patients (33%). Daily insulin requirements were approximately 2-fold greater in SICU patients compared with BICU patients ($P < .05$). Tight control in both SICU and BICU patients was associated with a decreased incidence of sepsis compared with poor glycemic control (10% vs 58% and 60% vs 70%, respectively) and a decreased mortality rate (0 vs 58% and 20% vs 50%; SICU vs BICU, respectively). The percentage of total body surface area burned in BICU patients was 10% and 45% in the ≤150 and >150 mg/dL groups. Mortality rate in the poor control group was >10-fold greater than that of the tight control group; for patients ≥65 years of age, mortality was nearly double than that of patients <65 years of age. The greatest mortality rate (62%) was seen in patients >65 years of age with poor control.

Conclusion.—Tight control with IIT is associated with an increased survival rate in both BICU and SICU patients. Age is associated with survival, with patients older than 65 years of age having the greatest mortality rate.

▶ The authors summarize the reasons for hyperglycemia in the burn patient and insulin resistance that may occur. Not surprisingly, the mortality rate was improved and sepsis decreased with tighter control of blood glucose. Similar survival benefits in burn patients versus trauma patients in the intensive care unit are certainly not surprising. The greatest problem is making staff understand and accept the definition of tight glucose control. Hyperglycemia as a potential cause of sepsis is certainly not a new concept. Unfortunately, once sepsis occurs, achieving blood glucose control is even more difficult and the end result more unpredictable.

R. E. Salisbury, MD

Burns pruritus—A study of current practices in the UK
Goutos I (Stoke Mandeville Hosp, Buckinghamshire, UK)
Burns 36:42-48, 2010

Pruritus is a universal symptom associated with burns healing. Little research has been conducted to assess physicians' attitudes and management principles in specialist units. A survey of UK burn units has identified a variety of opinions on the importance of various factors affecting the incidence of pruritus and a lack of a systematic approach in the assessment and treatment of this distressing symptom. A clear pattern emerged favouring the use of antihistaminergic agents for burns pruritus management with a low uptake of agents acting on the central nervous system as well as non-pharmacological adjuncts. The cumulative responses from the cohort of respondents are presented and issues pertinent to further research and clinical management are discussed.

▶ The value of this article is that it emphasizes the appalling lack of interest in studying the etiology and treatment of burn pruritus, even though it is a major issue for surviving burn patients. In the study of other burn units, it became apparent that there was no consensus on etiology or treatment. This study emphasizes that the reports of agents presently being used are preliminary at best. The bibliography is outstanding for anyone interested in this problem.

R. E. Salisbury, MD

Comparison of efficacy of silicone gel, silicone gel sheeting, and topical onion extract including heparin and allantoin for the treatment of postburn hypertrophic scars
Karagoz H, Yuksel F, Ulkur E, et al (Maresal Cakmak Military Hosp, Erzurum, Turkey; Haydarpasa Training Hosp, Istanbul, Turkey)
Burns 35:1097-1103, 2009

We compared the efficacy of silicone gel (Scarfade®), silicone gel sheet (Epi-Derm™), and topical onion extract including heparin and allantoin (Contractubex®) for the treatment of hypertrophic scars.

Forty-five postburn scars were included in the study. Patients with scars less than 6 months from injury were assigned at random to three groups each containing 15 scars, and their treatment was continued for 6 months. Scars were treated with Scarfade®, Epiderm™ and Contractubex®. Scar assessment was performed at the beginning of the treatment, and at the end of the sixth month when the treatment was completed by using the Vancouver scar scale.

The difference between before and after treatment scores for each three groups was statistically significant. The difference between Scarfade® group and Epi-Derm™ group was not significant; however, the differences of the other groups (Scarfade®-Contractubex®, Epiderm™-Contractubex®) were significant.

Silicone products, either in gel or sheet, are superior to Contractubex® in the treatment of the hypertrophic scar. The therapist should select the most appropriate agent according to the patient's need and guidelines of these signs.

▶ These authors attempt to do a very nice prospective study comparing the efficacy of 3 different modalities for the treatment of hypertrophic scars. Significantly, they used a world-recognized scar assessment: the Vancouver scale. While there was no control group, they rightly note that each of the 3 modalities of treatment had already been proven to be efficacious, and their goal was merely to compare and decide which was best. It is of interest that the silicone products, either gel or sheet, worked equally well and therefore use should be left to the discretion of the therapist. Epiderm was the most efficacious, but it had more complications than the gel products.

R. E. Salisbury, MD

A Ten-Year Experience With Hemodialysis in Burn Patients at Los Angeles County + USC Medical Center

Soltani A, Karsidag S, Garner W (Univ of Southern California, Los Angeles)
J Burn Care Res 30:832-835, 2009

Acute renal failure (ARF) is a rare, but serious, complication after burn injury that is commonly thought to be fatal. Before the modern era, there were few survivors of burn injuries who required dialysis. We report our 10-year experience with ARF and dialysis at the Los Angeles County + USC burn unit. During the period of August 1994 to February 2004, 3356 patients were admitted. Furthermore, 1143 patients were admitted to the intensive care unit and 1125 had burns >10% TBSA. Thirty-three patients developed ARF necessitating dialysis, equaling 0.98% of all admitted patients, and 2.7% of patients with TBSA > 10% burns, which is at the low end of published burn unit data. The average age of these patients requiring dialysis was 49 years, 91% were men, 24% were diabetic, and 39% were positive for substances of abuse at admission, and the average TBSA burned was 36%. This is compared with an average age of 31 years, 70% men, 7.3% diabetic, and 14.7% intoxicated in the general burned population at our burn unit. Furthermore, our overall mortality in the burn unit was 5% overall and 14% in patients with >10% TBSA burns during the study period. In patients requiring hemodialysis, the mortality rate was 69.7%. The average time to hemodialysis was 14 days in our series, and patients, on average, required 10.3 days of dialysis support. These mortality data are the lowest recorded for burned patients requiring dialysis and suggest that ARF is a survivable complication in some of these patients.

▶ This very nice retrospective study is important because it emphasizes the team effort and fortitude that is required to salvage patients previously thought unsalvageable. The authors work in an extremely busy burn center in an urban area that invariably collects the sickest patients. The authors carefully review the reasons for acute renal failure in thermally injured patients, and the mortality rate of 69.7% in this population is excellent. It is most important to note that the presence of acute renal failure should trigger a redoubling of efforts of the medical team, not a tacit admission of defeat. The low incidence of acute renal failure in their 10-year study is at least partially due to improved resuscitation and decreased incidence of sepsis resulting from improvements in diagnosis and care.

R. E. Salisbury, MD

A Follow-Up Study of Adults With Suicidal Burns: Psychosocial Adjustment and Quality of Life
Daigeler A, Langer S, Hüllmann K, et al (Ruhr-Univ Bochum, Germany)
J Burn Care Res 30:844-851, 2009

The severity of the burn injuries, accompanying injuries, and the often concomitant psychiatric disease complicate the treatment of patients with suicidal burns. Data from 45 patients who were treated for suicidal burn injuries from 1994 to 2005 were acquired from the patients' charts and interviews with standardized questionnaires (n = 11) concerning their psychological status pretrauma and posttrauma, as well as their quality of life with special reference to psychosocial adjustments. None of the patients survived more than 69% TBSA burns; no one with 41% or less died. Most of the patients had prediagnosed psychiatric disorders. The educational and social background of the patients and religious beliefs played a minor role for choosing this method of suicide. Aggression levels were above the average population, whereas self-direction was underdeveloped. Forty percent, albeit unsuccessfully, committed subsequent suicide attempts. Most patients felt only moderate social impairment by the burn wound residuals, the majority had intensified and improved their social contacts, and most felt no relevant decrease of quality of life compared with their personal situation before the suicide attempt. Patients who survive the suicide attempt can become integrated in social life again. More data are needed to reliably identify patients at risk in advance.

▶ This type of article should be discussed at staff conference involving the entire burn team. With the current difficulties in funding and cutbacks in resources for patient care, staff members have a right to question care for a subset of individuals who 40% of the time subsequently seek to kill themselves. Communication with family members and among the staff needs to be exquisitely clear. There are times when comfort care only is appropriate, and other times when a full effort should be mustered. Family and staff have to be in accord, otherwise a terrible situation turns into an obscenity.

R. E. Salisbury, MD

Nasal Reconstruction After Severe Facial Burns Using a Local Turndown Flap
Taylor HOB, Carty M, Driscoll D, et al (Shriner's Burn Hosp for Children and Harvard Med School, Boston, MA)
Ann Plast Surg 62:175-179, 2009

Reconstruction of the nose after severe burn injury is a challenging problem. There are usually associated facial burns, which limits the availability of local flaps. Reconstruction with unburned distant tissue is often not appropriate because of the resulting mismatch in color and texture. Successful nasal reconstruction can be accomplished in this group of challenging patients using a simple, inferiorly based flap from the nasal dorsum with subsequent skin grafting to the resulting defect.

We have used an inferiorly based nasal turndown flap to reconstruct severe nasal deformities after burn injury in 28 patients. The flap tissue consists of the dorsal surface of the nose, which is usually made up of skin graft and scar. The flap base is the scar transition zone between the dorsum of the nose and the lining mucosa. This is turned over to provide nasal length, projection, and to stimulate alar lobules. The resulting defect on the dorsum of the nose is then skin grafted. If further length or refinement is required, the procedure may be repeated. The records of all patients who underwent this procedure were reviewed for demographics, age at burn, percentage of total body surface area burned (%TBSA), availability of the forehead, number of procedures, and complications.

Twenty-eight patients underwent nasal reconstruction in our series using this local turndown flap. Most of these patients had severe burns, with an average %TBSA of 46%. The procedure was initially applied to patients with devastating injuries and %TBSA of 80%–95%, with extremely limited donor sites. As the success of the procedure was established, less severely burned patients were included in the series, thereby lowering the mean %TBSA. All patients had partial or complete destruction of their forehead donor site. All patients presented for multiple hospitalizations, with an average of 17 hospital admissions.

Using this local turndown flap, adequate nasal length and projection could be achieved. There were few complications. All of the flaps survived, although there were 2 cases of necrosis of the distal edge of the flaps (0.7%). This resulted in decreased length and projection but this problem was successfully addressed with additional staged procedures. Contraction of local scar tissue created bulk and support, eliminating the need for distant tissue transfer or cartilage grafting. Twelve of the 28 patients required repeat turndown flaps to achieve sufficient nasal length and projection. These results were durable over a follow-up period of up to several decades.

A simple, multistaged dorsal nasal flap can be used to reconstruct severe nasal deformities after facial burn injury. This can obviate the need for distant tissue transfer. Even in patients with subtotal nasal amputation and complete absence of cartilaginous support, the opportunistic use of scar tissue can restore nasal tip projection and alar lobule architecture without cartilage grafting. The resulting nasal reconstruction blends well into the surrounding facial appearance. This simple technique has been remarkably successful in this selected group of patients with challenging nasal deformities.

▶ This very fine article from the Shriners Burn Hospital for Children of Boston has a large series (28 patients) and long-term follow-up of nasal turndown flap and skin grafting for reconstruction of severe nasal deformities. The authors realized other choices are possible but demonstrate long-term results using a local technique that has a high chance of success. The need for a successful result with a low incidence of failure was certainly germane in this vulnerable and fragile population who have had life-threatening experiences and multiple surgeries. Photographic documentation of the long-term results is exemplary.

R. E. Salisbury, MD

Transplantation of cultivated oral mucosal epithelial cells for severe corneal burn

Ma DH-K, Kuo M-T, Tsai Y-J, et al (Chang Gung Memorial Hosp, Taoyuan, Taiwan; Chang Gung Memorial Hosp, Kaohsiung, Taiwan; et al)
Eye 23:1442-1450, 2009

Purpose.—To access the feasibility of using cultivated oral mucosal epithelial cell transplantation (COMET) for the management of severe corneal burn.

Methods.—COMET was performed to promote re-epithelialization in two eyes with acute alkaline burn and one eye with chronic alkaline burn, and to reconstruct the ocular surface in two eyes with chronic thermal burn. Autologous oral mucosal epithelial cells obtained from biopsy were cultivated on amniotic membrane. Immunoconfocal microscopy for keratins and progenitor cell markers was performed to characterize the cultivated epithelial sheet. Following transplantation, the clinical outcome and possible complications were documented. The patients were followed for an averaged 29.6 ± 3.6 (range: 26–34) months.

Results.—Cultivated oral mucosal epithelial sheet expressed keratin 3, 13, and progenitor cell markers p63, p75, and ABCG2. After COMET, all the corneas became less inflamed, and the corneal surface was completely re-epithelialized in 6.0 ± 3.2 (range: 3–10) days in all but one patients. Microperforation occurred in one patient, and a small persistent epithelial defect developed in another. Both were solved uneventfully. In all patients, superficial corneal blood vessels invariably developed, and to further improve vision, conjunctivo-limbal autografting ($N = 3$) and/or penetrating keratoplasty ($N = 3$) were performed subsequently. The vision of all patients showed substantial improvement after additional surgeries.

Conclusions.—This study showed the potential of COMET to promote re-epithelialization and reduce inflammation in acute corneal burn, and to reconstruct the corneal surface in chronic burn. COMET may, therefore, be considered an alternative treatment for severe corneal burn.

▶ The results of corneal burns secondary to Stevens-Johnson syndrome (SJS)/TENS are so catastrophic and seemingly irreversible that these studies are extremely exciting. The authors have found that cultivated oral mucosal epithelial cell transplants have decreased inflammation and improved vision without the need for immunosuppression necessary with allografts.

R. E. Salisbury, MD

Heterotopic ossification in burns: Our experience and literature reviews
Chen H-C, Yang J-Y, Chuang S-S, et al (Memorial Hosp and Univ, Linkou, Taiwan)
Burns 35:857-862, 2009

Purposes.—Heterotopic ossification (HO) is an uncommon, but high profile complication of burns. In this paper, a retrospective study was undertaken to evaluate our treatment and results of HO. Relevant literature was also reviewed to search for new advances in prevention and management for patients with HO after burns.

Materials and Methods.—A retrospective study was undertaken in Chang Gung Memorial Hospital, Linkou. We collected 12 patients who suffered from HO after burn and received operation in our hospital between June 2000 and September 2007. The data was expressed as mean.

Results.—Patients' gender distribution was 10 males and 2 females. The mean age was 43 years old (range, 30–59). Causes of burn were flame burn (75%), scald burn (8%), contact burn (8%), and high-voltage electrical burn (8%). Mean TBSA was 39% (range, 8–90%). Nine of 12 patients (75%) were admitted to intensive care unit (ICU) and 6 (50%) received mechanical ventilator support. The mean ICU stay was 82 days (range, 26–240 days). The elbow was the most commonly affected joint (92%). The outcome of surgery was acceptable in all elbows at the time of surgery. The mean ROMs before surgery were 31° (range, 0–75°). The mean ROMs after surgery were 99° (range, 70–115°); mean gain was 68° (range, 35–115°). One (8%) patients had recurrent HO after operation. The mean outpatient department follow-up time was 14.6 months (range, 1–40 months). The incidence of HO in our burn center is 0.15%.

Conclusion.—Although HO after burn is uncommon, physicians should keep the complication in mind. When burn patients complain decreased ROM or "locking sign" in their joints, X-ray examination is indicated to rule out HO. Surgery is the treatment of choice when the diagnosis of HO is confirmed.

▶ This literature review is excellent for one interested in this very rare complication of burn injuries. Unfortunately, little new knowledge has been shed on the problem in the last 25 years and the etiology still remains speculative. More importantly, the timing of surgical correction is also unclear. The authors do note that some suggest delaying surgical correction until the bone scan returns to normal, but other studies yield reasonable results with earlier surgical intervention. The final answers remain unclear because there is no good experimental model and the incidence is so low that no one has the opportunity to study the problem prospectively.

R. E. Salisbury, MD

Full-Thickness vs Split-Skin Grafting in Pediatric Hand Burns—A 10-Year Review of 174 Cases
Chandrasegaram MD, Harvey J (Children's Hosp Westmead, Sydney, Australia)
J Burn Care Res 30:867-871, 2009

This study was undertaken to assess the incidence of contractures following grafting of pediatric hand burns. Primary pediatric hand burns grafted between January 1997 and July 2007 were reviewed by three groups: A) hand grafts (palmar and/or dorsal grafts excluding digits); B) digit grafts; and C) hand and digit grafts (grafts to palm and/or dorsum including digits). The incidence of contractures and operative release in those with full-thickness grafting (FTG) versus split-skin grafting (SSG) was analyzed. There were 174 grafted pediatric hand burns. In group A, the incidence of contractures with SSG was 26 vs 11% with FTG. Subgroup analysis revealed comparable contracture rates between palmar and dorsal grafts treated with SSG, 24 vs 25%. The only FTG contracture was a palmar graft. The incidence of contractures in digit grafts or group B was low, 3 of 29 with SSG and 0 of 27 with FTG. In group C, the incidence of contractures in the SSG group was 43%, with none in the FTG group, $P \leq 0.019$. This was higher with SSG to the palm and digits at 67 vs 21% with dorsal grafts. The study revealed an overall 34 of 126 (27%) incidence of contractures with SSG and 1 of 45 (2%) with FTG, $P < 0.001$. The incidence of operative scar release was 15% in the SSG group and 2% in the FTG group, $P = 0.019$. This study supports the use of FTG in the treatment of primary hand burns particularly where the burn involves the surface of the palm and extends into the digits.

▶ This article is extremely even-handed in its approach to the problem of full-thickness burns requiring grafting in the pediatric population. The authors duly note that there were decreased contractures in the patients with full-thickness skin grafts, but recognize that the ability to do these grafts depends on the extent of total-body burn and also the depth of the burn on the hand. It is obvious that individuals with fourth-degree burns will not get a good result regardless of the type of graft that is applied; in fact this type of wound may require allowing granulation tissue to form followed by thin split-thickness skin grafts to get a take. Of interest, the authors compared the results of split-thickness skin grafting done by plastic surgeons versus general surgeons and the results were comparable. Thus, the good results with the full-thickness grafts were most likely due to the quality of the skin as opposed to the skill set of the surgeon (general surgeons prefer split-thickness skin grafting).

R. E. Salisbury, MD

Anatomical Study of Pectoral Intercostal Perforators and Clinical Study of the Pectoral Intercostal Perforator Flap for Hand Reconstruction
Oki K, Murakami M, Tanuma K, et al (Nippon Med School, Tokyo, Japan)
Plast Reconstr Surg 123:1789-1800, 2009

Background.—The authors have used pectoral intercostal perforator flaps to reconstruct burned or injured hands by staged transfer. This flap is designed with a narrow skin pedicle that includes intercostal perforators from the fifth to eighth intercostal spaces, with a wide flap area that lies on the upper abdomen. The distal area is thinned down to the subdermal vascular network level; thus, such flaps are called "superthin flaps" or subdermal vascular network flaps. In this article, the authors discuss the arterial networks associated with this flap and present clinical cases.

Methods.—The authors performed an anatomical study using 13 cadavers to obtain angiograms and dissect the anterior chest and abdominal region. Clinically, the authors retrospectively analyzed 21 cases over 13 years.

Results.—Anatomically, the anterior intercostal regions could be divided into three segments with regard to vascular supply to the skin and subcutaneous layer. In particular, in the fifth to eighth intercostal spaces, perforators communicated with one another to form a "latticework" pattern. In addition, the vascular territories participating in the pectoral intercostal perforator flap, that is, the intercostal perforators, the superior epigastric artery system, and the deep inferior epigastric artery system, linked with each other through choke vessels. In the authors' clinical cases, functional and aesthetic results were satisfactory.

Conclusions.—The pectoral intercostal perforator flap was supported by the arterial networks among perforators in the intercostal spaces and in the upper abdomen. This flap is one useful method for reconstruction of the hand region, providing good quality in terms of thinness and texture.

▶ This article is a beautifully done academic study of anatomy first done in cadavers and then used in the clinical situation. Obviously, the indications for this procedure are extremely limited (the authors only had 21 cases over 13 years). It is simply another possibility in the armamentarium of the surgeon that would require very careful study and practice before use.

R. E. Salisbury, MD

Reconstruction of the burned hand using a super-thin abdominal flap, with donor-site closure by an island deep inferior epigastric perforator flap
Liu Y, Song B, Zhu S, et al (Plastic Surgery Hosp, Beijing, The People's Republic of China)
J Plast Reconstr Aesthet Surg 63:e265-e268, 2010

A pedicled super-thin superficial inferior epigastric artery flap can provide a thin and pliable skin coverage for the hand dorsum, and debulking of the flap during elevation limits the need for secondary procedures. Simultaneously, an island deep inferior epigastric perforator flap transferred to reconstruct the flap donor site in the abdomen subsequently minimises donor-site morbidity.

▶ This article demonstrates technical virtuosity providing skin and soft tissue coverage for a contracted burned hand. Of greater significance, however, is the fact that the authors do not show the functional improvements achieved with their operation. Furthermore, they do not express in the body of the article whether the patient was improved or not with this flap technique. The point is that we have gone beyond simply being able to do a procedure. It is mandatory to pick the correct procedure and one that has an acceptable cost-benefit ratio. Would this patient have benefited from a lesser procedure? Would the improvement achieved be worth the performed operation? Would it have been possible to do something simpler and achieve gains that were not statistically different from those shown? These are the questions we must ask our residents in training. The ability to perform an operation is simply not an indication to do the operation.

R. E. Salisbury, MD

Reconstruction of Postburn Antebrachial Contractures Using Pedicled Thoracodorsal Artery Perforator Flaps

Uygur F, Sever C, Tuncer S, et al (Haydarpaşa Training Hosp, Istanbul, Ankara, Turkey; Gazi Univ Med School, Ankara, Turkey; Kocaeli Univ Med School, Turkey)
Plast Reconstr Surg 123:1544-1552, 2009

Background.—Full-thickness burns involving the antecubital area result in severe contractures. Functional impairment is inevitable if the affected areas are not managed properly. Proper treatment requires complete release and radical excision of the scar tissue, followed by reconstruction using durable tissue that will not contract during long-term follow-up.

Methods.—Nine patients with flexion contractures were reconstructed with pedicled thoracodorsal artery perforator flaps between 2004 and 2008. All of the patients were male, and their ages ranged from 20 to 23 years (mean, 21.4 years). The size and orientation of the skin islands were planned according to the defect size and orientation. The size of the flaps varied from 6.5 to 9.0 cm in width (mean, 8.0 cm) and 16.0 to 21.0 cm in length (mean, 20.0 cm). All of the patients were followed up for 6 to 12 months (mean, 9.3 months).

Results.—All of the flaps used on the postburn antecubital contractures survived completely. Minimal transient venous congestion occurred in two flaps during the early postoperative period. A complete range of motion at the elbow joint was achieved in all patients by the end of the reconstruction period.

Conclusions.—This study revealed that the pedicled thoracodorsal artery perforator flap is a suitable alternative for postburn elbow contractures. A very long pedicle can be obtained to transfer the flap to the antecubital area without tension. With its thin, pliable texture and large size, it adapts well to forearm skin and the donor-site scar is considered cosmetically acceptable.

▶ This elegant article clearly discusses the problems of postburn antebrachial contractures and possible surgical solutions. The particular choice of flaps used by the authors is well described, including potential complications. Significantly, the authors had no complications and all flaps were successfully performed. They emphasize that there is a steep learning curve and an experienced team is needed to achieve these good results. In fairness they discuss other methods of reconstruction, but unfortunately do not clearly point out when each should be used. Specifically, the 2 cases illustrated in the article had not had any previous attempts at reconstruction. Therefore, it would have seemed reasonable to do an incision/excision of a scar contracture and split the skin graft with postoperative splinting as a first alternative. Results are often excellent, the procedure is simpler, the postoperative complications less severe. The authors' demonstration of a 100% success rate is evidence that this flap belongs in the armamentarium of those who do burn reconstruction.

R. E. Salisbury, MD

Preventing Unintentional Scald Burns: Moving Beyond Tap Water
Lowell G, Quinlan K, Gottlieb LJ (Rush Univ Med Ctr, Chicago, IL; Univ of Chicago, IL)
Pediatrics 122:799-804, 2008

Objective.—The goal was to examine in detail the mechanisms of significant scald burns among children <5 years of age, to discover insights into prevention.

Methods.—Medical records for children <5 years of age who were admitted with scald burns between January 1, 2002, and December 31, 2004, were identified through the University of Chicago Burn Center database. Demographic data and details of the circumstances and mechanisms of injury were extracted from the medical records.

Results.—Of 640 admissions to the University of Chicago Burn Center during the 3-year study period, 140 (22%) involved children <5 years of age with scald burns. Of the 137 available charts reviewed, 118 involved unintentional injuries. Of those unintentional injuries, 14 were tap water scalds and 104 were non–tap water scalds. Of the non–tap water scalds, 94 scalds (90.4%) were related to hot cooking or drinking liquids. Two unexpected patterns of injury were discovered. Nine children (8.7%) between the ages of 18 months and 4 years were scalded after opening a microwave oven and removing the hot substance themselves. Seventeen children (16.3%) were scalded while an older child, 7 to 14 years of age, was cooking or carrying the scalding substance or supervising the younger child.

Conclusions.—Current prevention strategies and messages do not adequately address the most common mechanisms of scald injury requiring hospitalization. Easy access to a microwave oven poses a significant scald risk to children as young as 18 months of age, who can open the door and remove the hot contents. An engineering fix for microwave ovens could help protect young children from this mechanism of scalding. Involvement of older children in a subset of scald injuries is a new finding that may have prevention implications.

▶ It is well known that the home is the most dangerous place for a young child, and the authors once again highlight that the kitchen is not a playroom. It is astonishing that 104 out of their 640 admissions in a 3-year period were due to accidents in the kitchen of underage children. These numbers clearly suggest that current prevention programs are not achieving the desired effect.

R. E. Salisbury, MD

Randomized Controlled Trial to Determine the Efficacy of Long-Term Growth Hormone Treatment in Severely Burned Children

Branski LK, Herndon DN, Barrow RE, et al (Univ of Texas Med Branch and Shriners Hosps for Children, Galveston)
Ann Surg 250:514-523, 2009

Background.—Recovery from a massive burn is characterized by catabolic and hypermetabolic responses that persist up to 2 years and impair rehabilitation and reintegration. The objective of this study was to determine the effects of long-term treatment with recombinant human growth hormone (rhGH) on growth, hypermetabolism, body composition, bone metabolism, cardiac work, and scarring in a large prospective randomized single-center controlled clinical trial in pediatric patients with massive burns.

Patients and Methods.—A total of 205 pediatric patients with massive burns over 40% total body surface area were prospectively enrolled between 1998 and 2007 (clinicaltrials.gov ID NCT00675714). Patients were randomized to receive either placebo (n = 94) or long-term rhGH at 0.05, 0.1, or 0.2 mg/kg/d (n = 101). Changes in weight, body composition, bone metabolism, cardiac output, resting energy expenditure, hormones, and scar development were measured at patient discharge and at 6, 9, 12, 18, and 24 months postburn. Statistical analysis used Tukey t test or ANOVA followed by Bonferroni correction. Significance was accepted at $P < 0.05$.

Results.—RhGH administration markedly improved growth and lean body mass, whereas hypermetabolism was significantly attenuated. Serum growth hormone, insulin-like growth factor-I, and IGFBP-3 was significantly increased, whereas percent body fat content significantly decreased when compared with placebo, $P < 0.05$. A subset analysis revealed most lean body mass gain in the 0.2 mg/kg group, $P < 0.05$. Bone mineral content showed an unexpected decrease in the 0.2 mg/kg group, along with a decrease in PTH and increase in osteocalcin levels, $P < 0.05$. Resting energy expenditure improved with rhGH administration, most markedly in the 0.1 mg/kg/d rhGH group, $P < 0.05$. Cardiac output was decreased at 12 and 18 months postburn in the rhGH group. Long-term administration of 0.1 and 0.2 mg/kg/d rhGH significantly improved scarring at 12 months postburn, $P < 0.05$.

Conclusion.—This large prospective clinical trial showed that long-term treatment with rhGH effectively enhances recovery of severely burned pediatric patients.

▶ This article from the Galveston Shrine further documents the authors' extremely large experience with human growth hormone in burned children. Their prospective study revealed that long-term treatment with human growth hormone enhanced recovery of the pediatric burn patient. The reader is encouraged to review the entire series of articles by this superb group and their experience with metabolism in the thermally injured patient.

R. E. Salisbury, MD

Age Differences in Inflammatory and Hypermetabolic Postburn Responses

Jeschke MG, Norbury WB, Finnerty CC, et al (Shriners Hosps for Children, Galveston, TX; et al)
Pediatrics 121:497-507, 2008

Objective.—The aim of this study was to identify contributors to morbidity and death in severely burned patients <4 years of age.

Methods.—A total of 188 severely burned pediatric patients were divided into 3 age groups (0–3.9 years, 4–9.9 years, and 10–18 years of age). Resting energy expenditure was measured through oxygen consumption, body composition through dual-energy x-ray absorptiometry, liver size and cardiac function through ultrasonography, and levels of inflammatory markers, hormones, and acute-phase proteins through laboratory chemistry assays.

Results.—Resting energy expenditure was highest in the 10- to 18-year-old group, followed by the 4- to 9.9-year-old group, and was lowest in the 0- to 3.9-year-old group. Children 0 to 3.9 years of age maintained lean body mass and body weight during acute hospitalization, whereas children >4 years of age lost body weight and lean body mass. The inflammatory cytokine profile showed no differences between the 3 age groups, whereas liver size increased significantly in the 10- to 18-year-old group and was lowest in the 0- to 3.9-year-old group. Acute-phase protein and cortisol levels were significantly decreased in the toddler group, compared with the older children. Cardiac data indicated increased cardiac work and impaired function in the toddler group, compared with the other 2 age groups.

Conclusions.—Increased mortality rates for young children are associated with increased cardiac work and impaired cardiac function but not with the inflammatory and hypermetabolic responses.

▶ This article should be read in conjunction with the other fine work done on metabolism in burn patients by this group at the Galveston Shrine. The authors found that increased mortality rates for young children were associated with increased cardiac work, but not with inflammatory and hypermetabolic responses.

R. E. Salisbury, MD

Analysis of Upper Extremity Motion in Children After Axillary Burn Scar Contracture Release

Sison-Williamson M, Bagley A, Petuskey K, et al (Shriners Hosps for Children Northern California, Sacramento)
J Burn Care Res 30:1002-1006, 2009

Burns to the upper extremity and axilla frequently result in the formation of contractures that can impede shoulder range of motion. The purpose of this study was to determine the long-term effects of upper extremity burn scar contracture release on motion during activities of daily living in the first year postrelease. Upper extremity motion analysis was conducted on children aged 4 to 17 years before and 1, 3, 6, and 12 months after axillary contracture release surgery. Movements were analyzed during three functional tasks including high reach (reaching for an object), hand to head (combing hair), and hand to back pocket (toileting). A total of 23 subjects (34 axillary contractures; mean age 10 ± 3 years; mean TBSA burn 40 ± 6%) completed the study. Preoperatively, decreased shoulder mobility due to axillary contractures resulted in the use of compensatory motions to complete the tested activities. Surgical release of the contracture increased shoulder mobility and decreased compensatory movements. Improvements were maintained for 1 year after surgery with majority of the improvement involving shoulder flexion. Axillary contracture release surgery improves functional shoulder mobility and decreases compensatory motions used during activities of daily living in the first year postrelease. Additional follow-up is needed to evaluate the impact of growth on scar development.

▶ This article nicely emphasizes that in order to analyze the effectiveness of contracture release, one has to consider more than simple passive and active range of motion. The authors evaluate functional movement, range of motion, and the effect of surgery. The patients experienced a distinct increase in functional range of motion for a year following surgery. Very rightly they note that the children range from 4 to 17 years of age and cannot predict what effect the growth will have on their final outcome. Our criteria for evaluating the results of surgery must be more dynamic and functionally oriented.

R. E. Salisbury, MD

An Audit of First-Aid Treatment of Pediatric Burns Patients and Their Clinical Outcome
Cuttle L, Kravchuk O, Wallis B, et al (Univ of Queensland, Herston, Australia; Univ of Queensland, St Lucia, Australia)
J Burn Care Res 30:1028-1034, 2009

This study describes the first aid used and clinical outcomes of all patients who presented to the Royal Children's Hospital, Brisbane, Australia in 2005 with an acute burn injury. A retrospective audit was performed with the charts of 459 patients and information concerning burn injury, first-aid treatment, and clinical outcomes was collected. First aid was used on 86.1% of patients, with 8.7% receiving no first aid and unknown treatment in 5.2% of cases. A majority of patients had cold water as first aid (80.2%), however, only 12.1% applied the cold water for the recommended 20 minutes or longer. Recommended first aid (cold water for ≥20 minutes) was associated with significantly reduced reepithelialization time for children with contact injuries ($P = .011$). Superficial depth burns were significantly more likely to be associated with the use of recommended first aid ($P = .03$). Suboptimal treatment was more common for children younger than 3.5 years ($P < .001$) and for children with friction burns. This report is one of the few publications to relate first-aid treatment to clinical outcomes. Some positive clinical outcomes were associated with recommended first-aid use; however, wound outcomes were more strongly associated with burn depth and mechanism of injury. There is also a need for more public awareness of recommended first-aid treatment.

▶ The authors note that their publication is one of the very few to relate first-aid treatment to clinical outcomes. Although their attempt is a good one, the interpretation of the results always raises questions that one finds with any retrospective study. Not surprisingly, wound outcomes were more strongly associated with burn depth and mechanism of injury. The bibliography is excellent, however, and more work needs to be done with the publication of burn prevention articles to minimize mistakes by first responders.

R. E. Salisbury, MD

Incidence of Fractures Among Children With Burns With Concern Regarding Abuse

DeGraw M, Hicks RA, Lindberg D (St John's Hosp Children's Ctr, Detroit, MI; Indiana Univ, Indianapolis; Brigham and Women's Hosp, Boston, MA)
Pediatrics 125:e295-e299, 2010

Objective.—Consensus recommendations state that a radiographic skeletal survey is mandatory for all children <2 years of age with concern for physical abuse. It has been suggested that patients with burns may represent a special subgroup at lower risk for occult fractures, compared with other abused children. Our objective was to determine the prevalence of fractures in children referred for subspecialty abuse evaluations because of burns.

Methods.—We performed retrospective analyses of data collected as part of the Using Liver Transaminases to Recognize Abuse (ULTRA) research network. Data were collected for all children <5 years of age who were referred to 19 child protection teams for subspecialty child abuse evaluations over 1 year ($N = 1676$). We compared the rate of fractures in children presenting with burns with that in other children evaluated for abuse.

Results.—Of 97 children <24 months of age with burns, 18 (18.6%) were also found to have fractures. Among all 1203 children <24 months of age, 649 (53.9%) had fractures. Eleven children had multiple fractures, and 12 children had fractures with radiographic evidence of healing. Two children were noted to have classic metaphyseal fractures.

Conclusion.—The rate of fractures in children who present with burns and concerns regarding physical abuse is sufficient to support the recommendation for routinely performing skeletal surveys for children <2 years of age.

▶ The results of this study are not only surprising but also embarrassing. With all of the efforts in burn prevention, including films, presentations, and publications, the authors still found that 21 of 97 children who had burns were not evaluated for fractures. They found that among children less than 2 years of age, all of whom had been referred for evaluation for possible physical abuse, the children with burns were more likely not to have been evaluated for fractures. The American Academy of Pediatrics (AAP) has recommended that skeletal surveys be performed for all children less than 2 years of age with concerns for abuse, including those presenting with burns. It is absolutely inconceivable that those involved in emergency care of children have not gotten the message. One can only assume that learning must be by endless repetition ad nauseum to avoid needless deaths.

R. E. Salisbury, MD

Burn Therapists' Opinion on the Application and Essential Characteristics of a Burn Scar Outcome Measure

Forbes-Duchart L, Cooper J, Nedelec B, et al (Winnipeg Health Sciences Centre, Manitoba, Canada; Univ of Manitoba, Winnipeg, Canada; McGill Univ, Montreal, Quebec, Canada)
J Burn Care Res 30:792-800, 2009

Comprehensive burn rehabilitation requires the use of an appropriate burn scar outcome measure (BSOM). The literature reports many BSOMs; however, an objective, practical, inexpensive, valid, reliable, and responsive instrument eludes us. A problem in the development of such a measure is disagreement in which scar properties to include. The objective of this study was to determine the burn scar variables that therapists believe should be included in a BSOM. An Internet survey was administered to burn occupational and physical therapists. The response rate was 38.6% (105 surveys). Of the respondents, 38.1% use a BSOM; of those, 75% use the Vancouver Scar Scale. Reasons why respondents do not use a BSOM (61.9%) are because they are not familiar with available measures, have not found one that is clinically practical, or need more training. The majority (95%) believes that using a BSOM is important, and the following BSOM characteristics were reported as important: reliable, valid, quick, easy, and noninvasive. Respondents indicated that the following properties should be included in a BSOM: pliability (96.2%), vascularity (92.4%), height (87.6%), appearance (75.2%), skin breakdown (74.3%), itch (73.3%), surface texture (70.5%), pigmentation (68.6%), and pain (67.6%). This study suggests that using a BSOM is important despite its inconsistent use, and BSOM education may be valuable. The top three agreed-upon properties for inclusion are already incorporated into the most commonly used BSOM—the Vancouver Scar Scale—suggesting that modifications may be reasonable.

▶ This article is distressing for several reasons. The objective of the study was to determine burn scar variables that therapists believe should be included in a burn scar outcome measure. Unfortunately, there was only a 38.6% response to the survey. Surely therapists are not too busy to respond to such an important issue, leading one to question their commitment to science. Of the 38.6% that responded, only 38.1% used burn scar outcome measures. Thus, one must conclude that at most units there is no objective assessment of the success or failure of the management of burn scars. Lack of attention to this problem not only results in poor patient care but also the possibility of medical legal issues. Lastly, a cottage industry has grown up hawking products for burn scar management without true documentation of their efficacy.

R. E. Salisbury, MD

Aquacel® Ag with Vaseline gauze in the management of toxic epidermal necrolysis (TEN)
Huang S-H, Yang P-S, Wu S-H, et al (Kaohsiung Med Univ Hosp, Taiwan)
Burns 36:121-126, 2010

Toxic epidermal necrolysis (TEN) is a rare condition with potentially high mortality and involves severe exfoliative disease of the skin and mucous membranes induced by drugs. The reported fatality of TEN varies widely from 20% to 60%. The technique for TEN wound coverage described in this article involves the use of various dressings.

Patients and Methods.—Nine women with histologically confirmed TEN (>30% total body surface area, TBSA) were treated at our burn intensive care unit. All patients received hydrotherapy and wounds were covered with Aquacel® Ag and Vaseline gauzes onlay. Following this, elastic cotton bandage was wrapped around the dressing. The dressing was changed and the wound evaluated twice a week. Efficacy was established by the wound achieving ≥95% re-epithelialisation of the study area.

Results.—The mean age was 60.1 years (range from 7 to 88 years). The percentage of body surface area affected by epidermal slough ranged from 30% to 85% TBSA, with a mean of 51%. One patient expired due to severe sepsis on day 3. Eight patients achieved over 95% wound healing. All wounds healed well without the need for skin grafting. However, two of them expired on day 14 and day 20 because of pneumonia and retention of carbon dioxide, respectively. The average duration to achieve 95% wound healing was 10.4 days in eight cases (range from 7 to 14 days). No adverse reactions were noted.

Conclusion.—Aquacel® Ag dressing can be easily removed during hydrotherapy. The wound pain is reduced. By changing the dressing just twice a week, we were able to evaluate the wound directly, decrease the odour and increase the quality of life of the patients. In addition, lower frequency of dressing changes decreases the manpower requirements and is cost effective. Use of Aquacel® Ag with Vaseline gauze is a good alternative for the management of TEN wounds.

▶ The authors describe their experience with Aquacel Ag, providing a very effective treatment modality for patients with toxic epidermal necrolysis (TEN). This particular dressing is efficacious because it releases silver into the wound, thus controlling bacterial proliferation, decreasing the frequency of dressing changes, and not destroying the underlying regenerating epithelium when it is removed. Cost effectiveness of this dressing certainly should be evaluated as it seems to be an ideal dressing for treatment of these patients.

R. E. Salisbury, MD

Bacteremia in Stevens-Johnson Syndrome and Toxic Epidermal Necrolysis: Epidemiology, Risk Factors, and Predictive Value of Skin Cultures
de Prost N, Ingen-Housz-Oro S, Duong TA, et al (Université Paris XII, Créteil, France)
Medicine 89:28-36, 2010

Toxic epidermal necrolysis (TEN) is a rare drug-related life-threatening acute condition. Sepsis is the main cause of mortality. Skin colonization on top of impaired barrier function promotes bloodstream infections (BSI). We conducted this study to describe the epidemiology, identify early predictors of BSI, and assess the predictive value for bacteremia of routine skin surface cultures.

We retrospectively analyzed the charts of all patients with Stevens-Johnson syndrome (SJS) and TEN hospitalized over an 11-year period. Blood cultures and skin isolates were recovered from the microbiology laboratory database. Early predictors of BSI were identified using a Cox model. Sensitivity, specificity, and negative and positive predictive values of skin cultures for the etiology of BSI were assessed.

The study included 179 patients, classified as having SJS (n = 54; 30.2%), SJS/TEN overlap (n = 59; 33.0%), and TEN (n = 66; 36.9%). Forty-eight episodes of BSI occurred, yielding a rate of 15.5/1000 patient days. Inhospital mortality was 13.4% (24/179). Overall, 70 pathogens were recovered, mainly *Staphylococcus aureus* (n = 23/70; 32.8%), *Pseudomonas aeruginosa* (n = 15/70; 21.4%), and Enterobacteriaceae organisms (n = 17/70; 24.3%). Variables associated with BSI in multivariate analysis included age >40 years (hazard ratio [HR], 2.5; 95% confidence interval [CI], 1.35–4.63), white blood cell count >10,000/mm^3 (HR, 1.9; 95% CI, 0.96–3.61), and percentage of detached body surface area

≥30% (HR, 2.5; 95% CI, 1.13–5.47). Skin cultures had an excellent negative predictive value for bacteremia due to *S aureus* (especially methicillin-resistant strains) and *P aeruginosa*, but not for those due to Enterobacteriaceae organisms. In contrast, the positive predictive value was low for all pathogens studied.

To our knowledge, this is the largest study describing the epidemiology and risk factors of BSI in patients with SJS/TEN. The body surface area involved is the main predictor of BSI. Excellent negative predictive values of skin cultures for *S aureus* and *P aeruginosa* bacteremia should help clinicians consider targeted empirical antibiotic choices when appropriate.

▶ This article is interesting for several reasons. The authors have a long-standing interest in Stevens-Johnson syndrome (SJS) and toxic epidermal necrolysis (TEN) as reflected by a multitude of publications. The authors, however, seem intrigued by the fact that the results of the retrospective study show that the skin cultures yielded a very poor positive predictive value relating to bloodstream infection. Burn center scientists have known this fact since the 1960s. Quantitative culture and wound biopsy remain the standard of care for determining the bacteriologic status of the wound. Patients with SJS and TEN are extremely susceptible to invasive infection just like patients with burns. The most common source of wound infection remains a patient's colonic contents. Qualitative skin culture has been shown time and again to not reflect what is happening in the wound itself. The quantitative swab technique and wound biopsy clearly delineate that patients are only contaminated as opposed to infected. Growing greater than 10/5 organisms per gram of tissue has been best correlated with systemic sepsis. Routine wound surveillance several times per week is mandatory to avoid a lethal bacteremia and is used in most burn centers, explaining why patients with SJS and TEN are best served by being admitted to a burn center critical care unit.

R. E. Salisbury, MD

Role of tumor necrosis factor–α and matrix metalloproteinase–9 in blood-brain barrier disruption after peripheral thermal injury in rats: Laboratory investigation

Reyes R, Guo M, Swann K, et al (The Univ of Texas Health Science Ctr at San Antonio)
J Neurosurg 110:1218-1226, 2009

Object.—A relationship has been found between peripheral thermal injury and cerebral complications leading to injury and death. In the present study, the authors examined whether tumor necrosis factor–α (TNF–α) and matrix metalloproteinase–9 (MMP-9) play a causative role in blood-brain barrier (BBB) disruption after peripheral thermal injury.

Methods.—Thirty-two male Sprague-Dawley rats were subjected to thermal injury. One hour later, 8 rats were injected with TNF-α neutralizing antibody, and 8 were injected with doxycycline, an inhibitor of the MMP family proteins; 16 rats did not receive any treatment. Brain tissue samples obtained 7 hours after injury in the treated animals were examined for BBB function by using fluorescein isothiocyanate–dextran and by assessing parenchymal water content. Protein expression of basement membrane components (collagen IV, laminin, and fibronectin) was quantified on Western blot analysis, and MMP-9 protein expression and enzyme activity were determined using Western blot and gelatin zymography. Thermally injured rats that did not receive treatment were killed at 3, 7, or 24 hours after injury and tested for BBB functioning at each time point. Histological analysis for basement membrane proteins was also conducted in untreated rats killed at 7 hours after injury. Results of testing in injured rats were compared with those obtained in a control group of rats that did not undergo thermal injury.

Results.—At 7 hours after thermal injury, a significant increase in the fluorescein isothiocyanate–dextran and water content of the brain was found ($p < 0.05$), but BBB dysfunction was significantly decreased in the rats that received TNF-α antibody or doxycycline ($p < 0.05$). In addition, the components of the basal lamina were significantly decreased at 7 hours after thermal injury ($p < 0.01$), and there were significant increases in MMP-9 protein expression and enzyme activity ($p < 0.05$). The basal lamina damage was reversed by inhibition of TNF-α and MMP-9, and the increase in MMP-9 protein was reduced in the presence of doxycycline ($p < 0.05$). The authors found that MMP-9 enzyme activity was significantly increased after thermal injury ($p < 0.01$) but decreased in the presence of either TNF-α antibody or doxycycline ($p < 0.01$).

Conclusions.—The dual, inhibitory activity of both TNF-α and MMP-9 in brain injury suggests that a TNF-α and MMP-9 cascade may play a key role in BBB disruption. These results offer a better understanding of the pathophysiology of burn injuries, which may open new avenues for burn treatment beyond the level of current therapies.

▶ There has been an extraordinary lack of articles describing the effects of thermal injury on the neurosystem. This particular article is fascinating because it not only suggests that tumor necrosis-α and matrix metalloproteinase-9 (MMP-9) may play a key role in disrupting the blood brain barrier and causing increased cerebral edema following a burn injury, but also that there are several inhibitory drugs that can help prevent this phenomenon such as tumor necrosis-α neutralizing antibody and doxycycline.

It has been well known that significant burn injuries give a generalized increase in capillary permeability that lead to edema even in unburned areas of the body. The brain is obviously an organ at particular risk, and edema secondary to a large burn and subsequent vigorous volumes of intravenous resuscitation might well lead to burn encephalopathy. The present effort bears further investigation.

R. E. Salisbury, MD

4 Hand and Upper Extremity

Biomechanical Analysis of Surgical Correction of Syndactyly
Miyamoto J, Nagasao T, Miyamoto S (Keio Univ, Tokyo, Japan; Natl Cancer Ctr Hosp East, Chiba, Japan)
Plast Reconstr Surg 125:963-968, 2010

Background.—The dorsal rectangular flap technique has been widely used for the correction of syndactyly. In this method, however, the linear scar along the palmar border of the webspace may lead to secondary contracture and web creep. Some modifications have been advocated for breaking these linear scars. In this study, these modifications were evaluated biomechanically with the finite element method.

Methods.—Based on computed tomography findings of seven adult hands, three scar models were created: the dorsal rectangular flap, the dorsal flap with palmar-based triangular flap, and the dorsal flap with V-shaped tip. Forced displacements were applied to mimic the hand-opening motion, and scar stresses and web displacement were investigated.

Results.—The maximal stress of the scar was significantly greater in the dorsal rectangular flap group than in the other groups (dorsal flap with palmar-based triangular flap, $p = 0.046$; dorsal flap with V-shaped tip, $p = 0.018$). The web was displaced most distally in the dorsal rectangular flap group compared with the other groups (dorsal flap with palmar-based triangular flap, $p = 0.043$; dorsal flap with V-shaped tip, $p = 0.043$). There was no significant difference between the dorsal flap with a palmar-based triangular flap group and the dorsal flap with a V-shaped tip group.

Conclusions.—The authors' results indicate that both the palmar-based triangular flap and the V-shaped tip flap work well. It is strongly recommended that any break should be made in the palmar edge of the webspace for prevention of web creep.

▶ The authors present an intriguing way of illustrating and analyzing a frequently seen clinical finding after syndactyly reconstruction—web creep and scar contracture. Their results demonstrate that by disrupting the linear palmar scar, stress forces across the scar and distal web space displacement are reduced. The suggested modifications to the dorsal rectangular flap are straightforward and can be easily adapted to clinical practice. This article provides a good conceptual option for clinicians facing problems with web

creep following syndactyly reconstruction and can help in reducing the occurrence of this complication and the need for revision surgery later. I personally
really like the dorsal flap and have tried to compensate for the creep by deep-
ening the webspace by 2 to 3 mm. Maybe I should just switch flaps.

D. J. Smith, Jr, MD

Injectable Collagenase Clostridium Histolyticum for Dupuytren's Contracture

Hurst LC, Badalamente MA, Hentz VR, et al (State Univ of New York; Stanford
Hosps and Clinics, Palo Alto, CA; et al)
N Engl J Med 361:968-979, 2009

Background.—Dupuytren's disease limits hand function, diminishes the
quality of life, and may ultimately disable the hand. Surgery followed by
hand therapy is standard treatment, but it is associated with serious potential complications. Injection of collagenase clostridium histolyticum, an
office-based, nonsurgical option, may reduce joint contractures caused
by Dupuytren's disease.

Methods.—We enrolled 308 patients with joint contractures of 20
degrees or more in this prospective, randomized, double-blind, placebo-
controlled, multicenter trial. The primary metacarpophalangeal or proximal interphalangeal joints of these patients were randomly assigned to
receive up to three injections of collagenase clostridium histolyticum
(at a dose of 0.58 mg per injection) or placebo in the contracted collagen
cord at 30-day intervals. One day after injection, the joints were manipulated. The primary end point was a reduction in contracture to 0 to 5
degrees of full extension 30 days after the last injection. Twenty-six
secondary end points were evaluated, and data on adverse events were
collected.

Results.—Collagenase treatment significantly improved outcomes.
More cords that were injected with collagenase than cords injected with
placebo met the primary end point (64.0% vs. 6.8%, P<0.001), as well
as all secondary end points (P≤0.002). Overall, the range of motion in
the joints was significantly improved after injection with collagenase as
compared with placebo (from 43.9 to 80.7 degrees vs. from 45.3 to
49.5 degrees, P<0.001). The most commonly reported adverse events
were localized swelling, pain, bruising, pruritus, and transient regional
lymph-node enlargement and tenderness. Three treatment-related serious
adverse events were reported: two tendon ruptures and one case of
complex regional pain syndrome. No significant changes in flexion or
grip strength, no systemic allergic reactions, and no nerve injuries were
observed.

Conclusions.—Collagenase clostridium histolyticum significantly reduced contractures and improved the range of motion in joints affected by advanced Dupuytren's disease. (ClinicalTrials.gov number, NCT00528606).

▶ This treatment is receiving a lot of notoriety, and rightfully so. The data are very impressive and the complication rate is low. Unfortunately, it is not Food and Drug Administration (FDA) approved yet. Keep a close watch, as to date this seems like a very positive addition to the treatment armamentarium.

D. J. Smith Jr, MD

Collagenase Injection as Nonsurgical Treatment of Dupuytren's Disease: 8-Year Follow-Up
Watt AJ, Curtin CM, Hentz VR (Stanford Univ Hosps and Clinics, Palo Alto, CA)
J Hand Surg 35A:534-539, 2010

Purpose.—Collagenase has been investigated in phase II and phase III clinical trials for the treatment of Dupuytren's disease. The purpose of this study is to report 8-year follow-up results in a subset of patients who had collagenase injection for the treatment of Dupuytren's contracture.

Methods.—Twenty-three patients who participated in the phase II clinical trial of injectable collagenase were contacted by letter and phone. Eight patients were enrolled, completed a Dupuytren's disease questionnaire, and had independent examination of joint motion by a single examiner.

Results.—Eight patients completed the 8-year follow-up study: 6 had been treated for isolated metacarpophalangeal (MCP) joint contracture, and 2 had been treated for isolated proximal interphalangeal (PIP) joint contracture. Average preinjection contracture was 57° in the MCP group. Average contracture was 9° at 1 week, 11° at 1 year, and 23° at 8-year follow-up. Four of 6 patients experienced recurrence, and 2 of 6 had no evidence of disease recurrence at 8-year follow-up. Average preinjection contracture was 45° in the PIP group. Average contracture was 8° at 1 weeks, 15° at 1 year, and 60° at 8-year follow-up. Both patients experienced recurrence at 8-year follow-up. No patients had had further intervention on the treated finger in either the MCP or the PIP group. Patients subjectively rated the overall clinical success at 60%, and 88% of patients stated that they would pursue further injection for the treatment of their recurrent or progressive Dupuytren's disease.

Conclusions.—Enzymatic fasciotomy is safe and efficacious, with initial response to injection resulting in reduction of joint contracture to within 0°–5° of normal in 72 out of 80 patients. Initial evaluation of long-term recurrence rates suggests disease recurrence or progression in 4 out of 6 patients with MCP contractures and 2 patients with PIP contractures;

however, recurrence was generally less severe than the initial contracture in the MCP group. In addition, patient satisfaction was high.
Type of Study/Level of Evidence.—Therapeutic IV.

▶ This study is really exciting. Enzymatic fasciotomy appears to be a reality with excellent 8-year results. The bad news is that there is no uniform answer. The good news is that this is being reported by a highly respected and reliable group of investigators. Clearly, neither surgical fasciotomy nor enzymatic fasciotomy is a definitive cure. What appears evident is that collagenase injection offers a potential nonsurgical treatment for Dupuytren's disease. This appears poised to become a standard part of the algorithm for treatment of Dupuytren's disease.

D. J. Smith, Jr, MD

Arthroscopic Ganglionectomy Through an Intrafocal Cystic Portal for Wrist Ganglia
Chen AC-Y, Lee W-C, Hsu K-Y, et al (Chang Gung Univ, Taoyuan, Taiwan)
Arthroscopy 26:617-622, 2010

Purpose.—A retrospective study was conducted on arthroscopic ganglionectomy in wrists using a novel intrafocal cystic portal. The safety and efficacy of this technique were assessed by treatment of 15 wrists in 15 patients.
Methods.—Arthroscopic ganglionectomy was performed by the same surgeon with the patient under general anesthesia or regional block. Preoperative complaints, intraoperative findings, and postoperative results of all the patients were reported. The mean follow-up was 15.3 months. Functional assessment by use of modified Mayo wrist scores, patient satisfaction, and recurrence were included in the follow-up evaluation.
Results.—Two thirds of the patients acquired good to excellent results, whereas the results for the remaining third were fair. Complications included 1 recurrence and 1 case of transient paresthesia sensation. The most common arthroscopic findings were capsular and ligament lesions, rather than ganglionic stalks.
Conclusions.—Arthroscopic ganglionectomy through an intrafocal cystic portal is a safe and efficacious option for the treatment of painful wrist ganglia.
Level of Evidence.—Level IV, therapeutic case series.

▶ Wrist arthroscopy is gaining popularity as a diagnostic and treatment modality for wrist pathology from degenerative diseases to traumatic ligamentous injuries, with new indications emerging rapidly. The authors describe a new technique to address ganglion cysts through a less-invasive arthroscopic approach in a case study of 15 patients. Their results were fair to excellent, with only 1 recurrence in a 15-month follow-up period. This modality may be useful in the management of primary ganglion cysts; proficiency in wrist arthroscopy is an obvious prerequisite. The procedure itself will be more technically challenging, and the cost to benefit ratio for equipment use, operating time, and insurance reimbursement are all issues that need to be addressed. In cases of recurrent ganglion cysts, arthroscopy may have limited use. This does have appeal but does not seem to have immediate promise.

D. J. Smith Jr, MD

Blinded, Prospective, Randomized Clinical Trial Comparing Volar, Dorsal, and Custom Thermoplastic Splinting in Treatment of Acute Mallet Finger
Pike J, Mulpuri K, Metzger M, et al (Washington School of Medicine, St Louis, MO; British Columbia's Children's Hosp, Vancouver, Canada; St Paul's Hosp, Vancouver, British Columbia, Canada)
J Hand Surg 35A:580-588, 2010

Purpose.—To compare volar, dorsal, and custom splinting techniques in acute Doyle I mallet finger injuries.

Methods.—We developed a radiographic lag measurement using the contralateral normal digit as an internal control for establishing the approximate preinjury maximal extension of the mallet finger. The difference in maximal distal interphalangeal joint extension between the injured and contralateral normal digit was defined as the radiographic lag difference. We randomized 87 subjects meeting the inclusion criteria to one of 3 splint types: volar padded aluminum splint, dorsal padded aluminum splint, and custom thermoplastic. Splints were continued for 6 weeks full-time. A total of 77 subjects were available for measurement of the primary outcome measure: radiographic lag difference at week 12. Secondary outcome measures were recorded at weeks 7 and 24.

Results.—No lag difference was demonstrated at week 12 (p = .12), although a trend suggesting superiority (closest value to 0 difference) of the custom thermoplastic splint was observed. The mean radiographic lag differences were $-16.2°$ (95% confidence interval [CI], $-21.3°$ to $-11.0°$) for the dorsal padded aluminum splint, $-13.6°$ (95% CI, $-18.0°$ to $-9.2°$) for the volar padded aluminum splint, and $-9.0°$ (95% CI, $-14.5°$ to $3.4°$) for the custom thermoplastic splint. Secondary between-group analyses showed no differences for radiographic or clinical lag, Michigan Hand Outcome Questionnaire scores, or complications. Secondary analyses of the whole cohort suggested that clinical measurement overestimates true lag, increased lag occurs after discontinuation of splinting, and clinically measured improvement in lag is noted at week 24.

Conclusions.—No lag difference was demonstrated between custom thermoplastic, dorsal padded aluminum splint, and volar padded aluminum splinting for Doyle I acute mallet fingers. Clinical measurement overestimates true lag in mallet injuries. Increased lag occurs after discontinuation of splinting. Increased age and complications correlate with worse radiographic lag.

Type of Study/Level of Evidence.—Therapeutic II.

▶ With a type I mallet finger in which there is a closed rupture of the extensor tendon insertion, distal interphalangeal (DIP) joint immobilization in full extension for 6 weeks is the recommended treatment. This study showed there was no lag difference (measured radiographically) with the 3 different splint types, although a trend suggesting superiority of the custom splint was observed after 6 weeks. Based on these findings, I would tend to treat my patients with a custom thermoplastic splint and continue splinting at night for an additional 4 to 6 weeks because increased lag occurred after discontinuation of splinting.

D. J. Smith, Jr, MD

Complications of Open Trigger Finger Release
Will R, Lubahn J (Hamot Med Ctr, Erie, PA)
J Hand Surg 35A:594-596, 2010

Purpose.—Open release of A1 pulleys for trigger finger has been thought of as a relatively benign procedure with a low complication rate. Few studies have examined the rate of complications in trigger finger release. The objective of this study was to retrospectively review the complications documented for a cohort of patients who received open trigger finger releases.

Methods.—We conducted a retrospective chart review of 43 patients who had had 78 open trigger finger releases by a single surgeon. Any postoperative complications that were documented were recorded. Complications were then divided into major and minor. Major complications required further surgery or resulted in significant limitations of activities of daily living; minor complications hindered recovery, responded to treatment (if applicable), and either resolved or had little impact on function.

Results.—Two major complications were noted: a synovial fistula that required excision, and proximal interphalangeal joint arthrofibrosis that required cast application for pain relief. The major complication rate was 3% per trigger release (2/78). Twenty-seven minor complications in 22 digits were documented for these cases, including decreased range of motion, scar tenderness, pain, and wound erythema. The minor complication rate was 28% (22/78). The overall, combined complication rate for these primary interventions was 31% (24/78).

Conclusions.—Open trigger finger release is thought to be a low-risk procedure by most practitioners. In this study, we found that major complications do occur infrequently; however, the rate of minor complications was surprisingly high and related mostly to wound complications or loss of finger range of motion. The surgeon performing open trigger finger releases should inform the patient of the likelihood of having these minor complications.

▶ The authors report a retrospective review of 78 trigger finger releases in 43 patients. Complications, major with 3% and minor with 31%, are surprisingly high—that is, until the literature is reviewed. The retrospective reviews that exist show complications ranging from 11% to 43%. While this review is on the high side, it is still well within the bounds of the refereed literature. Thus, we have a dilemma. The published results show higher than expected complications, but there is no prospective trial. A more definitive study is needed. Otherwise, we will continue along with the impression that this procedure has few complications when, in reality, minor complications are high.

D. J. Smith, Jr, MD

Using Evidence to Minimize the Cost of Trigger Finger Care
Kerrigan CL, Stanwix MG (Dartmouth Hitchcock Med Ctr, Lebanon, NH)
J Hand Surg 34A:997-1005, 2009

Purpose.—Critics of U.S. health care cite both underuse and overuse of resources. With more than one third of Americans paying for medical care out of pocket, optimizing the cost-benefit ratio of care is a high priority. Clinical trials have established the success of the different treatment options for patients who present with trigger finger. The economic impact of these differing strategies has not been established. The aim of this study was to perform a cost-minimization analysis to identify the least costly strategy for effective treatment of trigger finger using existing evidence in the literature.

Methods.—Five strategies for the treatment of trigger finger were identified: (1) a steroid injection followed by surgical release for failure or recurrence, (2) a steroid injection followed by a second injection for failures or recurrence, followed by definitive surgery if needed, (3) 3 steroid injections before definitive surgery if needed, (4) surgical release, and (5) percutaneous release with definitive open surgery if needed. To reflect the costs, we used 2 sources of data: our institution's billing charges to private payers and our institution's reimbursements from Medicare. A literature review identified median success rates of the different treatment strategies. We conducted a series of analyses to evaluate the effect of varying individual costs and success rates.

Results.—The second strategy is the least costly treatment of those considered in this study. The most costly treatment, surgical release, costs between 248% and 340% more than the second strategy. For surgical or percutaneous release to cost less than the second strategy, the surgical billing charge would need to be lower than $742 for private payers or less than $305 of Medicare reimbursement.

Conclusions.—Trigger finger is a common problem with many acceptable treatment algorithms. Management of trigger finger with 2 steroid injections before surgery is the least costly treatment strategy.
Type of Study/Level of Evidence.—Decision Analysis II.

▶ This article is one of the better articles I have seen showing what the future may hold. It could be that we are going to be told which treatment to use based on cost. Most surgeons I work with attempt 1 or 2 steroid injections prior to surgery, so this will probably not impact many practices. However, cost may become a higher priority in considering future care decisions. Overall, this is a good article regarding cost analysis.

D. J. Smith, Jr, MD

Barbed Suture Tenorrhaphy: An Ex Vivo Biomechanical Analysis
Parikh PM, Davison SP, Higgins JP (Georgetown Univ Hosp, Washington, DC; Union Memorial Hosp, Baltimore, MD)
Plast Reconstr Surg 124:1551-1558, 2009

Background.—Using barbed suture for flexor tenorrhaphy could permit knotless repair with tendon-barb adherence along the suture's entire length. The purpose of this study was to evaluate the tensile strength and repair-site profile of a technique of barbed suture tenorrhaphy.
Methods.—Thirty-eight cadaveric flexor digitorum profundus tendons were randomized to polypropylene barbed suture repair in a knotless three-strand or six-strand configuration, or to unbarbed four-strand cruciate repair. For each repair, the authors recorded the repair site cross-sectional area before and after tenorrhaphy. Tendons were distracted to failure, and data regarding load at failure and mode of failure were recorded.
Results.—The mean cross-sectional area ratio of control repairs was 1.5 ± 0.3, whereas that of three-strand and six-strand barbed repairs was 1.2 ± 0.2 ($p = 0.009$) and 1.2 ± 0.1 ($p = 0.005$), respectively. Mean load to failure of control repairs was 29 ± 7 N, whereas that of three-strand and six-strand barbed repairs was 36 ± 7 N ($p = 0.32$) and 88 ± 4 N ($p < 0.001$), respectively. All cruciate repairs failed by knot rupture or suture pullout, whereas barbed repairs failed by suture breakage in 13 of 14 repairs ($p < 0.001$).
Conclusions.—In an ex vivo model of flexor tenorrhaphy, a three-strand barbed suture technique achieved tensile strength comparable to that of four-strand cruciate repairs and demonstrated significantly less repair-site bunching. A six-strand barbed suture technique demonstrated increased tensile strength compared with four-strand cruciate controls and significantly less repair-site bunching. Barbed suture repair may

offer several advantages in flexor tenorrhaphy, and further in vivo testing is warranted.

▶ I wondered how long it would be before articles like this started appearing. The use of the barbed suture for tendon repair has many attractive advantages. How the barb is set in the tendon will be interesting. Whether there is increased resistance because of the barbed suture should be considered. Keep an eye on this. It may be useful in the future but not now.

D. J. Smith, Jr, MD

Fascial Flap Reconstruction of the Hand: A Single Surgeon's 30-Year Experience
Carty MJ, Taghinia A, Upton J (Brigham and Women's/Faulkner Hosp, Boston, MA; Harvard Med School, Boston, MA)
Plast Reconstr Surg 125:953-962, 2010

Background.—The reconstruction of complex hand wounds is challenging due to the requirements for thin and pliable coverage with a reliable vascular supply, potential for sensibility, and provision of a gliding surface. Fascial flaps represent an excellent option for the reconstruction of these complicated defects.

Methods.—A retrospective review of fascial flap reconstructive procedures to the hand undertaken by a single microsurgeon was performed for operations occurring between 1979 and 2009. Both pedicled and free tissue transfer procedures were included in both pediatric and adult patients. Data were culled from a combination of patient charts, hospital records, radiographic studies, and clinical photographs.

Results.—Sixty fascial flap reconstructive procedures to the hand were analyzed in 60 patients from the defined 30-year period. The most common pathological process necessitating reconstruction was acute trauma ($n = 32$, 53 percent). Most of the soft-tissue injuries included in the study sample were located on the dorsal hand and wrist ($n = 27$, 45 percent). The most commonly utilized reconstructive modality was the temporoparietal fascial flap ($n = 35$, 58 percent). Most reconstructions were completed as free tissue transfers ($n = 46$, 77 percent). Perioperative complications were relatively minor; no flap losses were recorded. All cases studied demonstrated excellent long-term coverage with no evidence of underlying tendon adhesion or contracture.

Conclusion.—Fascial flaps represent an excellent option for coverage of soft-tissue defects of the hand that are not amenable to reconstruction with skin grafting alone, particularly for localized defects with denuded tendons or exposed joints.

▶ When faced with a complex hand defect, it is necessary to find coverage that is thin and pliable and will allow for joint mobility and/or tendon gliding. If skin graft coverage is inadequate, biosynthetic materials are often espoused because traditional muscle or fasciocutaneous flaps tend to be bulky and require secondary revisions. However, materials such as Integra are expensive and require 2 stages, this article is especially relevant in today's practice because it presents a single-stage option of covering complex hand wounds. This study is also one of the first long-term patient outcome studies for the use of fascial flaps in the hand. I really expected to see more large series of these flaps at an earlier time.

D. J. Smith, Jr, MD

Acellular Dermal Regeneration Template for Soft Tissue Reconstruction of the Digits

Taras JS, Sapienza A, Roach JB, et al (Jefferson Med College of Thomas Jefferson Univ, Philadelphia, PA; Drexel Univ, Philadelphia, PA; The Philadelphia Hand Ctr, PA)
J Hand Surg 35A:415-421, 2010

Purpose.—Trauma to the digits often leaves soft tissue defects with exposed bone, joint, and/or tendon that require soft tissue replacement. The objective of this study was to evaluate the effectiveness of acellular dermal regeneration template combined with full-thickness skin grafting for soft tissue reconstruction in digital injuries with soft tissue defects.

Methods.—Acellular dermal regeneration template was used to reconstruct digital injuries with exposed bone, joint, tendon, and/or hardware not amenable to treatment with healing by secondary intention, rotation flaps, or primary skin grafts. Acellular dermal regeneration template was applied to 21 digits in 17 patients. Nineteen digits had exposed bone, 8 digits had exposed tendon, 6 digits had exposed joints, and 2 digits had exposed hardware. The acellular dermal regeneration template was sutured over the soft tissue defect. Over 3 weeks, a neodermis formed. The superficial silicone layer of the acellular dermal regeneration template was removed, and the digits received full-thickness epidermal autografting with cotton bolster.

Results.—The duration of postoperative follow-up extended to a minimum of 12 months. For the injury sites where acellular dermal regeneration template was applied, the total area of application ranged from 1 cm^2 to 24 cm^2, with the largest individual site measuring 12 cm^2. Twenty of 21 digits demonstrated 100% incorporation of the acellular dermal regeneration template skin substitute. One digit that had sustained multilevel trauma developed necrosis requiring revision amputation. Full-thickness epidermal autografting was performed an average of 24 days after acellular dermal regeneration template skin substitute application and demonstrated a 100% take in 16 of 20 digits and partial graft loss of 15% to 25% in 4 of 20 digits that did not require further treatment.

Conclusions.—Acellular dermal regeneration template combined with secondary full-thickness skin grafting is an effective method of skin reconstruction in complex digital injuries with soft tissue defects involving exposed bone, tendon, and joint. The neodermis increases tissue bulk and facilitates epidermal autografting with digital injuries that otherwise would require flap coverage or skeletal shortening of the digit.

Type of Study/Level of Evidence.—Therapeutic IV.

▶ I picked this because there are increased reports of use of synthetic products for difficult wound coverage. This may be helpful with significant burns and may even be preferable to bulkier flaps in selected circumstances. I am not sure whether there is an advantage of one product over another. The important thing will be to feel comfortable with a product and use it appropriately.

D. J. Smith, Jr, MD

Rate of Infection After Carpal Tunnel Release Surgery and Effect of Antibiotic Prophylaxis

Harness NG, Inacio MC, Pfeil FF, et al (Kaiser Anaheim Med Ctr, CA; Univ of California Irvine, Anaheim)
J Hand Surg 35A:189-196, 2010

Purpose.—To determine the rate of postoperative wound infection and the association with prophylactic antibiotic use in uncomplicated carpal tunnel release surgery.

Methods.—We performed a multicenter, retrospective review of all the carpal tunnel release procedures performed between January 1, 2005, and August 30, 2007. Data reviewed included the use of prophylactic antibiotics, diabetic status, and the occurrence of postoperative wound infection. We determined the overall antibiotic usage rate and analyzed the correlation between antibiotic use and the development of postoperative wound infection.

Results.—The rate of surgical site infections in the 3003 patients who underwent carpal tunnel release surgery (group A) was 11. Antibiotic usage data were available for 2336 patients (group B). Six patients without prophylactic antibiotics had infection, as did 5 patients with prophylactic antibiotics. This difference was not statistically significant. Of the 11 surgical site infections, 4 were deep (organ/space) and 7 superficial (incisional). The number of patients with diabetes in the overall study population was 546, 3 of whom had infections. This was not statistically different from the nondiabetic population infection rate (8 patients).

Conclusions.—The overall infection rate after carpal tunnel release surgery is low. In addition, the deep (organ/space) infection rate is much lower than previously reported. Antibiotic use did not decrease the risk of infection in this study population, including patients with diabetes. The routine use of antibiotic prophylaxis in carpal tunnel release surgery is not indicated. Surgeons should carefully consider the risks and benefits of routinely using prophylactic antibiotics in carpal tunnel release surgery.

Type of Study/Level of Evidence.—Therapeutic III.

▶ I am really glad to see an article like this. So frequently studies equivocate and still recommend the use of antibiotics—probably as a legal deterrent. Here we have substantive data to support that antibiotics are not needed even for patients with diabetes. The real test will be whether we will implement the recommendation.

D. J. Smith, Jr, MD

Five-Year Follow-Up of Carpal Tunnel Release in Patients Over Age 65
Weber RA, DeSalvo DJ, Rude MJ (Scott and White Memorial Hosp, Temple, TX; Scott, Sherwood and Brindley Foundation, Temple, TX; The Texas A&M Univ System Health Science Ctr College of Medicine, Temple)
J Hand Surg 35A:207-211, 2010

Purpose.—In 2005, a prospective clinical trial with a 6-month follow-up demonstrated the efficacy of carpal tunnel release in patients 65 years and older and showed that age is not a contraindication to surgery. The purpose of this study was to determine whether there was any further improvement, maintenance of results, or recurrence of carpal tunnel symptoms 5 years after surgery.

Methods.—We contacted all 66 patients (with a total of 92 hands involved) from the original study to be enrolled for re-evaluation. Of the original cohort, 12 were unavailable because of death or severe neurologic impairment. Of the remaining 54 patients, 19 agreed to participate in this follow-up study of their 29 hands. For the 5-year follow-up, patients underwent a repeat history and physical examination with particular emphasis on the status of their hands over the past 5 years. The Michigan Hand Outcome Questionnaire was again used to determine overall hand function, activities of daily living, work performance, pain, aesthetics, and satisfaction with hand function.

Results.—The mean age of patients available for 5-year follow-up was 78 ± 3 years. The patients maintained their symptom improvement, demonstrating no significant difference between the 6-month and 5-year follow-up data; their physical findings, except for grip strength, were likewise unchanged. The patients also retained their improved 2-point discrimination. Scar tenderness decreased over the 5 years. The Michigan Hand Outcome Questionnaire confirmed the fact that initial postoperative improvement in all parameters persisted at least 5 years. One patient underwent repeat carpal tunnel release of 1 hand for recurrent symptoms. Overall, 94% of patients were either very or completely satisfied with their results.

Conclusions.—Patients who were 65 years of age or older at the time of surgery maintained their clinical improvement for at least 5 years after surgery.

Type of Study/Level of Evidence.—Therapeutic IV.

▶ This is a well-designed study with interesting confirmatory findings. The fact that results were stable after 6 months and maintained over 5 years is encouraging. The fact that only 19 of 54 patients agreed to be reinterviewed is disturbing. Were they originally put off by the study? Were they really no better and did not want to waste their time? The results are encouraging, but the unknown needs to be clarified.

D. J. Smith, Jr, MD

Intra- and Inter-Examiner Variability in Performing Tinel's Test
Lifchez SD, Means KR Jr, Dunn RE, et al (Johns Hopkins Univ, Baltimore, MD; Raymond M. Curtis Natl Hand Ctr, Baltimore, MD; Medstar Res Ctr, Baltimore, MD; et al)
J Hand Surg 35A:212-216, 2010

Purpose.—The Tinel sign was adopted in the early 1950s to detect sites of nerve compression. There have been few attempts to standardize how one elicits Tinel's sign. The goal of this study was to evaluate intra- and inter-examiner variability in the force generated using different techniques to elicit Tinel's sign.

Methods.—Nine clinicians, consisting of 3 experienced hand and peripheral nerve surgeons, 3 junior hand and peripheral nerve surgeons, and 3 surgeons in training were included in the study. Three different Tinel-type maneuvers were evaluated: (1) striking the load cell using the dominant middle finger only ("single-finger strike"), (2) using the dominant index and middle finger together ("double-finger strike"), and (3) preloading with the nondominant thumb and then striking the thumb with the dominant middle finger ("preload"). Test subjects were instructed to use their customary range of force during the testing. Each subject performed 3 sets of 5 strikes per technique.

Results.—There was a significant difference in nearly all subjects between the range of force generated with single- or double-finger techniques and preload technique. There was also a difference in nearly all subjects when comparing the range of forces using the single-and double-finger techniques. In addition, there were large differences in the range of forces produced by the examiners for each technique.

Conclusions.—There is no standardization for eliciting the Tinel sign. This study demonstrates considerable intra- and inter-examiner differences in the range of forces generated by the different Tinel's techniques that are used in clinical practice. This variability might explain clinical differences between examiners in the ability to obtain a Tinel sign in a patient and might explain the inconsistency of sensitivity and specificity reported for

Tinel's sign. Further research on standardization is needed, and future study protocols using Tinel's sign should take these findings into account.

► This is a long-overdue study comparing rater variability, but a routine text, used by all and yet with no standardization. Hopefully, the authors will follow up with how to make it standard. This study won't change your practice but should make you suspicious of results, including the Tinel's sign.

D. J. Smith, Jr, MD

Patient-Rated Outcome of Ulnar Nerve Decompression: A Comparison of Endoscopic and Open *In Situ* Decompression

Watts AC, Bain GI (Modbury Public Hosp, North Adelaide, South Australia, Australia; Univ of Adelaide, South Australia, Australia; Royal Adelaide Hosp, South Australia, Australia; et al)
J Hand Surg 34A:1492-1498, 2009

Purpose.—To report patient-rated outcomes after ulnar nerve decompression at the elbow and to compare the outcome after open *in situ* decompression with that after endoscopic *in situ* decompression.

Methods.—Patients having ulnar nerve decompression were evaluated using patient-rated outcome measures. Fifty-five patients were recruited; 3 were lost to follow-up, and 18 were excluded because they had anterior transposition. Of the thirty-four patients followed up for 12 months, 19 had endoscopic decompression and 15 had open *in situ* decompression. Patient demographics, presenting symptoms, range of elbow movement, grip and pinch strength, and sensation were recorded preoperatively and at 12 months by an independent observer. Postoperative patient satisfaction, pain, and ongoing paresthesia were recorded using visual analog scales. Subgroup analysis was performed to compare the outcome of open *in situ* decompression with that of endoscopic *in situ* decompression.

Results.—At 12 months after surgery, the proportion of patients satisfied with the outcome was 9 of 15 (60%) for open *in situ* surgery and 15 of 19 (79%) for endoscopic *in situ* surgery. The postoperative complication rate was significantly higher after open *in situ* decompression than that after endoscopic *in situ* decompression surgery (10%). Preoperative function scores were predictive of patient-rated satisfaction and were related to McGowan grade.

Conclusions.—The patient-reported outcome of surgical treatment of cubital tunnel syndrome is good but is affected by preoperative symptom severity. Outcomes after open and endoscopic *in situ* decompression, including the proportion of patients reporting satisfaction and functional improvement, are equivalent, but more patients reported complications after open decompression.

Type of Study/Level of Evidence.—Therapeutic III.

▶ This is a well-designed but small study. Hopefully, a prospective randomized trial will be initiated. The only difference in complications is in scar tenderness and numbness of the elbow. I will bet these resolve with time. With no significant difference, the endoscopic approach is probably significantly more expensive. It is hard to beat the traditional approach based on this information.

D. J. Smith, Jr, MD

Recurrence of Giant Cell Tumors in the Hand: A Prospective Study
Williams J, Hodari A, Janevski P, et al (Henry Ford Hosp, Detroit, MI)
J Hand Surg 35A:451-456, 2010

Purpose.—Giant cell tumors of the hand remain a treatment dilemma: treatment requires a balance between extensive dissections for excision versus risk of recurrence. There is no consensus regarding how best to manage this balance. The purpose of this study was to identify the recurrence rate of giant cell tumors of the hand, as well as the correlation with the specific tissue type involved.

Methods.—Two hundred thirteen cases of giant cell tumor of the hand were recorded in a prospectively designed, anatomically based registry that identified tumor location and surgical planes entered and tissues excised during the procedure. Mean follow-up was 51 months. Demographic and follow-up data were also tracked. The primary outcome tracked was tumor recurrence. Statistical analysis was conducted using chi-square analysis and the Fisher exact test to determine which perioperative and intraoperative factors were associated with tumor recurrence.

Results.—There were 27 recurrences among our cases. Tumors involving the extensor tendon, flexor tendon, or joint capsule had the strongest correlation with recurrence: 12, 8, and 12 cases, respectively. Conversely, there was only one recurrence among the patients who did not have any involvement of either the flexor or extensor tendons or joint capsules. There was no association for involvement of skin, neurovascular bundle, tendon sheath, or bone at the initial excision. No identifiable preoperative or postoperative factors were linked to recurrence.

Conclusions.—Our study shows that direct involvement of the extensor tendons, flexor tendons, or joint capsule puts patients in a high-risk category with respect to recurrence. Based on these findings, efforts regarding close monitoring and the role of adjuvant therapy should be directed at the high-risk population. This information may be helpful for hand surgeons developing evidence-based treatment algorithms for giant cell tumor in the hand.

Type of Study/Level of Evidence.—Prognostic III.

▶ This study is an excellent prospective evaluation of the treatment of giant cell tumors. The fact that there is a higher recurrence rate among those tumors that involved extensor or flexor tendons or joint capsules makes sense. Only 1 recurrence did not involve any of these structures. This provides excellent criteria for those patients who require closer follow-up and possible adjuvant therapy.

D. J. Smith, Jr, MD

5 Aesthetic

General

Benchmarking Outcomes in Plastic Surgery: National Complication Rates for Abdominoplasty and Breast Augmentation
Alderman AK, Collins ED, Streu R, et al (The Univ of Michigan Med Ctr, Ann Arbor; Dartmouth Med School, Hanover, NH; St Joseph Mercy Hosp, Ypsilanti, MI; et al)
Plast Reconstr Surg 124:2127-2133, 2009

Background.—The authors evaluated the use of national databases to track surgical complications among abdominoplasty and breast augmentation patients.

Methods.—Their study population included all patients with abdominoplasty or breast augmentation in the Tracking Operations and Outcomes for Plastic Surgeons (TOPS) and CosmetAssure databases from 2003 to 2007. They evaluated the incidence of hematoma, infection, and/or deep venous thrombosis/pulmonary embolism. Chi-square and t tests were used for the analyses.

Results.—The TOPS and CosmetAssure databases included 7310 and 3350 patients with abdominoplasty and 30,831 and 14,227 patients with breast augmentation, respectively. In the TOPS and CosmetAssure populations, the complication rates for abdominoplasty were 0.9 percent and 0.5 percent with hematoma ($p = 0.29$), 3.5 percent and 0.7 percent with infection ($p < 0.001$), and 0.3 percent and 0.1 percent with deep venous thrombosis/pulmonary embolism ($p = 0.05$), respectively. The complication rates for breast augmentation in TOPS and CosmetAssure were 0.6 percent and 0.7 percent with hematoma ($p = 0.21$), 0.3 percent and 0.1 percent with infection ($p < 0.001$), and 0.02 percent and less than 0.01 percent with deep venous thrombosis/pulmonary embolism ($p = 0.31$), respectively.

Conclusions.—Complication rates for abdominoplasty and breast augmentation were similar in TOPS and CosmetAssure, providing a measure of cross-validation. The low complication rates support the safety of these procedures when they are performed by plastic surgeons.

These data should be used by individual practitioners for outcomes benchmarking.

▶ Accurate outcome measures have been difficult to measure as most plastic surgery studies are single-institution reports of a relatively small number of patients. By using data from these 2 large databases, more accurate complication rates can be measured. Plastic surgeons can use these complication rates to benchmark their own results and look aggressively for improvement—that is, if their own rates are higher than expected. In addition, there was also a 5- to 6-fold increase in venous thromboembolism when abdominoplasty was combined with breast augmentation compared with either procedure being done alone.

K. A. Gutowski, MD

Benchmarking Outcomes in Plastic Surgery: National Complication Rates for Abdominoplasty and Breast Augmentation
Alderman AK, Collins ED, Streu R, et al (The Univ of Michigan Med Ctr, Ann Arbor; Dartmouth Med School, Hanover, NH; St Joseph Mercy Hosp, Ypsilanti, MI; et al)
Plast Reconstr Surg 124:2127-2133, 2009

Background.—The authors evaluated the use of national databases to track surgical complications among abdominoplasty and breast augmentation patients.

Methods.—Their study population included all patients with abdominoplasty or breast augmentation in the Tracking Operations and Outcomes for Plastic Surgeons (TOPS) and CosmetAssure databases from 2003 to 2007. They evaluated the incidence of hematoma, infection, and/or deep venous thrombosis/pulmonary embolism. Chi-square and t tests were used for the analyses.

Results.—The TOPS and CosmetAssure databases included 7310 and 3350 patients with abdominoplasty and 30,831 and 14,227 patients with breast augmentation, respectively. In the TOPS and CosmetAssure populations, the complication rates for abdominoplasty were 0.9 percent and 0.5 percent with hematoma ($p = 0.29$), 3.5 percent and 0.7 percent with infection ($p < 0.001$), and 0.3 percent and 0.1 percent with deep venous thrombosis/pulmonary embolism ($p = 0.05$), respectively. The complication rates for breast augmentation in TOPS and CosmetAssure were 0.6 percent and 0.7 percent with hematoma ($p = 0.21$), 0.3 percent and 0.1 percent with infection ($p < 0.001$), and 0.02 percent and less than 0.01 percent with deep venous thrombosis/pulmonary embolism ($p = 0.31$), respectively.

Conclusions.—Complication rates for abdominoplasty and breast augmentation were similar in TOPS and CosmetAssure, providing a measure of cross-validation. The low complication rates support the safety of these procedures when they are performed by plastic surgeons. These data should be used by individual practitioners for outcomes benchmarking.

▶ This article has significance on many different levels. First of all, the article provides useful, validated data regarding the incidence of specific complications for the 2 cosmetic procedures that were studied. Although there are some differences between the complication rates found in the 2 databases, these differences are not particularly important when it comes to counseling patients. The surgeon can easily describe a range of reported complication rates (not necessarily a single, specific rate) and effectively facilitate patient understanding of the magnitude of the complication risk (which is actually quite small) for each of these procedures. More importantly, the study shows valuable cross-validation of the 2 different databases, giving much more credence to the described complication rates found in each source. But most importantly, this study, reinforces the value of benchmarked data for determining the safety, validity, and value of specific plastic surgical procedures—even cosmetic procedures. In the future, these and other databases can and should be used to extract information that can be used to benchmark outcomes for virtually every plastic surgical procedure. The potential value of this benchmarked data in terms of influencing insurance companies, convincing the public about safety and efficacy, etc, will be enormous.

R. L. Ruberg, MD

The Effect of Electroacustimulation on Postoperative Nausea, Vomiting, and Pain in Outpatient Plastic Surgery Patients: A Prospective, Randomized, Blinded, Clinical Trial

Larson JD, Gutowski KA, Marcus BC, et al (Univ of Wisconsin Hosps and Clinics, Madison; NorthShore Univ HealthSystem, Chicago, IL)
Plast Reconstr Surg 125:989-994, 2010

Background.—Current rates of postoperative nausea and vomiting experienced by outpatient surgery patients are as high as 20 to 30 percent. Electroacustimulation therapy has been demonstrated to be effective in controlling these symptoms, but trials identifying its efficacy in the outpatient surgery population are lacking.

Methods.—One hundred twenty-two patients undergoing surgical procedures at an outpatient surgery center were randomized to two treatment arms. The first arm received the standardized pharmacologic postoperative nausea and vomiting prevention typical for patients undergoing outpatient surgery, whereas in the second arm, the ReliefBand and pharmacologic measures were used. The ReliefBand is a U.S. Food and Drug Administration–approved electroacustimulation device. Electroacustimulation is a derivative of acupuncture therapy that uses a small electrical current to stimulate acupuncture points on the human body and is thought to relieve nausea, vomiting, and pain. Outcomes measured were pain and nausea symptoms, emetic events, the need for rescue medications, and the time to discharge.

Results.—The electroacustimulation arm reported statistically significant lower nausea scores at 30 minutes and 120 minutes postoperatively ($p < 0.05$). In addition, subgroup analysis demonstrated significant findings in favor of the experimental group, with anatomical subsets of surgical patients requiring less pain medication and shorter times from surgery to discharge when compared with the standard treatment. However, electroacustimulation did not have a significant effect on the amount of pain experienced by patients in any group.

Conclusion.—The authors' study demonstrates that electroacustimulation offers added protection against symptoms of postoperative nausea and vomiting in an outpatient cosmetic surgery population, representing a safe and cost-effective addition to current pharmacologic preventive measures.

▶ With rates of 20% to 30% in outpatient surgery, reliable preventative measures to reduce the incidence of postoperative nausea and vomiting (PONV) can improve patient outcomes, decrease costs, and minimize postoperative readmissions. The Food and Drug Administration (FDA)-approved device used in this study is placed on the patient's wrist at the start of surgery, appears similar to a wrist watch, costs about $150, is reusable, and does not have any reported side effects. It may be considered a useful adjunct to standard pharmacologic PONV prophylaxis in an outpatient surgery setting.

K. A. Gutowski, MD

Skin, Soft Tissues, and Hair

Combination Jessner's Solution and Trichloroacetic Acid Chemical Peel: Technique and Outcomes

Herbig K, Trussler AP, Khosla RK, et al (Univ of Texas Southwestern Med Ctr, Dallas; Univ of Washington Med Ctr, Seattle)
Plast Reconstr Surg 124:955-964, 2009

Background.—Trichloroacetic acid is a commonly utilized agent for chemical resurfacing of the face. Jessner's solution in combination with trichloroacetic acid has been previously described for the treatment of facial rhytids in the dermatology literature. The purpose of this study was to describe the application technique and examine the clinical results of Jessner's solution in combination with trichloroacetic acid in a diverse plastic surgery patient population.

Method.—A retrospective chart evaluation of 105 patients undergoing combination Jessner's and 35% trichloroacetic acid facial peel procedures by the senior author was performed. Patient demographics, anatomic location of peel, concomitant surgical procedures, and postoperative complications were noted. Technique and endpoints are described.

Results.—Between January of 2000 and April of 2007, 115 chemical peels were performed by the senior author. All patients were female, ranging in age from 32 to 83 years (mean, 54 years). Of the 115 chemical peels performed, 104 were done with concomitant procedures. Eleven peels were performed alone. The most significant complications related to the combination peel were fungal infections (7.8 percent overall rate). In addition, the senior author performed 27 face/neck lifts with superficial musculoaponeurotic system (SMAS)-ectomy or SMAS plication along with full face combination peel, with minimal postoperative complications and no evidence of hypertrophic scarring.

Conclusions.—The combination of Jessner's solution and 35% trichloroacetic acid is an effective, safe resurfacing tool that can treat superficial to moderate rhytids. Despite the apparent simplicity of the procedure, there is a significant learning curve to understand the intricacies of chemical penetration in the skin. Consistency in results is achieved with experience and proper preoperative patient evaluation and selection.

▶ The ability to offer patients a medium depth (papillary dermis) peel can grow a physician's facial aesthetic practice without investing in expensive resurfacing devices. The trichloroacetic acid (TCA) peel is relatively easy to learn and can be performed in the office setting as an isolated procedure or in the operating room as a component of more extensive facial rejuvenation. The addition of Jessner's solution can extend the depth of the peel to the reticular dermis when correction of more significant rhytids is needed. The step-by-step patient evaluation and preparation protocol and specific peel technique described in this article should be reviewed by those who wish to incorporate medium depth peels into their practice.

K. A. Gutowski, MD

Fractional Photothermolysis for Skin Rejuvenation
Cohen SR, Henssler C, Johnston J (Univ of California, San Diego)
Plast Reconstr Surg 124:281-290, 2009

Background.—Fractional photothermolysis has become an important laser modality in management of a number of skin conditions and photoaging. The authors describe the scientific basis of fractional photothermolysis, report on most of the available devices, discuss their clinical uses and techniques, and attempt to decipher their relative efficacy.

Methods.—The authors reviewed as best as possible all fractional lasers currently approved by the Food and Drug Administration for distribution into the United States. Laser wavelength, means of delivery, depth of penetration, and special features were collated.

Results.—Nine fractional lasers were evaluated. Main differences in outcome were related to type of laser wavelength. In general, scanning technologies are faster and more precise. Deeper injuries result in more collagen remodeling. Variations in laser wavelengths, depth of injury, type of delivery system, consumables, and architecture of the fractionated laser light are important considerations when evaluating fractional lasers. Little scientific research comparing the injury, healing, and outcomes of the various fractional lasers is available.

Conclusions.—Fractional photothermolysis represents a breakthrough in laser treatment for a wide array of skin problems. The safety profile has been improved over conventional ablative lasers, and the range of skin types and treatment areas have been expanded. Unlike full-surface flat beam resurfacing, fractional resurfacing damages specific microtreatment zones within the target area. Nonablative fractionals do not achieve results similar to those of the fractional ablative lasers, but certain conditions may respond better to nonablative fractional treatments. More data are needed on the comparative effects of the various types of lasers and their best indications.

▶ In the last 3 years, more laser manufacturers started offering devices with fractional delivery of laser energy in an effort to decrease the side effects associated with ablative lasers. Using fractional technology, only a small portion of the treatment area is targeted by the laser, creating a pattern of small treated areas with surrounding viable epidermis and untreated dermis. The results of skin rejuvenation are typically not as good as the results seen after using nonfractional treatment, but there are fewer complications, less aftercare, and recovery is faster. This article provides a good overview for those considering introducing this technology to their practice, particularly those who avoided ablative lasers due to long recovery times and complications. Financial implications of the various devices are not detailed because there is room for price negotiation when making these purchases. However, a prospective buyer should be aware of repeating disposable and maintenance costs that need to be compared between devices.

K. A. Gutowski, MD

Treatment of Striae Distensae with Fractional Photothermolysis
Bak H, Kim BJ, Lee WJ, et al (Univ of Ulsan, Seoul, Korea; Chung-Ang Univ, Seoul, Korea; et al)
Dermatol Surg 35:1215-1220, 2009

Background.—Striae distensae are dermal scars characterized by flattening and atrophy of the epidermis. Although many treatment modalities have been tried with variable results, most have been disappointing.

Objective.—To determine whether striae distensae might respond to fractional photothermolysis.

Methods.—Twenty-two women with striae distensae were treated with two sessions each of fractional photothermolysis at a pulse energy of 30 mJ, a density level of 6, and eight passes at intervals of 4 weeks.

Response to treatment was assessed by comparing pre- and post-treatment clinical photography and skin biopsy samples.

Results.—Six of the 22 patients (27%) showed good to excellent clinical improvement from baseline, whereas the other 16 (63%) showed various degrees of improvement. Most of the lesions with excellent results were white in color and of long duration. Skin biopsy revealed that average epidermal thickness and dermal thickness were greater than at baseline. The immunoreactivity of procollagen type 1 increased after treatment. There were no significant side effects except erythema and mild pigmentation.

Conclusion.—Fractional photothermolysis may be effective in treating striae distensae, without significant side effects. Treatment outcomes were better in patients with white rather than red striae.

▶ Reliable and predictable treatment of striae distensae remains elusive. While some patients showed improvement after treatment with fractional photothermolysis using a Fraxel SR 1500 laser, the results were modest at best and limited to those who had white rather than pink colored striae.

K. A. Gutowski, MD

Ultrasound tightening of facial and neck skin: A rater-blinded prospective cohort study
Alam M, White LE, Martin N, et al (Northwestern Univ, Chicago, IL)
J Am Acad Dermatol 62:262-269, 2010

Background.—Nonablative skin tightening technologies offer the prospect of reduction of wrinkles and skin sagging with minimal downtime, discomfort, and risk of adverse events. The excellent safety profile is mitigated by the limited efficacy of such procedures.

Objective.—We sought to assess the efficacy of ultrasound skin tightening for brow-lift in the context of a procedure treating the full face and neck.

Methods.—This was a rater-blinded, prospective cohort study at a dermatology clinic in an urban academic medical center. Subjects were medicated with topical anesthetic and then treated with an investigational focused intense ultrasound tightening device to the forehead, temples, cheeks, submental region, and side of neck using the following probes: 4 MHz, 4.5-mm focal depth; 7 MHz, 4.5-mm focal depth; and 7 MHz, 3.0-mm focal depth. Standardized photographs of front and side views were obtained at 2, 7, 28, 60, and 90 days; rating scales of pain, adverse events, physical findings, and patient satisfaction were also completed. Primary outcome measure was detection of improvement in paired comparison of pretreatment and posttreatment (day 90) photographs by 3 masked expert physician assessors, cosmetic and laser dermatologists, and plastic surgeons who were not authors. Second primary outcome measure was objective brow elevation as quantitated by a standard procedure using fixed landmarks. Secondary outcomes measure was patient satisfaction as measured by a questionnaire.

Results.—A total of 36 subjects (34 female) were enrolled, one subject dropped out, and 35 subjects were evaluated. Median age was 44 years (range 32-62). On the first primary outcome measure, 30 of 35 subjects (86%) were judged by the 3 masked experienced clinician raters to show clinically significant brow-lift 90 days after treatment ($P = .00001$). On the second primary outcome measure, mean value of average change in eyebrow height as assessed by measurement of photographs at 90 days was 1.7 mm.

Limitations.—Limitations of this study include the inability to quantitatively measure lower face tightening because of the lack of fixed anatomic landmarks in this area.

Conclusion.—Ultrasound appears to be a safe and effective modality for facial skin tightening. A single ultrasound treatment of the forehead produced on average brow height elevation of slightly less than 2 mm. Most treated individuals responded, commonly with accompanying transitory mild erythema and edema.

▶ This small preliminary study demonstrated an almost 2-mm brow elevation in most, but not all, patients 90 days after treatment with a focused intense ultrasound device (Ulthera). Due to difficulty in objectively measuring the amount of tissue contraction in the cheek, jowls, and neck, a formal analysis of these areas was not done. Unlike other externally applied tissue tightening devices, Ulthera offers ultrasound visualization of the subcutaneous tissue targeted for thermal coagulation, and the depth of treatment can be varied by using different ultrasound probes. While 2 mm of brow elevation may not be clinically beneficial for many patients seeking brow and forehead rejuvenation, it does offer a nonsurgical option to patients with lesser degrees of brow ptosis. This technology will most likely continue to evolve and possibly improve to the point of offering significant skin improvements in selected patients.

K. A. Gutowski, MD

Treatment of Surgical Scars with Nonablative Fractional Laser Versus Pulsed Dye Laser: A Randomized Controlled Trial
Tierney E, Mahmoud BH, Srivastava D, et al (Laser and Skin Surgery Ctr, Carmel, Indiana; Henry Ford Health System, Detroit, MI)
Dermatol Surg 35:1172-1180, 2009

Objective.—Comparison of the efficacy of nonablative fractional laser (NAFL) and the V-beam pulsed dye laser (PDL) for improvement of surgical scars.

Methods.—A randomized blinded split-scar study. Fifteen scars in 12 patients were treated a minimum of 2 months after Mohs surgery. Patients were treated on half of the scar with a 1,550-nm NAFL and on the contra-lateral half with the 595 nm PDL.

Main Outcome Measure(s).—A nontreating physician investigator eval-uated the outcome of the scar in terms of scar dyspigmentation, thickness, texture, and overall cosmetic appearance (5-point grading scale).

Results.—After a series of four treatments at 2-week intervals, greater improvements were noted in the portion of surgical scars treated with NAFL (overall mean improvement 75.6%, range 60–100%, vs. PDL, 53.9%, range 20–80%; $p < .001$).

Conclusion.—These data support the use of NAFL as a highly effective treatment modality for surgical scars, with greater improvement in scar appearance than with PDL. It is likely that the greater depth of penetration and focal microthermal zones of injury with NAFL, inducing neocollagen-esis and collagenolysis, account for its greater improvement in scar remod-eling. These encouraging results lead us to recommend that NAFL be added to the current treatment armamentarium for surgical scars.

▶ Many options exist for aesthetic improvement of surgical scars. This well-designed study demonstrated nicely the advantage of a nonablative fractional laser (NAFL) (1550-nm erbium doped fiber laser, Fraxel RS, Reliant Technol-ogies) over the commonly used pulsed dye laser (PDL) (595 nm V-beam PDL, Candela Corporation Inc). Of particular improvement was scar hypopig-mentation by NAFL, which was not seen at all in the scars treated by PDL. Most of the improvement in each group was seen after 1 or 2 treatments with only small incremental improvements with subsequent treatments. Given the study design (scars treated shortly after Mohs surgery), the findings may not be applicable to larger scars, traumatic scars, scars with significant thickness and texture, or longer standing scars.

K. A. Gutowski, MD

Fractionated CO_2 Laser Resurfacing: Our Experience With More Than 2000 Treatments
Hunzeker CM, Weiss ET, Geronemus RG
Aesthet Surg J 29:317-322, 2009

Fractionated carbon dioxide (CO_2) laser resurfacing combines the concept of fractional photothermolysis with an ablative 10600-nm wave-length. This technology allows for the effective treatment of rhytides, photodamage, and scars, with shorter recovery periods and a significantly reduced side effect profile as compared to traditional CO_2 laser resurfac-ing. In this article, the authors review the concept of fractional

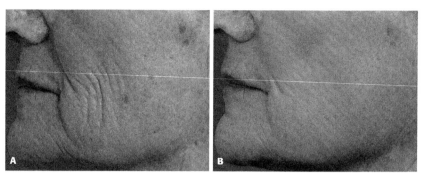

FIGURE 2.—**A,** Pretreatment view of a 68-year-old woman. **B,** Three months after the second full-face ablative fractional resurfacing treatment, demonstrating an improvement in skin tone and reduction of facial rhytides. (Reprinted from Hunzeker CM, Weiss ET, Geronemus RG. Fractionated CO2 laser resurfacing: our experience with more than 2000 treatments. *Aesthet Surg J.* 2009;29:317-322, with permission from Elsevier.)

photothermolysis, the expanding array of indications for use of fractionated CO_2 lasers, and their preferred treatment technique (Fig 2).

▶ The introduction of fractional laser technology is reintroducing the CO_2 laser with most of its benefits but few of the side effects. Using ablative fractional resurfacing (AFR) with a CO_2 laser, hypopigmentation (a common late complication of nonfractional CO_2 laser treatments), and scarring are nearly eliminated. With full-face AFR, complete re-epithelialization occurs in only 2 to 6 days, compared with 2 to 3 weeks of recovery following full-face traditional CO_2 laser resurfacing. The faster re-epithelialization after AFR results in fewer infections, less days of occlusive ointment application (which reduces acneiform eruptions), faster resolution of erythema, and more patient satisfaction.

The authors' experience is primarily with the Fraxel repair laser (Solta Medical) but other systems are available.[1] The most common indications are treatment of facial rhytides (Fig 2A & B), sun-damaged skin, and acne scarring, all of which can have improvement after 1 or 2 treatments. Unlike traditional CO_2 lasers, AFR can be used safely on the entire face, neck, and chest without significant concerns for pigment changes. AFR also provides good results for scar treatments, including hypertrophic and hypopigmented scars as well as atrophic acne scars. There is also evidence of improvement of mild lower eyelid dermatochalasis and pigment disorders. Like all new technologies, the duration of improvement needs to be determined. However, given that repeat treatments seem to be well tolerated, it is possible that patients will be willing to undergo maintenance AFR as needed if more improvement is needed.

K. A. Gutowski, MD

Reference

1. Cohen SR, Henssler C, Johnston J. Fractional photothermolysis for skin rejuvenation. *Plast Reconstr Surg.* 2009;24:281-290.

Advanced Laser Techniques for Filler-Induced Complications

Cassuto D, Marangoni O, De Santis G, et al (Univ of Catania, Italy; Fondazione Glauco Bassi, Trieste, Italy; Univ of Modena and Reggio Emilia, Italy; et al)
Dermatol Surg 35:1689-1695, 2009

Background.—The increasing use of injectable fillers has been increasing the occurrence of disfiguring anaerobic infection or granulomas. This study presents two types of laser-assisted evacuation of filler material and inflammatory and necrotic tissue that were used to treat disfiguring facial nodules after different types of gel fillers.

Materials and Methods.—Infectious lesions after hydrogels were drained using a lithium triborate laser at 532 nm, with subsequent removal of infected gel and pus (laser assisted evacuation). Granuloma after gels containing microparticles were treated using an 808-nm diode laser using intralesional laser technique. The latter melted and liquefied the organic and synthetic components of the granulomas, facilitating subsequent evacuation. Both lasers had an easily controllable thin laser beam, which enabled the physician to control tissue damage and minimize discomfort and pain.

Results.—All 20 patients experienced reduction or complete resolution, the latter increasing with repeated treatments.

Conclusion.—Laser-assisted treatment offers a successful solution for patients who have been suffering from disfiguring nodules from injected fillers—often for many years. The procedure broadens the range of treatment options in cases of untoward reactions to fillers, in line with surgical removal but with lower morbidity and less cosmetic disfigurement.

▶ Treatment of injectable filler-associated complications continues to evolve. Prevention of granuloma- and bioflim-related subclinical infections can be achieved by the use of proper injection techniques and appropriate patient selection and filler selection based on anatomical site. Most injectable filler users should be familiar with the common treatments for related complications, including steroid injections, antibiotics, incision/drainage, and lesion excision. The availability of a laser appears to expand treatment options, which in this series was most commonly used on lesions following injections of products with microspheres and not hyaluronic acid products. Furthermore, the outcome was typically a partial cure—few cases had a complete cure.

K. A. Gutowski, MD

The Spectrum of Adverse Reactions After Treatment with Injectable Fillers in the Glabellar Region: Results from the Injectable Filler Safety Study

Bachmann F, Erdmann R, Hartmann V, et al (Charité-Universitätsmedizin Berlin, Germany; et al)
Dermatol Surg 35:1629-1634, 2009

Background.—For the glabellar region, severe partly vascular adverse events have been reported after treatment with injectable fillers.

Methods and Materials.—For this study, data from the Injectable Filler Safety Study, a German-based registry for those reactions, was analyzed to characterize adverse events seen in the glabellar region. Patients were analyzed descriptively.

Results.—Forty of 139 registered patients reported adverse events in the glabellar region. All patients were female, with an average age of 52.3. Nineteen patients with adverse reactions to hydroxyethylmethacrylate (HEMA) and ethylmethacrylate (EMA) in a fixed combination with hyaluronic acid (HA) and 10 patients with adverse reactions to different hyaluronic acid products were reported; five patients reacted to poly-L-lactic acid (PLA). The most common adverse reactions to HEMA/EMA in HA and PLA were nodules and hardening. In HA-treated patients, erythema and inflammation, swelling, and pain were most frequent. The adverse reactions to HEMA/EMA in HA were severe in 50% of the patients. Severe adverse reactions were found to a lesser extent in patients treated with HA and PLA. Potential vascular complications were documented in only two patients.

Conclusion.—Adverse reactions seen in the glabella are overwhelmingly product associated and to a lesser extent location associated. Vascular complications with necrosis and ulceration were rare.

▶ Although their use continues to grow in popularity, injectable soft tissue fillers are not without side effects and complications. Even though serious and nontransient unintended results are rare, patient education of the risks and physician's knowledge of how to prevent, identify, and manage complications need to be stressed. This large series of complications from a German-based registry offers a glimpse of rare but disfiguring complications following filler injections in the glabella. Not all the fillers described are available in the United States, but the commonly used hyaluronic acid (HA) and polylactic acid (PLA) products were implicated in significant morbidity.

Recommendations for prevention and treatment of complications include the following:

(1) Overcorrection should be avoided. Repeated treatments with smaller volumes and pretreatment with botulinum toxin A to reduce the volume needed for correction may be advisable.

(2) If a vascular complication seems likely (a significant area of blanching occurs while injecting), the injection should be discontinued immediately.

Application of nitroglycerin paste and possibly heparin injections has been recommended to increase vasodilation.

(3) If signs of impending injection necrosis occur after injection of HA-based fillers, hyaluronidase may be used to diffuse the HA gel. (Hyaluronidase may be associated with allergic reactions.)

(4) Once necrosis has occurred, it is important to minimize scarring by providing diligent wound care.

(5) No surgical treatments for scar revision should be attempted during the first 3 months to allow time for scar maturation and the establishment of collateral circulation.

K. A. Gutowski, MD

Detection of Bacteria by Fluorescence in Situ Hybridization in Culture-Negative Soft Tissue Filler Lesions

Bjarnsholt T, Tolker-Nielsen T, Givskov M, et al (Univ of Copenhagen, Denmark; et al)

Dermatol Surg 35:1620-1624, 2009

Background.—Adverse reactions to polyacrylamide gel occur as swellings or nodules, and controversy exists whether these are due to bacterial infection or an autoimmune reaction to the filler.

Objectives.—Biopsies from culture-negative long-lasting nodules after injection with different types of polyacrylamide gel were examined with a combination of Gram stain and fluorescence in situ hybridization.

Results.—Bacteria were detected in biopsies from seven of eight patients. They inhabited gel and intervening tissue and tended to lie in aggregates.

Conclusion.—This study supports the assumption that infection with bacteria in aggregates causes culture-negative late adverse reactions to polyacrylamide gel, suggesting a biofilm environment.

▶ The polyacrylamide gel injectable filler (Aquamid), associated with most of the infections in the report, is not approved for use in the United States at this time. However, the conclusions may be applicable to complications associated with other fillers currently in use. Inflammatory reactions following filler injections frequently are culture negative and are treated with steroid injections. If undetected bacteria are present, the steroid administration may cause a more severe reaction with fistula formation and pus drainage.

When injecting a permanent filler such as polyacrylamide gel, extreme care must be taken to avoid bacterial contamination, and in case of injecting through sites with known high numbers of skin and mucosal bacteria (lips, skin with acne, or many hair follicles), prophylactic treatment with a high dose of relevant broad-spectrum antibiotics (eg, a single-dose combination of moxifloxacin, 400 mg and azithromycin, 500 mg) 2 to 6 hours before treatment is recommended.

Steroid administration alone or in combination with antibiotics favors the assembly of bacteria into a biofilm mode of growth. Therefore, bacterial infections of homogenous polymer gels must be recognized as such as soon as they develop (within 14 days) and treated accordingly with antibiotics (eg, clarithromycin 500 mg and moxifloxacin 400 mg, twice daily for 10 days) and not with steroids or substantial doses of nonsteroidal anti-inflammatory drugs.

K. A. Gutowski, MD

A Prospective Evaluation of the Efficacy of Topical Adhesive Pads for the Reduction of Facial Rhytids
Ryan WR, Most SP (Stanford School of Medicine, CA)
Arch Facial Plast Surg 11:252-256, 2009

Objective.—To determine the efficacy of an over-the-counter topical skin adhesive pad for reducing central forehead and glabellar rhytids over a 4-week period.

Design.—Prospective series involving 30 healthy volunteers with central forehead and glabellar rhytids at a tertiary care academic medical center. The participants used topical skin adhesive pads over the central forehead area and the glabella for 4 weeks in an effort to reduce rhytids. Before and after treatment, the participants had facial photographs taken and completed a questionnaire assessing the severity of their rhytids. Blinded to the timing of the photographs, 2 independent facial plastic surgeons scored the pretreatment and posttreatment rhytid severity using the Glogau scale (1-4) and a wrinkle severity scale (1-10) to evaluate treatment effect.

Results.—Twenty-six participants (87%) completed follow-up with an average of 7.4 hours of use of the topical adhesive pads per night. The independent evaluators found minimal improvements in the Glogau scores (mean [SD], 0.12 [0.33] [$P = .08$] and 0.06 [0.22] [$P = .18$] for the central forehead area and the glabella, respectively). The same evaluators also found minimal change in the wrinkle severity scores (mean [SD], 0.21 [1.28] [$P = .41$] and 0.25 [0.75] [$P = .10$] out of 10 for central forehead rhytids and glabellar rhytids, respectively). None of these measures were statistically significant. The study participants' self-evaluations demonstrated changes in the wrinkle severity scores of 0.35 (2.10) ($P = .41$) in the central forehead area and 0.73 (1.7) ($P = .04$) in the glabella.

Conclusions.—Subjective self-evaluation of topical adhesive pads demonstrates improvement in glabellar rhytids but may be affected by bias. Independent, blinded evaluation by facial plastic surgeons showed no statistical benefit in the reduction of rhytids in the central forehead area or the glabella.

▶ As patients look to noninvasive, more convenient, and less costly ways to reverse facial aging, it is not surprising that over-the-counter products will compete with treatments offered by physicians. The efficacy of such products is typically not tested in a scientific method, so physicians need to be knowledgeable to advise their patients appropriately.

K. A. Gutowski, MD

Long-term Safety and Efficacy of a New Botulinum Toxin Type A in Treating Glabellar Lines

Moy R, for the Reloxin Investigational Group (Moy-Fincher Med Group, Los Angeles, CA; et al)

Arch Facial Plast Surg 11:77-83, 2009

Objective.—To evaluate the long-term safety of repeated administrations of a new botulinum toxin type A (Reloxin; Medicis Pharmaceutical Corp, Scottsdale, Arizona) in the treatment of moderate to severe glabellar lines.

Methods.—Open-label assessment of 1200 patients receiving as many as 5 treatments of Reloxin over a 13-month period. The product was diluted in 2.5-mL sterile physiologic saline solution, 0.9%, without preservative to a concentration of 50 U of Reloxin per 0.25 mL of solution. Investigators injected 0.05 mL of the solution (10 U each) into each of 5 injection sites in the glabellar area on day 0 of each treatment cycle. There was a minimum 85-day gap between treatments. Postinjection clinical evaluation was performed on days 14 and 30 and monthly thereafter until retreatment, study completion, or early termination. The patients were telephoned on day 7 to check for adverse events (AEs) and concomitant medications, and patient diaries were used to document the onset of treatment effect.

Results.—The majority (72%) of treatment-emergent AEs were considered unlikely or not related to study treatment. Probably or possibly related treatment-emergent AEs occurred in 36% of patients. The most frequently occurring related AEs were injection site disorders (18%), nervous system disorders (14% and 12% headache), and eye disorders (9%). Related AEs around the injection site or eyes were usually reported by day 7 and then resolved. Reported ptosis does not differentiate between brow ptosis and eyelid ptosis. A total of 45 patients had a total of 55 instances of ptosis across all cycles, with most episodes lasting less than 3 weeks. The rates of ptosis decreased during successive cycles from 2.4% in cycle 1 to 0.6% in cycle 5. The proportion of patients reporting an onset of response by day 7 ranged from 93% to 95%. By investigator assessment, the response rate (patients reporting none or mild glabellar line severity scale scores on day 30) ranged from 80% to 91% during cycles 1 to 5.

Conclusions.—There was no evidence of cumulative AEs or tachyphylaxis with multiple Reloxin treatments over a period of 13 months. The treatments were well tolerated. The rates of ptosis decreased over successive cycles, and the proportion of responders by day 7 ranged from 93% to 95%.

▶ As new formulations of botulinum toxin enter the market place, practitioners will need to understand the differences between the various products available. The units of product required at each site, time to effect, duration of action, and product tissue diffusion vary between the products. This study demonstrates that Reloxin has a low adverse-effect profile. However, as with most injectable treatments, the results are user dependant and tend to improve with experience.

K. A. Gutowski, MD

A single-center, dose-comparison, pilot study of botulinum neurotoxin type A in female patients with upper facial rhytids: Safety and efficacy
Carruthers A, Carruthers J (Univ of British Columbia, Vancouver)
J Am Acad Dermatol 60:972-979, 2009

Background.—Treating multiple upper facial rhytids at one time is common, but has not been researched extensively.

Objective.—We sought to compare the safety, efficacy, and effect duration of 3 botulinum neurotoxin type A (BoNTA) doses in treating multiple upper facial rhytids.

Method.—Sixty women, randomized to 32, 64, or 96 U total doses, were assessed at baseline, week 2, week 4, then every 4 weeks. The primary efficacy measure was proportion of responders on the patient global assessment of improvement. Adverse events (AEs) were monitored.

Results.—All BoNTA doses were effective and safe. Significant between-group differences occurred in the percentage of responders (96 U: 71%, 64 U: 61%, 32 U: 26%; $P = .0007$). Adverse events did not differ significantly among groups; no serious treatment-related adverse events occurred.

Limitations.—BoNTA doses were fixed and not tailored to individuals.

Conclusion.—These results confirm the efficacy and safety of 3 doses of BoNTA for treating upper facial rhytids in female patients; higher doses afforded greater benefit (Fig 6).

▶ An interesting well-performed prospective double-blind year long study is to test the safety and efficacy of various doses of botulism-type A as manufactured by Allergan Inc. The authors state that their results might not be generalized to other versions or formulations of botulism toxin. Overall, the results document that treating multiple areas of the upper face, forehead wrinkles, glabella, and lateral crow's feet with 1 of 3 total doses (32, 64, and 96 U), in 16 injections, resulted in a dose-response curve such that the highest doses provided statistically significant more and longer desirable effects as judged by experts and patients. Adverse events between the 3 treatment groups were not significantly different. It would be of interest to determine whether the degree and duration

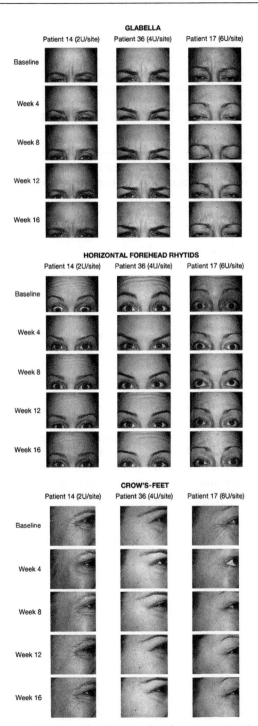

FIGURE 6.—Representative images of patients in each study arm, at various time points. (Reprinted from Carruthers A, Carruthers J. A single-center, dose-comparison, pilot study of botulinum neurotoxin type A in female patients with upper facial rhytids: safety and efficacy. *J Am Acad Dermatol*. 2009;60:972-979, with permission from the American Academy of Dermatology, Inc.)

of the effects were due solely to the doses used or whether the number of injection sites treated was also a factor. The authors conclude that although 96 U provided more of an effect, and did so for a longer time period, 64 U was a better dose, likely due to cost considerations. However, if that was the rationale for their recommendation, no cost effectiveness data were presented in this study, nor referenced in the article.

S. H. Miller, MD, MPH

Six-Year Experience Using 1,000-Centistoke Silicone Oil in 916 Patients for Soft-Tissue Augmentation in a Private Practice Setting
Hevia O (Univ of Miami, FL)
Dermatol Surg 35:1646-1652, 2009

Background.—There are no previously published reports focusing exclusively on the use of 1,000-centistoke purified polydimethylsiloxane (PDMS-1000) for cosmetic soft-tissue augmentation.

Objective.—To provide clinical experience with its cosmetic use, solely and in conjunction with other nonpermanent fillers, in a private practice setting.

Methods and Materials.—A retrospective chart review was conducted for patients treated by the author over 6 years, beginning in 2003. Treatments were tabulated according to facial region and arbitrarily designated as rhytides, acne scars, lips, infraorbital, nasolabial, and general contour. Therefore, up to six treatments were possible with any visit. Concomitant treatment with nonpermanent fillers, as well as any significant adverse events, was noted as well.

Results.—Nine hundred sixteen patients were treated (816 (89%) female, 100 (11%) male). There were 5,246 treatments over 3,307 visits, with an average of 3.5 visits per patient and 1.6 treatments per visit. Adverse events were limited to overcorrection in 11 patients (1%). Of the 916 patients, 257 (28%) were also treated with other (nonpermanent) fillers without incident.

Conclusion.—Over the 6-year period, PDMS-1000 was found to be effective and safe in the cosmetic practice setting. Other (nonpermanent) fillers were also used without incident.

▶ Purified polydimethylsiloxane (PDMS-1000, Silikon 1000) is a medical-grade silicone oil that was approved by the Food and Drug Administration (FDA) in 1997 for treatment of selected cases of retinal detachment. It has been used more recently as an off-label soft tissue filler. For better or worse, injectable silicone has an unfavorable history dating back to the 1940s and 1950s when nonmedical grade silicone oil was injected in large amounts as a soft tissue filler and for breast augmentation. Short- and long-term results were poor and dramatic complications followed. However, the highly purified medical grade product described has a more favorable safety profile and, when used properly in small volumes, appears to have reasonable long-term results. The ideal patient would be interested in a permanent correction, with as few treatments as possible. Typical injection volumes varied from 0.5 to 1.0 mL (for general contouring) to 0.01 to 0.05 mL (for fine line correction) using a microdroplet technique with 27-G or 30-G needles. The complication rate was surprisingly low (perhaps because of the retrospective chart review study design) and cannot be compared with complication rates seen in prospective trials of contemporary soft tissue fillers. Other than overcorrection in 11 patients and 1 patient who developed hyperpigmentation, there were no other complications (no cases of granulomatous reaction, cellulitis, edema, or persistent erythema). Given the unfavorable history of silicone injection and lack of FDA approval for this indication, it is understandable that most surgeons would not want to incorporate this into their practice. However, as more studies emerge, perhaps the use of silicone injections may be reevaluated and become accepted.

K. A. Gutowski, MD

Late-Onset Immune-Mediated Adverse Effects after Poly-ʟ-Lactic Acid Injection in Non-HIV Patients: Clinical Findings and Long-Term Follow-Up
Alijotas-Reig J, Garcia-Gimenez V, Vilardell-Tarres M (Vall d'Hebron Univ Hosp, Barcelona, Spain)
Dermatology 219:303-308, 2009

Background.—It has been thought that poly-ʟ-lactic acid (PLLA) injections do not have inflammatory side effects. Recent evidence shows that local/regional/systemic delayed adverse effects may appear with its use.

Objective.—To evaluate the clinical complaints, treatment response and long-term follow-up of non-HIV patients with delayed immune-mediated adverse effects related to PLLA injections.

Methods.—Prospective, case series study of 10 patients with delayed adverse effects related to PLLA injections. The inclusion criterion was defined as the onset at least 6 months after PLLA use, with 1 or more of the following clinical signs: oedema, skin induration, swelling/tender nodules with or without discharge of pus or filler material. Several systemic manifestations were also included. Patients with immediate side effects were excluded. Patients underwent clinical management and long-term follow-up.

Results.—The average latency period to the onset of symptoms was 19.2 months (range: 6–60). Tender, inflammatory nodules and facial oedema were commonly seen. One case presented a systemic granulomatous disorder as a complication. After 50.2 months of average follow-up (range: 38–78), 5 patients are in remission, 4 have recurrent bouts and the last case has been lost to follow-up.

Conclusion.—Although infrequently, local and/or regional and/or systemic delayed and recurrent granulomatous reactions may complicate PLLA gel injections.

▶ This is an important study for all who inject patients with different types of permanent and nonpermanent fillers. Unfortunately the expectation that these substances are totally innocuous is unrealistic, and it is incumbent upon everyone who treats patients with them to conduct long-term follow-up. It is equally important to maintain records of the treatment protocols and subsequent events, which might enable future physicians to identify patients who might be at greater risk for complications. Although poly-L-lactic acid (PLLA) is said to be a biodegradable gel in which the solution portion disappears quickly, the more solid component is counted on to produce a bulking effect. It does so by creating a reactive tissue response in the host. It is obvious that in some patients this response can and does go awry and may lead to late granulomatous complications. Most of the patients were treated with nonsteroidal anti-inflammatory drugs (NSAIDs) and steroids. One patient was lost to follow-up, and 4 patients had varying degrees of recurrence.

S. H. Miller, MD, MPH

Poly-L-Lactic Acid for Neck and Chest Rejuvenation
Mazzuco R, Hexsel D (Brazilian Ctr for Studies in Dermatology, Porto Alegre, Brazil; Univ of Passo Fundo, Brazil)
Dermatol Surg 35:1228-1237, 2009

Background.—Poly-L-lactic acid (PLLA) has been widely used in the enhancement of facial contours, but its use in nonfacial areas is rarely cited.

Objectives.—To demonstrate the efficacy and safety of PLLA for neck and chest rejuvenation.

Methods.—Thirty-six patients with different degrees of cutaneous flaccidity, atrophy, and wrinkles in the neck and chest were treated with PLLA. The technical details and the methods of evaluation (photographic analysis by three independent evaluators in the 21 patients who had alterations visible in the photographs taken before treatment and satisfaction questionnaire at the end of the treatment in all 36 patients) are described in this article.

Results.—In the photographic analysis, improvement was found in 81% to 100% of the 21 cases ($p < .001$). In the questionnaire regarding the degree of satisfaction, 91.6% said they were pleased with the result of the procedure and stated they would do it again. After 18 months of follow-up, the results were maintained. Only one of the 36 patients (3%) had early-onset subcutaneous nodules as a complication.

Conclusion.—Injection of PLLA seems to be a safe and efficacious treatment for the correction of some aspects of aging in the neck and chest.

▶ The fine lines and transverse creases of the neck are not suitable for treatment by common resurfacing procedures. Some improvement can be seen with intense pulsed light (IPL) treatments and other collagen-stimulating energy devices. This new use of poly-L-lactic acid (PLLA), a soft tissue volumizing product, offers a reasonable option in improving an otherwise hard to treat area. Combined with a botulinum toxin for platysmal bands, this PLLA application can offer an alternative to a surgical neck lift (although with less improvement, only temporary results and commonly the need for more than 1 treatment session). Important points in using PLLA include a higher dilution than previously recommended (10-12 mL of sterile water per vial) and reconstitution 2 to 3 days before injection (as opposed to 4-24 hours).

K. A. Gutowski, MD

Efficacy and Tolerability of Admixing 0.3% Lidocaine with Dermicol-P35 27G for the Treatment of Nasolabial Folds

Weinkle S (Private Practice, Bradenton, FL)
Dermatol Surg 36:316-320, 2010

Background.—Dermicol-P35 27G, an advanced collagen dermal filler, is effective for nasolabial fold (NLF) correction.

Objectives.—To compare the efficacy and tolerance of Dermicol-P35 27G premixed with lidocaine with that of Dermicol-P35 27G injected after topical anesthesia for NLF correction.

Materials and Methods.—In a split-face protocol, 10 patients were injected with Dermicol-P35 27G/topical anesthesia or Dermicol-P35 27G/0.3% lidocaine. Patients were monitored for adverse events and for pain using the Thermometer Pain Scale (TPS) and a visual analog scale (VAS). Efficacy was measured using the Modified Fitzpatrick Wrinkle Scale and the Global Aesthetic Improvement Scale.

Results.—Patients experienced significantly less pain with Dermicol-P35 27G/0.3% lidocaine than with Dermicol-P35 27G/topical anesthesia (mean clinician-assessed TPS scores ± standard deviation: 2.0 ± 0.8 and 5.2 ± 2.1, respectively, $p < .001$). Patients reported less discomfort with Dermicol-P35 27G/0.3% lidocaine than with Dermicol-P35 27G/topical anesthesia (mean VAS scores: 2.0 ± 1.0 and 6.3 ± 2.0, respectively, $p < 001$; TPS scores: 2.3 ± 0.6 and 5.4 ± 1.2, respectively, $p < 001$). Both treatments yielded similar efficacy scores and were well tolerated. Adverse events were mild.

Conclusion.—Dermicol-P35 27G/0.3% lidocaine resulted in less pain than Dermicol-P35 27G/topical anesthesia, with no observed reduction in efficacy.

▶ Not all patients require anesthetics during soft tissue filler injections of the nasolabial folds. For those who do, a few options are available. Topical anesthetics take time to reach a significant level of anesthesia and nerve blocks affect a much larger area than needs to be treated. Skin cooling does not last long and may require frequent reapplication during filler injection. The addition of lidocaine to the filler appears to offer a significant reduction in immediate pain. In this case, Dermicol-P35 27G (Evolence, a porcine-based collagen filler) was mixed with 0.18 mL of 2% lidocaine in a 3 cc syringe, and the plungers were alternately depressed for 10 mixing strokes before injection with a 27G needle. While patients will still feel the needle penetrating the skin, the injection of the filler product is better tolerated. This is the first study demonstrating improved tolerability of a collagen-based filler when mixed with lidocaine. (Please note that Evolence manufacturer Johnson & Johnson removed the filler from the US market in November 2009.)

K. A. Gutowski, MD

Reduced Pain with Use of Proprietary Hyaluronic Acid with Lidocaine for Correction of Nasolabial Folds: A Patient-Blinded, Prospective, Randomized Controlled Trial
Monheit GD, Campbell RM, Neugent H, et al (Univ of Alabama at Birmingham, UK; Georgia Skin Cancer and Aesthetic Dermatology, Athens; Total Skin and Beauty Dermatology Ctr, Birmingham, Alabama; et al)
Dermatol Surg 36:94-101, 2010

Background.—Pain during and after implantation of dermal gel fillers is a consistent complaint of patients undergoing soft tissue augmentation. Reduction of pain during injection would increase patient comfort and improve the overall patient experience.

Objective.—To evaluate pain at the injection site during and after the injection of Prevelle SILK or Captique and to evaluate outcomes after 2 weeks.

Methods & Materials.—In a patient-blinded, prospective, randomized, split-face design trial, a nonanimal-derived hyaluronic acid based filler formulated with lidocaine (Prevelle SILK) was injected in one nasolabial fold (NLF), and the same filler without lidocaine (Captique) was injected in the contralateral NLF of 45 enrolled patients. Injection site pain was measured using a visual analogue scale at injection (time 0) and 15, 30, 45, and 60 minutes after injection. Patients were asked to return for an evaluation after 2 weeks and to complete a self-assessment questionnaire during the follow-up visit.

Results.—There was more than 50% less pain associated with the dermal gel with lidocaine than with the same filler without lidocaine at all time points ($p < .05$). The greatest difference in pain was recorded at the time of injection, and then the effect gradually declined over the 60-minute period. Both fillers were well tolerated, and there was no difference in outcome after 2 weeks.

Conclusion.—Addition of lidocaine to a filler resulted in significantly less pain associated with the procedure without compromising outcomes.

▶ The addition of a local anesthetic to a soft tissue filler decreases patient discomfort—in this case, for up to 45 minutes after injection. This is the first randomized, controlled, patient-blinded study showing the benefit of adding lidocaine to a hyaluronic acid dermal filler.

K. A. Gutowski, MD

Controlled, Randomized Study of Pain Levels in Subjects Treated with Calcium Hydroxylapatite Premixed with Lidocaine for Correction of Nasolabial Folds

Marmur E, Green L, Busso M (Mount Sinai Med Ctr New York; George Washington Univ; Univ of Miami, Coral Gables, FL)
Dermatol Surg 36:309-315, 2010

Background.—Calcium hydroxylapatite (CaHA) has been administered after nerve block injection of anesthetic agents.

Objectives.—This prospective, randomized, split-face, single-blind study (50 subjects) assessed the pain reduction, safety, and effectiveness of premixing CaHA with 2% lidocaine for the treatment of nasolabial folds (NLFs).

Methods and Materials.—Subjects were randomized to receive treatment with CaHA alone in one NLF (control) and with CaHA premixed with lidocaine in the other NLF (treatment). Subjects completed pain assessments using a validated visual analog scale at specified time points immediately after injection, 1 hour after injection, and 1 month later. Subjects also indicated relative pain experience and preference assessments. Investigators completed aesthetic assessments at 2 weeks and 1 month. Subjects and investigators recorded adverse events.

Results.—Subjects reported statistically significantly less pain in the treatment fold than in the control fold and expressed unanimous preference for the treatment injection over the control. Aesthetic results were essentially equivalent for both treatments.

Conclusion.—Investigators concluded that CaHA premixed with lidocaine results in significant pain reduction during dermal filler injection while maintaining the aesthetic improvement of CaHA without lidocaine and demonstrating comparable local transient adverse events for treatment and control.

▶ This randomized study of a local anesthetic mixed with a soft tissue filler showed a 4-point reduction (on a 0 to 10 scale) in pain measurement after mixing 0.2 cc of 2% lidocaine with Radiesse. The mixture can be done 24 hours in advance and does not affect the final outcome when injected in nasolabial folds.

K. A. Gutowski, MD

Eyelid

A Retrospective Review of Calcium Hydroxylapatite for Correction of Volume Loss in the Infraorbital Region
Hevia O (Univ of Miami, FL)
Dermatol Surg 35:1487-1494, 2009

Background.—The correction of infraorbital volume loss with dermal fillers results in a natural, youthful, rested appearance. Defects in this facial region should be treated for optimal patient satisfaction.

Objective.—This retrospective review describes large-scale use of injection of calcium hydroxylapatite (CaHA) and a technique for injection into the infraorbital region.

Methods and Materials.—Using a 30-gauge, 0.5 needle, CaHA was injected into the infraorbital region of 301 patients. Neat CaHA was initially twice diluted with lidocaine 2% solution in 85 patients. Subsequently, 216 patients were treated with single-dilution CaHA and 0.15 mL of 2% lidocaine.

Results.—Injection of CaHa through a 30-gauge, 0.5 needle resulted in minimal bruising, discomfort, or pain. Infraorbital volume restoration was achieved efficiently and effectively, with natural results. Patients were satisfied with the longevity of correction. Adverse events were few and confined to ecchymosis (10%), edema (2%), and erythema (1%). Three of six patients reported edema lasting beyond 7 days. No overcorrection was observed.

Conclusion.—Using a 30-gauge, 0.5 needle, diluted CaHA can be safely injected into the infraorbital region with minimal adverse events and high patient satisfaction.

▶ The use of soft tissue fillers in the periorbital region should be done with caution, as the thin skin and superficial bone are not forgiving if proper technique is not used. However, in this large series the results were reported as favorable and complications were minimal. The modifications described (dilution of the CaHA product, use of a 30 G needle, very small injection volumes, delivery of the product at the level of the periosteum, total injection volumes of less than 0.6 mL of CaHA for both eyes and no injections above the infraorbital rim) most likely contribute to the favorable outcomes. As with many of the

newer clinical applications of injectable fillers, the use of calcium hydroxylapatite (CaHA) (Artefill in this case) is an off-label use of the product.

K. A. Gutowski, MD

Correction of Nasojugal Groove With Tunnelled Fat Graft
de la Cruz L, Berenguer B, García T (Madrid, Spain)
Aesthetic Surg J 29:194-198, 2009

Background.—Pronounced nasojugal sulcus (tear trough deformity) is
a frequent and distressing symptom in aesthetic palpebral surgery. The
sliding fat technique using the transcutaneous or transconjunctival
approach has proven to be considerably useful in patients with clinically
evident fat bags. In the absence of fat bags, commonly used techniques
can lead to unpredictable (and frequently less than optimal) results.

Objective.—The authors report their experience with correcting the
nasojugal groove in the absence of palpebral fat bags by use of a one-
piece, free fat graft as an alternative to autologous fat injections or the
placement of alloplastic materials.

Methods.—The authors conducted a retrospective study of a consecutive
series of 34 patients (33 women and one man) between 42 and 57 years of
age. In all cases, small, free fat grafts harvested from the medial fat
compartment of the upper eyelid were placed precisely under the depression through two stab incisions in the suborbicularis plane, filling in the
groove.

Results.—Results were considered excellent in 24 out of the 34 patients.
Results in the remaining 10 patients were rated as good, in most cases
because of mild undercorrection. All patients expressed a high degree of
satisfaction. Recovery time was very short and no eye or eyelid complications were observed.

Conclusions.—Correction of the nasojugal groove with a tunnelled fat
graft causes minimal tissue trauma and allows exact placement of the

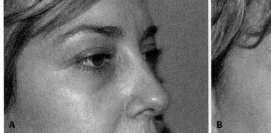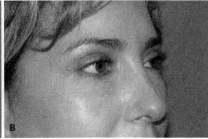

FIGURE 5.—**A,** Pretreatment view of a 44-year-old woman with pronounced congenital nasojugal
groove (or tear trough deformity). **B,** Posttreatment view six months after undergoing upper blepharoplasty and tunnelled fat graft. (Reprinted from de la Cruz L, Berenguer B, García T. Correction of nasojugal groove with tunnelled fat graft. *Aesthetic Surg J*. 2009;29:194-198.)

graft. The upper palpebral fat has unique characteristics that render it an ideal graft material for correction of the nasojugal groove in patients with no concomitant lower fat bags. This procedure offers more predictable results and a lower incidence of adverse effects than more commonly used techniques (Fig 5).

▶ Correction of the nasojugal groove (tear trough deformity) has been done with inferior orbital fat repositioning, fat graft injections, fat pearl grafts, prosthetic implants, and now direct percutaneous placement of fat grafts harvested from the upper orbit compartments. The results are good (Fig 5) and patient satisfaction is rated as high, but the length of follow-up is not presented. As with other fat graft procedures, it is important to watch for graft lump and cyst formation over time, which in the thin-skinned infraorbital area can be problematic.

K. A. Gutowski, MD

Blending of the eyelid–cheek junction and removal of protruding fat: an intraoral approach to blepharoplasty of the lower eyelid
Zhang H, Liu C, Peng C, et al (PLA General Hosp, Beijing, PR China)
Br J Oral Maxillofac Surg 47:541-544, 2009

Blepharoplasty is one of the most common aesthetic procedures done today. The protruding fat and lid–cheek junction are the most conspicuous signs of aging that need attention. During zygomatic reduction by an intraoral approach we found occasionally that the orbital fat can be exposed through the perforated periosteum at the inferior obital rim. We therefore developed a new blepharoplasty procedure using an oral approach.

Seventeen patients aged from 26 to 38 years, of whom six had had a previous unsuccessful blepharoplasty and one had a history of injury to the lower lid, were studied. The operation was done under an infraorbital nerve block and local anaesthesia through an intraoral incision at the upper vestibular groove. The periosteum was raised on the surface of the maxilla to the infraorbital rim, and the infraorbital nerve preserved. The periosteum and the orbital septum were incised along the whole length of the infraorbital rim. The fat that was exposed through the incision was either removed or preserved and fixed to the outer soft tissue with sutures.

Cosmetic results were good and the oral incision healed without infection. Six patients developed numbness in the infraorbital region, five of whom recovered within 3 months; the other recovered by 6 months postoperatively.

▶ The intraoral approach to fat resection and repositioning offers another way to treat fat bulges in the lower eyelid. The technique seems simple and can be done using a nerve block and a lighted retractor. While a transconjunctival approach may be easier, there are cases where it may be preferable to avoid an eyelid incision (adhesive scars caused by injury to the eyelids; thick and fragile conjunctiva caused by chronic infection that will result in difficult exposure and bleeding; and scars from previous blepharoplasty which will increase the risk of retraction of the eyelid). The main drawback is the 18% incidence of temporary infraorbital injury, which could be decreased with more surgical experience.

K. A. Gutowski, MD

Treatment of infraorbital dark circles by autologous fat transplantation: a pilot study
Roh MR, Kim T-K, Chung KY (Yonsei Univ College of Medicine, Seoul, Korea)
Br J Dermatol 160:1022-1025, 2009

Background.—Infraorbital dark circles are a cosmetic concern for a large number of individuals. However, the exact definition and precise cause has not been elucidated clearly. In our experience infraorbital dark circles due to thin and translucent lower eyelid skin overlying the orbicularis oculi muscle can be treated successfully with autologous fat transplantation.

Objectives.—This study was conducted to clarify the nature of dark circles under the eyes and determine the efficacy of autologous fat transplantation.

Patients and Methods.—Ten patients with dark circles due to increased vascularity and translucency of the skin were included. They received at least one autologous fat transplantation and follow-up evaluations were conducted at least 3 months after the last treatment.

Results.—An average of 1·6 autologous fat transplantations were done in both infraorbital areas. Patients showed an average of 78% improvement (average grading scale: 2·6 out of 4). Most of the patients showed improvement in the infraorbital darkening and contour of the lower eyelids.

Conclusions.—Autologous fat transplantation is an effective method for the treatment of infraorbital dark circles due to thin and translucent lower eyelid skin overlying the orbicularis oculi muscle.

▶ Improvement of dark circles under the eyes depends on identifying the underlying cause and applying the correct treatment. When due to infraorbital hyperpigmentation, bleaching agents and laser treatments may be useful. If the dark circles are due to volume loss, and have an associated tear trough, then volume replacement (or fat repositioning) should be a better option. However, volume replacement in the infraorbital area with fat or soft tissue fillers is prone to suboptimal results due to the thin skin, making any minor contour irregularity noticeable. Fat grafts in this area can become palpable and visible. While the concept of fat grafting is correct, one should proceed with caution as the potential complications are significant. The results are seen in Fig 1 in the original article. Note that the patient in Fig 1e and f may have been better served by having a lower eyelid blepharoplasty with fat repositioning and a small skin resection.

K. A. Gutowski, MD

Face, Neck and Brow

Prediction of Face-Lift Outcomes Using the Preoperative Supine Test

Hsu C, Gruber RP, Dosanjh A (Stanford Univ Med Ctr, Palo Alto, CA; Univ of California (SF), San Francisco)

Aesth Plast Surg 33:828-831, 2009

Background.—Patients considering a facelift (facial rhytidectomy) need some means of predicting their surgical outcomes. This will help them decide whether to proceed with the operation.

Methods.—A total of 50 consecutive patients were asked to examine themselves with a hand-held mirror while lying supine on an examining table to give them a reasonable approximation of their postoperative result.

Results.—The tissues of the face redrape in a very aesthetic manner when lying completely supine. The appearance that the patient sees of himself or herself during the "supine test" correlated very well with the actual postop result after rhytidectomy consisting of subcutaneous undermining, SMAS plication, and platysmaplasty.

Conclusion.—This supine test may be useful in helping patients preoperatively predict their facelift outcomes and may serve as a good adjunct to imaging.

▶ It is common for patients seeking a facelift to demonstrate what they wish to have lifted by pushing on their facial tissue with their fingers in a superior lateral direction. The appearance of their face when they do this is not necessarily what the result will be as usually patients pull their skin tighter than is done during surgery. The supine test is a simple maneuver allowing a prospective patient to see the appearance of their facial tissues without the pull of gravity. Patients do need to be cautioned that the result seen demonstrates improvement only to the sides of the face, jowl area, and neck, not in the periocular or perioral regions. The correlation between the results seen during the test and actual postoperative results will be surgeon and technique dependent, but the authors feel that there is high reliability in predicting results when a submucosal aponeurotic system (SMAS) plication/platysmaplasty is done. The test results may not be applicable when substantial malar elevation is done. If a minimal access cranial suspension (MACS) facelift is being considered, then Tonnard suggests a true preoperative vertical lift simulation by having the patient stand on their head and photographing their face while they are upside down. Although the supine test is low tech, it may be a fast, inexpensive, simple, and perhaps more reliable way of demonstrating postoperative results compared with the currently evolving high-tech digital imaging systems.

K. A. Gutowski, MD

Use of the Harmonic Blade in Face Lifting: A Report Based on 420 Operations
Firmin FO, Marchac AC, Lotz NC (Clinique Georges Bizet, Paris, France; Royal North Shore Hospital and Sydney, Australia)
Plast Reconstr Surg 124:245-255, 2009

Background.—An important concern for patients who undergo a face lift is the recovery time. Use of the Harmonic blade (Ethicon Endo-Surgery, Cincinnati, Ohio) for surgical dissection and hemostasis in face lift has improved recovery time and greatly reduced the risk of hematomas in the senior author's practice.

Methods.—A retrospective study evaluated the complication rate using the Harmonic blade in face and neck lifting ($n = 420$) between 2001 and 2007. A prospective study was conducted on 100 cases (October of 2006 to May of 2008) to evaluate the mean operative time, drainage, and recovery time. Results at day 8 were evaluated using a scale of 1 to 4 (1 = nil tracking to 4 = marked tracking).

Results.—The complication rate in 420 cases was low and decreased with experience. Complications included hematoma ($n = 5$), temporary facial paresis ($n = 4$), submental lipolysis ($n = 3$), skin perforation ($n = 1$), minor skin burn ($n = 1$), skin necrosis ($n = 0$), and hair loss ($n = 0$). Mean operative time for face lift with a superficial musculoaponeurotic system procedure and anterior platysmaplasty was 180 minutes (range, 140 to 210 minutes). Drainage at day 1 was 20 cc (range, 0 to 30 cc). Average return to normal social life was by day 8 (range, 5 to 20 days). Results at day 8 were graded 1 for edema and ecchymosis.

Conclusions.—The beneficial effects of the Harmonic blade are obvious objectively and subjectively to both the surgeon and the patients. Understanding the key technical details involved with its use will improve the learning curve for the surgeon as this technology becomes an asset in face lifting.

▶ The harmonic device uses energy to produce high frequency vibration at the tip of the blade, which causes tissue cavitation and protein denaturation, allowing for tissue dissection and coagulation, respectively. Unlike traditional electrocautery, no electrical current is transmitted, and there is minimal thermal injury to surrounding tissue. These physical properties of harmonic technology seem to provide good results in facelift procedures as bruising and edema appear to be less at 8 days after surgery compared with traditional electrocautery technology. In addition, infiltration with a vasoconstrictive agent was not necessary. While there is a short learning curve and additional equipment cost, the faster recovery may be worthwhile.

K. A. Gutowski, MD

Composite Platysmaplasty and Closed Percutaneous Platysma Myotomy: A Simple Way to Treat Deformities of the Neck Caused by Aging
Gonzalez R (UNAERP Medicine School, Ribeirao Preto, Brazil)
Aesthet Surg J 29:344-354, 2009

Background.—Although cervical skin and platysmal laxity are more apparent at the lateral area of the neck, the reported treatments focus on performing plication on the anterior midline or releasing the muscle's lateral border and tractioning it back. Because of the ineffectiveness of such methods in solving more complex cases, surgeons have been trying more efficient procedures that are also riskier and could therefore increase the complication rate.

Objective.—The author describes a simple method for treating cervical laxity using composite platysmaplasty. He also reports on the use of closed platysma myotomy to treat remaining or recurrent platsymal bands.

Methods.—A vertical incision was made on the platysma, parallel to the midline, followed by the creation of a flap made of skin and platysma at the area where tone loss was more evident. When this flap was pulled back, it formed a double muscle layer that pressed on the submandibular gland, pushing it back into its original position. The tightening achieved by the fixation of the flap provided excellent definition of the mandible line. The platysma bands were approached by a method of percutaneous incision of the platysma.

Results.—Between October 2005 and December 2008, 129 patients underwent surgery. Seventeen patients underwent closed percutaneous platysma myotomy in conjunction with platysmaplasty. Four patients underwent platysma myotomy to treat platysmal bands in a secondary procedure from two to eight months after the original surgery. All patients were satisfied with the aesthetic results of treatment. The only serious complications were two cases of temporary neuropraxia of the cervical branch and one hematoma with partial necrosis of retroauricular skin.

Conclusions.—Composite platysmaplasty, combined with closed platysma myotomy when indicated, has a short learning curve and provides satisfactory results with a low complication rate and fast recovery. While closed platysma myotomy has been performed by the author as an independent procedure, those operations are not covered in this report and deserve a separate study.

▶ This procedure is a combination of a new and an old technique to correct platysmal bands. The new component involves the creation of a composite platysma/skin flap anterior to the danger zone containing the mandibular marginal and cervical nerves (Fig 2C in the original article). This flap is then pulled posteriorly and sutured at a level below the mandibular angle. Using this technique, 4.5% of patients who did not have any treatment of medial platysmal bands required subsequent closed platysmal myotomy. This older myotomy technique involves simple band transection using a percutaneously placed suture saw through the bands at 1- to 2-cm intervals in a serial fashion. Based on the results shown, it is difficult to judge whether the composite platysma/skin flap offers an improved result compared with a traditional skin flap with platysmal tightening. The results of the percutaneous myotomies seem to offer a reasonable correction of platysmal bands and could easily be performed in an office setting with local anesthetic. The duration of improvement with this myotomy technique needs to be reported.

K. A. Gutowski, MD

Identical Twin Face Lifts with Differing Techniques: A 10-Year Follow-Up
Alpert BS, Baker DC, Hamra ST, et al (The California Pacific Med Ctr Davies Campus, San Francisco)
Plast Reconstr Surg 123:1025-1033, 2009

To evaluate the efficacies of four different surgical techniques in facial rejuvenation, two sets of identical twins were operated on by four different surgeons. The technical approaches to facial rejuvenation included lateral superficial musculoaponeurotic system (SMAS)-ectomy with extensive skin undermining, composite rhytidectomy, SMAS-platysma flap with bidirectional lift, and endoscopic midface lift with an open anterior platysmaplasty. All patients were photographed by an independent surgeon at 1, 6, and 10 years postoperatively. At the same time interval, the cases were presented and discussed in a panel format at the annual meeting of the American Society for Aesthetic Plastic Surgery. Each operating surgeon was allowed to critique the results and discuss how his methods had changed over the intervening 10-year interval. Postoperative photographs at 1, 6, and 10 years after surgery are included to allow the reader to examine long-term results utilizing various approaches to facial rejuvenation in identical twins (Fig 1).

▶ While the question of which facelift technique is best has not been answered, some observations can be made:

1. Each of the techniques used yielded a dramatic improvement in facial appearance.
2. After 10 years, each patient looked better than before surgery, regardless of technique.
3. While the identical twins did not look identical 10 years after surgery, it is hard to determine whether this is due to facelift technique or other (environmental) factors.
4. It is difficult to determine which differences in twin appearance after 10 years are attributable to the differences in surgical technique.

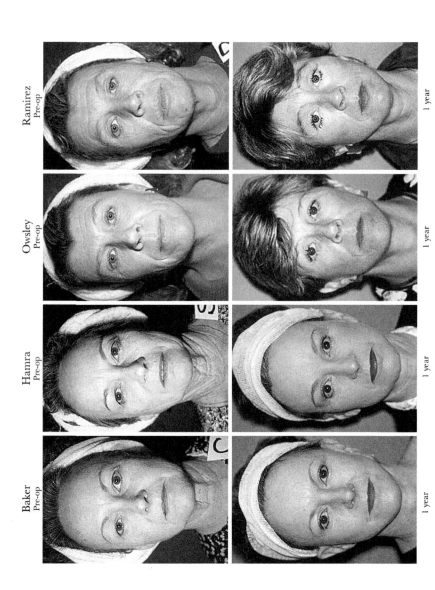

FIGURE 1.—Four patients. Preoperative and 1-year, 6-year, and 10-year postoperative views. (Reprinted from Alpert BS, Baker DC, Hamra ST, et al. Identical twin face lifts with differing techniques: a 10-year follow-up. *Plast Reconstr Surg.* 2009;123:1025-1033, with permission from the American Society of Plastic Surgeons.)

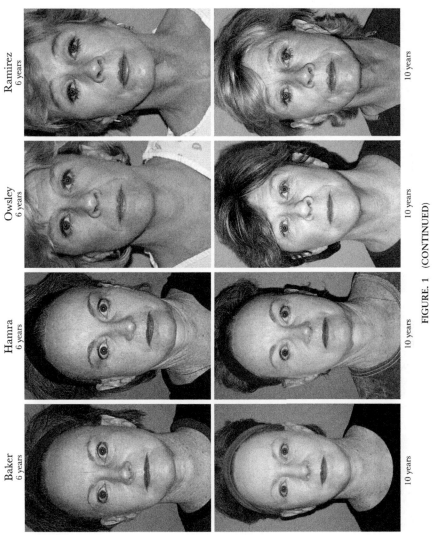

FIGURE. 1 (CONTINUED)

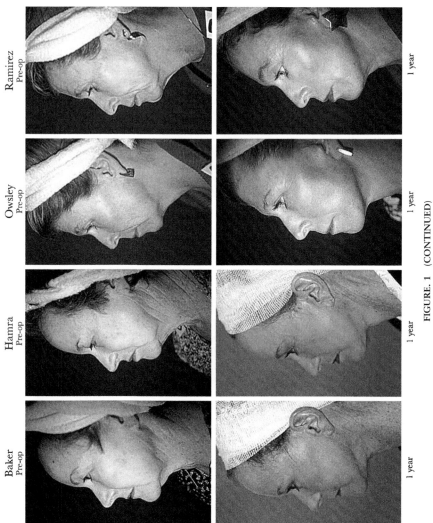

FIGURE. 1 (CONTINUED)

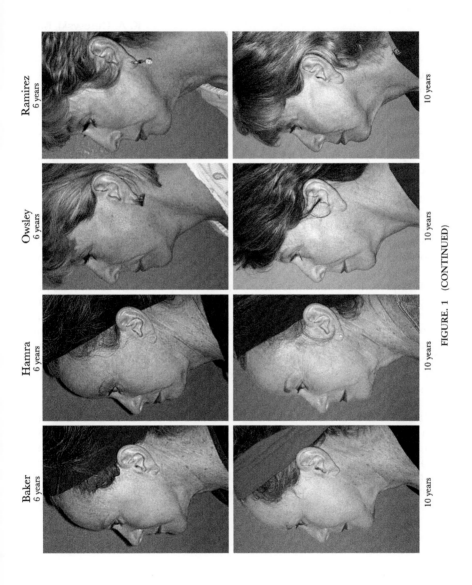

FIGURE. 1 (CONTINUED)

What conclusions should one draw from this report? It seems that between these 4 facelift techniques there is not a great difference 10 years after surgery. If this is true then each individual surgeon should consider other factors and focus on choosing a technique that is safe, reproducible, and offers a reasonable recovery time.

K. A. Gutowski, MD

Suture Suspension Technique for Midface and Neck Rejuvenation

Gamboa GM, Vasconez LO (Med College of Georgia, Augusta; Univ of Alabama at Birmingham)
Ann Plast Surg 62:478-481, 2009

Seventeen patients averaging 51 years of age underwent 23 surgical procedures, including suture suspension for both midface and neck rejuvenations. A 3/0 polypropylene thread with bioabsorbable cones with multiple point fixations in addition to 2×0.5-cm polypropylene surgical mesh are used in this technique. The mean postoperative, follow-up time was 9 months. Of the 17 patients, 12 underwent this procedure for midface rejuvenations, 3 for facial palsy, 5 for neck aesthetic procedures, 2 for brow ptosis, and 1 for brow asymmetry. The average number of sutures used for each face was 4 and 2 were used for each neck. The authors present an anatomic study for the safe placement of sutures, the surgical technique, and a microscopic photo documentation of the fibrosis around the suture knot and cone. All patients developed temporary edema. Two patients had a moderate aesthetic improvement of the face, and 1 patient underwent resuspension of the sutures 4 months postsurgery. Overall early patient satisfaction at 9 months was 90%. This technique has the potential to be a useful and effective clinical tool for minimally invasive face and neck rejuvenations.

▶ The Silhouette Lift is a variation on other minimally invasive facial suspension techniques that uses a polypropylene suture with bioabsorbable cones and multiple point fixation. While patient satisfaction was high at 9 months, long-term results are not known. As with other similar techniques (discussed in articles that follow), patients should be advised on the limited results and short-lived improvements that are typically seen.

K. A. Gutowski, MD

Outcomes in Threadlift for Facial Rejuvenation
Garvey PB, Ricciardelli EJ, Gampper T (Univ of Virginia Health System, Charlottesville; Summit Cosmetic Surgery and Skin Care, Wilmington, NC)
Ann Plast Surg 62:482-485, 2009

The search for less invasive surgical techniques to address the effects of facial aging led to the development of barbed polypropylene sutures for facial suspension. Theoretical advantages of these "threadlifts" included limited scarring, rapid recovery, relative safety, and reduced cost when compared with a standard rhytidectomy. The goal of this study was to evaluate the outcomes of patients undergoing threadlifts to determine the actual complication rates, the durability of results, and the rates of reoperative surgery. A single surgeon's initial 2-year experience with 72 patients undergoing threadlifts was retrospectively reviewed. Preoperative patient demographical and clinical data, operative information, and postoperative outcomes data were compiled and evaluated.

A total of 72 thread lifts were performed by 1 surgeon over a 24-month period. Of these patients, 76% underwent threadlift alone, whereas concomitant procedures were performed in 24% of patients. Minor complications were common and usually self-limited. Forty-two percent of patients underwent a secondary procedure after primary threadlift, an average of 8.4 months after the original surgery. Thirty-one percent of patients required revisional surgery for cosmetic reasons an average of 8.7 months after their threadlift. Eleven percent of the patients ultimately required removal of palpable threads.

Threadlift is a safe procedure associated with minor complications. Rates of revisional surgery for cosmesis are high after threadlift. Time to revisional surgery for cosmesis is short. Results achieved by threadlift are subtle and short-lived. Threadlift is not a minimally invasive replacement of surgical rhytidectomy. Patients should understand the limitations of this technique and its high rates of revisional surgery.

▶ This report of 72 patients who underwent facial rejuvenation with Contour Threads (barbed, unidirectional clear polypropylene suture) shows that the results are short lasting and revisions are common within the first year. Most patients had 8 or 12 sutures placed, typically in the malar and jowl regions. Despite the purported advantage of a fast recovery, many patients developed a lateral cheek "chevron" deformity which lasted from days to weeks, making a return to social activities difficult. While patient reported outcomes and satisfaction were not measured, potential patients should be told to expect that this minimally invasive technique is not a substitute for traditional surgical procedures. Because the average age of the patients was 57 years, it is possible that younger patients may have somewhat better results.

K. A. Gutowski, MD

Thread-lift for Facial Rejuvenation: Assessment of Long-term Results

Abraham RF, Defatta RJ, Williams EF III (Albany Med College, NY)
Arch Facial Plast Surg 11:178-183, 2009

Objective.—To evaluate the long-term success of the thread-lift procedure for facial rejuvenation.

Methods.—Thirty-three patients underwent a thread- lift procedure alone or in combination with other facial rejuvenation procedures to the brow, midface, jowl, and neck. Ten patients underwent thread-lifts only, and 23 had thread-lifts with other procedures. Ten additional patients having had non–thread-lift rejuvenation procedures, including lipotransfer, chemical peels, and rhytidectomies, were randomly designated as controls. The mean follow-up period was 21 months (range, 12-31 months). Photodocumentation was obtained at each visit. Long-term aesthetic results were evaluated by 4 independent, blinded, and board-certified facial plastic surgeons. Each result was graded on a scale of 0 to 3, with 0 indicating no change; 1, minimal improvement; 2, moderate improvement; and 3, considerable improvement. The population was divided into 3 groups for comparison. Two-tailed t test ($P = .05$) was used for statistical analysis of aesthetic outcomes.

Results.—Although aesthetic improvement was noted in all groups at 1 month, measurable results persisted to the end of the study for all but the group that underwent the thread-lift procedure only. Aesthetic improvement scores of the non–thread-lift control group were better than the group that underwent thread-lift only. Similarly, when the thread-lift was combined with other procedures, scores were better than when thread-lift was used alone. Statistical significance was demonstrated in both of these comparisons ($P < .01$).

Conclusions.—The thread-lift provides only limited short- term improvement that may be largely attributed to postprocedural edema and inflammation. Our results objectively demonstrate the poor long-term sustainability of the thread-lift procedure. Given these findings, as well as the measurable risk of adverse events and patient discomfort, we cannot justify further use of this procedure for facial rejuvenation.

▶ Another report on the use on Contour Threads (but with blinded, independent evaluators) supports previous conclusions that the results are modest and short-lived. While not typically discussed, the occasional serious complications of these procedures may not be easily overcome because fibrosis around the suture may make removal difficult.

K. A. Gutowski, MD

A Novel Bioabsorbable Device for Facial Suspension and Rejuvenation

Knott PD, Newman J, Keller GS, et al (Head and Neck Inst, Cleveland, OH; Stanford Univ Med Ctr, Palo Alto, CA; UCLA (Univ of California, Los Angeles) Med Ctr)
Arch Facial Plast Surg 11:129-135, 2009

To evaluate the safety and efficacy of a novel bioabsorbable suspension device made of a polymer of polylactic acid polyglycolic acid (Endotine Ribbon), we performed a retrospective multi-institutional case study of 21 patients who underwent minimally invasive or open rhytidectomy with the use of the device in an ambulatory surgery center setting. Twelve patients had an excellent result, 7 a good result, and 2 a fair result. Early complications were corrected with technical modifications. Patient satisfaction was high. The Ribbon is a safe and effective adjunct for performing both minimally invasive and open rhytidectomy and cervical lifting.

▶ This suspension device differs from thread lift suspension (which has now been shown to have only short-term improvement), in that tissue undermining is done that allows for tissue fibrosis after suspension with the hope that the results will be longer lasting. Depending on how the suspension is done, both jowls and the neckline can be improved. While it is difficult to predict how long these results will last, it appears that this device may be limited to patients who are willing to accept a less than ideal result and not willing to have a prolonged recovery. Anterior platysmal bands should not be expected to improve with this device, and it should be avoided in patients with thin skin due to the potential for palpability and visibility.

K. A. Gutowski, MD

Extremity and Trunk

Abdominoplasty With Progressive Tension Closure Using A Barbed Suture Technique

Warner JP, Gutowski KA (Univ of Wisconsin–Madison)
Aesthetic Surg J 29:221-225, 2009

Background.—Seroma and skin necrosis are potential complications following abdominoplasty. Many methods have been employed to prevent these complications, including the progressive tension suture technique.

Objective.—The authors evaluate a progressive tension suture technique modification using the Quill barbed suture (Angiotech Pharmaceuticals, Inc., Vancouver, British Columbia, Canada) to determine whether the original benefits of this classic technique can be obtained in a shorter operative period.

Methods.—The modified progressive tension closure technique with Quill sutures uses barbed sutures to plicate the abdominoplasty flap to the underlying abdominal wall. The placement of the suture is performed with a running suture technique and provides progressive tension, resulting in minimal tension along the incision line. Data from 58 patients undergoing abdominoplasty using this technique are examined, including time to insert the sutures and complications such as seroma, hematoma, and skin necrosis.

Results.—There was a marked reduction in the time necessary to perform the modified progressive tension suture technique using barbed sutures compared to previously published data. The authors' average time was nine minutes to complete plication of the entire abdominal flap. One seroma is reported, which was resolved with one aspiration. No hematomas or skin necrosis complications are reported.

Conclusions.—Using barbed sutures to perform progressive tension suture closure in abdominoplasty is a safe and effective way to considerably reduce operative time and retain all of the benefits of the original progressive tension suture technique.

▶ While the use of progressive tension sutures (PTS) to eliminate postoperative drains in abdominoplasty is not new, this modification of the PTS method allows for faster suture placement using "barbed" suture technology. The technique does take a bit more time than the standard abdominoplasty without PTS, and has a short learning curve. However, there seems to be increased patient satisfaction when drains can be avoided.

For further reading on this subject I suggest an article by Pollock et al.[1]

K. A. Gutowski, MD

Reference

1. Pollock H, Pollock T. Progressive tension sutures: a technique to reduce local complications in abdominoplasty. *Plast Reconstr Surg.* 2000;105:2583-2586.

Abdominoplasty Flap Elevation in a More Superficial Plane: Decreasing the Need for Drains
Fang RC, Lin SJ, Mustoe TA (Northwestern Univ Feinberg School of Medicine, Chicago, IL; Beth Israel Deaconess Med Ctr, Boston, MA)
Plast Reconstr Surg 125:677-682, 2010

Background.—Abdominoplasty has continued to become more frequently performed in the post–bariatric surgery and aesthetic patient populations. With the increase in these procedures, there is a need to decrease the length of drains for patient comfort and postoperative recovery. The authors' hypothesis was that a more superficial plane of abdominal flap elevation during abdominoplasty would decrease the postoperative need for drains.

Methods.—The authors reviewed 202 consecutive abdominoplasties with 99 procedures performed using a standard suprafascial dissection (group I) and 103 procedures using a modified plane of flap elevation that preserves the thin areolar tissue along the abdominal wall (group II). Patient demographics, perioperative complications, and drain data were recorded.

Results.—Patient characteristics did not differ significantly, with the mean age of group I and group II (44 ± 8.9 years and 44 ± 9.6 years, respectively) and body mass index of group I and group II (24 ± 3.8 and 24 ± 3.8, respectively) being similar. Perioperative complications included seven seromas in group I and two seromas in group II. There were two minor hematomas in group I and two minor hematomas in group II. The drains for patients in group II met criteria for removal 3 days earlier than those for group I ($p < 0.0001$). On average, patients in group II had drains removed at postoperative days 4 to 5.

Conclusions.—Flap elevation in a plane superficial to the standard suprafascial approach during abdominoplasty may decrease the length of time required for drains in the postoperative period in the abdominoplasty patient. Decreasing the length of time for postoperative drains may improve patient comfort and expedite recovery.

▶ This simple modification of a standard abdominoplasty technique seems to allow for earlier drain removal and presumably less patient discomfort due to drains. While easy to incorporate into one's practice, a surgeon wishing to completely eliminate the need for drains in abdominoplasty patients should consider using progressive tension sutures,[1,2] which have been demonstrated in multiple studies to be effective.

K. A. Gutowski, MD

References

1. Warner JP, Gutowski KA. Abdominoplasty with progressive tension closure using a barbed suture technique. *Aesthet Surg J.* 2009;29:221-225.
2. Pollock H, Pollock T. Progressive tension sutures: a technique to reduce local complications in abdominoplasty. *Plast Reconstr Surg.* 2000;105:2583.

Infection Risk From the Use of Continuous Local-Anesthetic Infusion Pain Pumps in Aesthetic and Reconstructive Abdominal Procedures

Hovsepian RV, Smith MM, Markarian MK, et al (Aesthetic and Plastic Surgery Inst, Orange, CA; et al)
Ann Plast Surg 62:237-239, 2009

Postoperative pain control after abdominal procedures can be an area of significant concern. Continuous local-anesthetic infusion pain pumps have been clearly documented in recent literature to provide effective early postoperative pain control, in addition to other benefits. Our goal was to evaluate any increase in the risk of infection with the use of pain pumps with aesthetic and reconstructive abdominal procedures.

A retrospective chart review evaluated 159 patients who underwent abdominoplasty (with or without suction-assisted lipectomy), panniculectomy, or a transverse rectus abdominis myocutaneous (TRAM) flap for breast reconstruction. Information was collected on descriptive and demographic information, and the incidence of postoperative infection. Of the 159 patients who underwent abdominal procedures, 100 (62.9%) received the pain pump for postoperative pain control. None of those 100 patients developed an infection. Fifty-nine patients did not receive a pain pump, and 2 of those patients (3.3%) developed an infection. Overall, 1.3% (2 of 159) of patients in our study developed a postoperative infection.

There is no increase in the risk of postoperative infection with the use of continuous local-anesthetic infusion pain pumps used after aesthetic and reconstructive abdominal procedures.

▶ The use of temporary portable local anesthetic infusion devices (pain pumps) is a validated method of improved pain control in many surgical procedures. Despite the indwelling nature of the infusion catheters, no studies have demonstrated an increased infection rate; this also appears to be true for plastic surgery procedures of the abdominal wall (abdominoplasty, panniculectomy, and transverse rectus abdominis myocutaneous [TRAM]). Of these 3 procedures, it is questionable if there is really a benefit to the use of a pain pump in a panniculectomy where there is only skin excision and no abdominal wall dissection or plication.

K. A. Gutowski, MD

Outpatient Abdominoplasty Facilitated by Rib Blocks
Michaels BM, Eko FN (Berkshire Cosmetic and Reconstructive Surgery Ctr, Pittsfield, MA)
Plast Reconstr Surg 124:635-642, 2009

Background.—Striving to increase patient comfort and feasibility of performing abdominoplasties as outpatient procedures, investigators have been exploring alternative methods of anesthesia to safely avoid general anesthesia. These techniques may result in decreased narcotic administration, and decreased postoperative nausea and vomiting. The authors have added the use of preoperative local anesthesia rib blocks with sedation to replace general anesthesia in abdominoplasties.

Methods.—All cases of abdominoplasty performed by the senior author (B.M.M.) were reviewed from 1999 to 2006 and divided into two groups. Group 1 was composed of 39 operations performed using general anesthesia. Group 2 was composed of 29 operations performed using rib blocks placed by the surgeon and supplemented by intravenous sedation. Chart review collected data on time in the operating and recovery rooms, use of narcotics and antiemetics, frequency of postoperative nausea and vomiting, and patient-reported pain. Possible confounding factors, additional procedures, anesthetic and surgical complications, and the need for hospitalization were also recorded. Statistical analysis with two-tailed Mann-Whitney and chi-square testing was used to reject the null hypothesis when comparing the two groups.

Results.—Statistically significant decreases in recovery room time, postoperative narcotics, postoperative nausea and vomiting, and pain were achieved using rib blocks. All other measures were similar for both groups. There were no hospitalizations, pneumothoraxes, major complications or deaths.

Conclusion.—Rib blocks placed before the start of surgery result in decreased recovery room times, pain, and postoperative nausea and vomiting, achieving increased patient comfort and feasibility of performing abdominoplasties in the outpatient setting.

▶ To facilitate safe outpatient abdominoplasty, proper postoperative pain control and reduction of postoperative nausea and vomiting is needed. The addition of rib blocks appears to achieve these goals. In this series, bilateral fourth through twelfth rib blocks (using a 2 cc injection of an equal mixture of 0.25% bupivacaine and 1% lidocaine with 1:100 000 of epinephrine) were made at each block site. An additional injection of local anesthetic was used in the suprapubic area.

This technique offers another option in performing an abdominoplasty using conscious sedation instead of general anesthesia. In place of using a local anesthetic injection with a tumescent technique, a rib block can provide a similar level of analgesia. The rib block also provides pre-emptive analgesia that prevents establishment of altered sensory processing that amplifies postoperative pain. This well documented effect may minimize intraoperative and postoperative narcotic requirements. When using rib blocks, the surgeon should be prepared for supplementary measures of anesthesia if the rib block does not work (as was the case in a few patients) and carefully monitor for signs of pneumothorax.

K. A. Gutowski, MD

Lipoabdominoplasty
Saldanha OR, Federico R, Daher PF, et al (Santa Cecília Univ, São Paulo, Brazil)
Plast Reconstr Surg 124:934-942, 2009

Background.—Abdominoplasty is one of the most common aesthetic operations. Wide bibliographic research has revealed that there is a safe method whereby two techniques—liposuction and abdominoplasty—can be associated in the same procedure. The authors present a new abdominoplasty technique combining a selective undermining with complete abdominal liposuction.

Methods.—The authors standardized steps with which to perform a safe association of traditional abdominoplasty with liposuction of the entire abdomen and infracostal areas. Using selective undermining, it is possible to preserve at least 80 percent of the blood supply in the abdominal wall, causing little nervous trauma, preserving the great majority of the

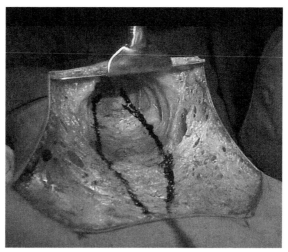

FIGURE 3.—Selective undermining, diastasis demarcation, preservation of the Scarpa facia, and the inferior fuse demarcation to be removed. (Reprinted from Saldanha OR, Federico R, Daher PF, et al. Lipoabdominoplasty. *Plast Reconstr Surg*. 2009;124:934-942, with permission from the American Society of Plastic Surgeons.)

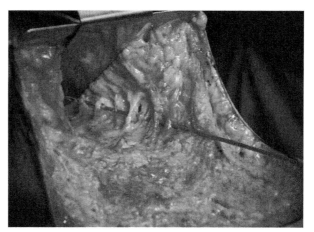

FIGURE 4.—Perforating vessels. (Reprinted from Saldanha OR, Federico R, Daher PF, et al. Lipoabdominoplasty. *Plast Reconstr Surg*. 2009;124:934-942, with permission from the American Society of Plastic Surgeons.)

lymphatic vessels, and resulting in few complications compared with traditional abdominoplasty, including post–bariatric surgery procedures. In this study, lipoabdominoplasty was performed on 445 patients: eight male patients and 437 female patients, from 2000 to 2007.

Results.—The authors consider the results good and excellent, especially regarding patient evaluation, better body contour, abdominal rejuvenation, shorter scars, the form of the umbilicus, and a decrease in the abdominal measures.

Conclusion.—With a progressive adaptation of this technique, it is possible to achieve a harmonious body contour using a safe liposuction method on the abdominal and costal areas, with fast recovery and good to excellent results (Figs 3 and 4).

▶ Until recently, the recommendations by Matarasso from the early 1990s (not to perform liposuction in the central abdomen) were respected when performing abdominoplasty together with liposuction. As the procedure evolved, technical variations allowed for more aggressive epigastric liposuction deep to Scarpa's fascia while limiting the amount of upper abdominal undermining to preserve vascularity. The continuous undermining of a traditional abdominoplasty is replaced by blunt cannula undermining as a way to minimize disruption of the perforating abdominal blood vessels. In the upper abdomen, a tunnel is created just slightly wider than the width of the rectus diastasis, again to minimize vessel disruption. The figures show the limited extent of dissection and the effects of discontinuous cannula undermining. While this technique appears useful for improving the central abdomen, the patients in the results shown did not appear to have a strong indication for central abdominal liposuction. It would be more interesting to see the results in those with more prominent central abdomen fat distribution. However, the complication rates for this procedure were very low and tended to be lower than for traditional liposuction.

K. A. Gutowski, MD

Abdominoplasty with Direct Resection of Deep Fat
Brink RR, Beck JB, Anderson CM, et al (The San Mateo Surgery Ctr, CA)
Plast Reconstr Surg 123:1597-1603, 2009

Background.—Suction-assisted lipectomy is an integral component of abdominoplasty for many surgeons. Its potential to affect the vascularity of the abdominal flap is usually offset by limiting the extent of undermining and not suctioning the central flap. The authors address whether these guidelines apply to direct excision of subscarpal fat and whether direct excision provides aesthetically superior abdominoplasty results with fewer complications.

Methods.—A 10-year review of consecutive abdominoplasty patients ($n = 181$) was conducted. Undermining was done to the xyphoid and just beyond the lower rib margins superiorly and at least as far as the anterior axillary line laterally. Fat deep to Scarpa's fascia was removed by tangential excision in all zones of the abdominal flap, including those considered at high risk for vascular compromise if subjected to liposuction after similar undermining. Concurrent liposuction of the abdominal flap was not done. Thirty patients had concurrent flank liposuction.

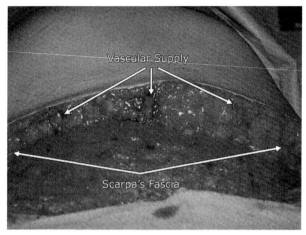

FIGURE 1.—The two sets of *arrows* show Scarpa's fascia and the large blood vessels running in the superficial fatty layer. There is no significant blood supply deep to Scarpa's fascia. This photograph was taken after the deep fat was removed from the right half of the abdominoplasty flap in the zone considered at risk for liposuction ("terrible abdominoplasty triangle"), leaving the superficial fat in pristine condition. (Reprinted from Brink RR, Beck JB, Anderson CM, et al. Abdominoplasty with direct resection of deep fat. *Plast Reconstr Surg.* 2009;123:1597-1603.)

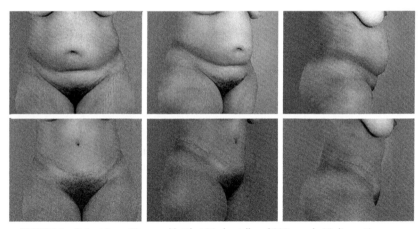

FIGURE 4.—Patient 3 was 38 years old, 5 feet 8 inches tall, and 205 pounds. No liposuction was performed. Even in obesepatients, removal of just the deep fat is sufficient to slenderize the abdomen. (Reprinted from Brink RR, Beck JB, Anderson CM, et al. Abdominoplasty with direct resection of deep fat. *Plast Reconstr Surg.* 2009;123:1597-1603.)

Results.—No patients experienced major full-thickness tissue loss. The incidence of limited necrosis at the incision line requiring subsequent scar revision was 0.7 percent in the 151 patients having abdominoplasty and 6.7 percent in the 30 patients having abdominoplasty combined with flank liposuction. Erythema and/or epidermolysis was seen in 4.8 percent of the abdominoplasty patients and 10 percent of the abdominoplasty/ flank liposuction group. The rate of seroma formation in both groups was approximately 16.5 percent.

Conclusions.—Direct excision of subscarpal fat does not subject any zone of the abdominoplasty flap to increased risks of vascular compromise. It is a safe technique that provides excellent abdominoplasty results (Figs 1 and 4).

▶ Advances in abdominal contouring have resulted in more aggressive use of liposuction in treating the anterior abdomen. Once considered off limits, the central abdominoplasty flap can be thinned deep to Scarpa's fascia without a compromise in complications (Fig 1). While perhaps more technique dependent, direct excision (as opposed to liposuction) of the fat deep to Scarpa's fascia appears to offer good results with minimal complications (Fig 4). This additional step may be best suited for those patients with central upper abdominal fat deposition that is out of proportion to fat deposition in the lateral abdomen.

K. A. Gutowski, MD

Lipoabdominoplasty: Revisiting the Superior Pull-Down Abdominal Flap and New Approaches
Uebel CO (Pontificia Universidade Catolica, Rio Grande Sul – PUCRS, Brazil)
Aesthetic Plast Surg 33:366-376, 2009

Abdominoplasty is a very common procedure, especially for patients with abdominal laxness, striaes, and muscle rectus diastases. With the advent of liposuction 28 years ago, we can improve body contouring by treating lipodystrophies in the epigastric, flank, trochanteric, and buttocks areas. The procedure combining abdominoplasty and liposuction is called lipoabdominoplasty. Many new techniques have been proposed since these procedures were introduced; we now revisit the superior pull-down abdominal flap technique with several new modifications and improvements.

▶ Advances in anterior abdominal contouring have produced a range of procedures using a combination of liposuction and less extensive abdominal flap undermining. The technical details described are worthwhile to review as follow:

• Using the sitting position to delineate the inferior curved incision.

• Supracondrocostal liposuction to loosen the inframammary area.

• Undermining of the epigastic area only enough to bring down the flap, protecting the lateral neurovascular pedicles.

• Exteriorizing and fixing the umbilicus 2 cm above its point of projection.

• Adhesion stitches (progressive tension sutures) to prevent seromas.

K. A. Gutowski, MD

Tensioned reverse abdominoplasty

Deos MF, Arnt RA, Gus El (Mauro Deos–Clínica de Cirurgia Plástica, Porto Alegre, Brazil)
Plast Reconstr Surg 124:2134-2141, 2009

Background.—Deformities of the upper portion of the abdominal wall can be difficult to solve, as in many cases abdominoplasties or mini-abdominoplasties lead to unsatisfactory results. Direct approaches to this region through inframammary incisions can be a good therapeutic option, once adequate patient selection has been performed and certain surgical principles are followed.

Methods.—This technique should be primarily indicated for patients complaining of skin laxity predominantly in the upper abdomen and for patients who will have such excess after liposuction. In patients who require resection of a large amount of tissue, a single, broad, U-shaped dissection should be used, associated with midline fascia plication, when required (group 1). In patients with a smaller amount of tissue to be resected, two oblique tunnels can be made toward the navel, with no incision unification at the midline, to provide less evident scars (group 2).

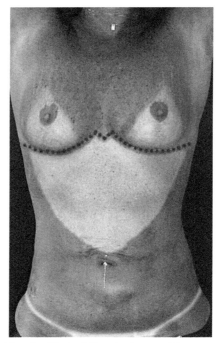

FIGURE 1.—Incision (*dotted red line*) and dissection (*gray area*) in a group 1 patient. For interpretation of the references to color in this figure legend, the reader is referred to web version of this article. (Reprinted from Deos MF, Arnt RA, Gus EI. Tensioned reverse abdominoplasty. *Plast Reconstr Surg.* 2009;124:2134-2141, with permission from the American Society of Plastic Surgeons.)

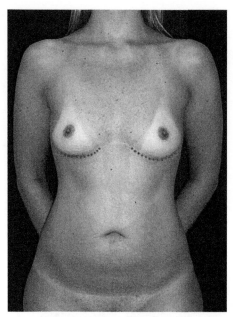

FIGURE 2.—Incision (*dotted red line*) and dissection (*gray area*) in a group 2 patient. For interpretation of the references to color in this figure legend, the reader is referred to web version of this article. (Reprinted from Deos MF, Arnt RA, Gus EI. Tensioned reverse abdominoplasty. *Plast Reconstr Surg.* 2009;124:2134-2141, with permission from the American Society of Plastic Surgeons.)

Results.—Eighteen procedures were performed: 12 in group 1 and six in group 2. Patients and surgeons were satisfied with the results Only minor complications occurred, and they did not result in definitive sequelae.

Conclusions.—The principle of progressive tension suture, previously utilized in conventional abdominoplasties, is now originally employed in reverse abdominoplasties as a continuous suture, enabling proper flap positioning, keeping the inframammary sulcus at its original position, and preventing tension on the resulting scar. Tensioned reverse abdominoplasty is an easily applicable technique that provides good results and should be considered in cases of abdominal laxity predominantly in the upper abdomen (Figs 1, 2 and 10).

▶ Failure to remove excess skin and fat of the upper abdomen has often resulted in disappointment on the part of patients who have undergone classic abdominoplasty with or without liposuction. It is not possible to control and tailor the skin of the upper abdomen as high as the inframammary crease, especially in women with wide-based and flaring rib cages, through a classic lower abdominoplasty incision. The authors propose a modification of the techniques described in the past.[1,2] For patients with minor upper and lower abdominal excess, they use a modification of the upper abdominoplasty and a miniabdominoplasty, when they might just as easily have used the more extensive upper inframammary. When using this technique, it is necessary to keep in mind

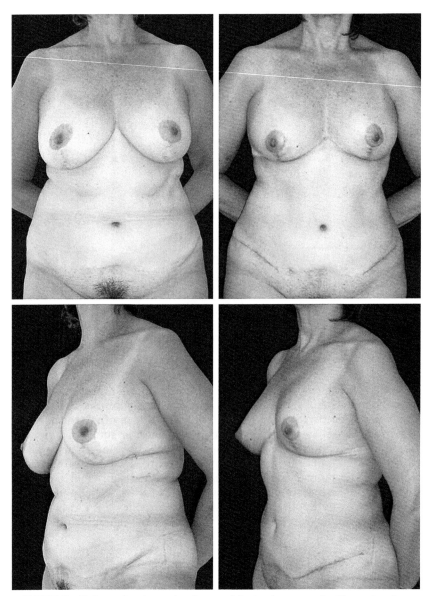

FIGURE 10.—Patient undergoing tensioned reverse abdominoplasty, group 1, with resection of excess skin on the breasts and lower abdomen. (*Left*) Preoperative views. (*Right*) Three-month postoperative results. (Reprinted from Deos MF, Arnt RA, Gus EI. Tensioned reverse abdominoplasty. *Plast Reconstr Surg.* 2009;124:2134-2141, with permission from the American Society of Plastic Surgeons.)

that careful reconstruction of the inframammary fold is important as the scars are quite visible should the patient wear a two-piece bathing suit.[3] In 2 of the 12 patients in the more extensive procedure group, complications of redundancy were noted, and in 2 of 6 less extensive procedures, inadequate correction occurred. The authors do note that the learning curve for the procedure is steep and stress the importance of using progressive tension sutures to support the movement of the flaps in a superior direction.

S. H. Miller, MD, MPH

References

1. Akbas H, Guneren E, Eroglu A, et al. The combined use of classic and reverse abdominoplasty on the same patient. *Plast Reconstr Surg*. 2002;109:2595-2596.
2. Rebello C, Franco T. Abdominoplasty through a submammary incision. *Int Surg*. 1977;62:462-463.
3. Baroudi R, Keppe EM, Carvalho CG. Mammary reduction combined with reverse abdominoplasty. *Ann Plast Surg*. 1979;2:368-373.

Effect of quilting sutures on seroma formation post-abdominoplasty
Ovens L, Pickford MA (McIndoe Surgical Centre, East Grinstead, UK)
Eur J Plast Surg 32:177-180, 2009

Quilting sutures have been shown to be effective in reducing seroma in latissimus dorsi donor wounds. This technique has been adapted to the closure of abdominoplasty flaps. Seventy-four female patients aged 25 to 76 who underwent abdominoplasty over eight years were reviewed retrospectively. In the first 40 consecutive patients, no quilting sutures were used, in the subsequent 34 patients, abdominal closure was performed with quilting sutures. Primary outcome measures were the incidence of seroma, number of times aspirated and total volume aspirated. Secondary outcome measures were haematoma formation, return to theatre, necrosis, dehiscence, infection and late revision. Six of 34 (17.6%) patients who had quilting sutures placed developed clinically obvious seroma compared to ten of 40 (25%) not quilted. There was no significant difference in the number of times the seroma was aspirated or the volume aspirated between the two groups. Three patients in the 'quilted' group developed small postoperative haematomas, managed conservatively. All four patients who developed a haematoma in the 'non-quilted' group returned to theatre for evacuation. There is no statistically significant difference in the incidence of seroma formation after abdominoplasty with or without quilting sutures.

▶ Since Pollock and Pollock's report that progressive tension sutures (PTS) can decrease clinically significant seroma formation after abdominoplasty, other studies have confirmed these findings. However, seromas identified by ultrasound may still be seen when PTS are used. In this report, quilting sutures did not have a significant effect on seroma formation despite also using drains. Interestingly, the seroma rates were high in both groups (17% and 25%), perhaps higher than most surgeons experience in their own practice. It may be that intraoperative technique and postoperative measures may have played a role. While this series did not demonstrate an advantage in using quilting sutures (perhaps due to the small sample size), other larger reports do support the use of PTS in minimizing seromas and eliminating the need for drains.

K. A. Gutowski, MD

Does Abdominoplasty With Liposuction of the Love Handles Yield a Shorter Scar? An Analysis With Abdominal 3D Laser Scanning
Rieger UM, Erba P, Wettstein R, et al (Univ Hosp of Basel, Switzerland; et al)
Ann Plast Surg 61:359-363, 2008

The aim of this study was to evaluate the combination of abdominoplasty with liposuction of both flanks with regards to length of scar, complications, and patient's satisfaction. A retrospective analysis of 35 patients who underwent esthetic abdominoplasty at our institution between 2002 and 2004 was performed. Thirteen patients underwent abdominoplasty with liposuction of both flanks, 22 patients underwent conventional abdominoplasty. Liposuction of the flanks did not increase the rate of complications of the abdominoplasty procedures. We found a tendency toward shorter scars in patients who underwent abdominoplasty combined with liposuction of the flanks. Implementation of 3-dimensional laser surface scanning to objectify the postoperative outcomes, documented a comparable degree of flatness of the achieved body contouring in both procedures. 3-dimensional laser surface scanning can be a valuable tool to objectify assessment of postoperative results.

▶ Lateral abdominal liposuction as an adjunct to abdominoplasty is commonly done to give an additional improvement in trunk contour. The safety of this combination of techniques is confirmed, and there was no increase in seroma formation. The use of 3-dimensional imaging technology demonstrated that the same level of contour "flatness" can be achieved with a shorter abdominal scar by using liposuction together with abdominoplasty. The rate of scar revisions and dog-ears was similar between the 2 groups, but the small sample size does not allow for commenting on the statistical significance of these observations.

K. A. Gutowski, MD

Does Thighplasty for Upper Thigh Laxity After Massive Weight Loss Require a Vertical Incision?

Shermak MA, Mallalieu J, Chang D (Johns Hopkins Bayview Med Ctr, Baltimore, MD; Johns Hopkins School of Medicine, Baltimore, MD)
Aesthet Surg J 29:513-522, 2009

Background.—After massive weight loss (MWL), many patients present with concerns about skin excess and laxity. The thigh is one of the more complex regions to address in MWL patients because of the differing degree, location, and quality of skin excess and fatty tissue, as well as surgical risk factors.

Objective.—The authors describe a technique called the anterior proximal extended (APEX) thighlift to effectively treat upper thigh skin excess with a hidden scar while also enhancing adjacent body regions.

Methods.—A review was performed of 97 MWL patients who underwent thighlift surgery between March 1998 and October 2007. Eighty-six women and 11 men, with average weight loss of 146 lb and average body mass index (BMI) at contouring of 29.8, were included in the study. The risk factors that were assessed included age, gender, medical conditions, tobacco use, BMI, weight of skin excised, and surgery

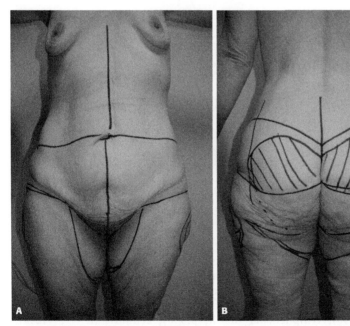

FIGURE 2.—**A**, Preoperative inner thigh crescent markings. The degree of excision is measured with a pinch test and no commitment is made until the surgeon is assured that closure is possible through step-wise excision and closure. **B**, Inner thigh crescent markings. Also planned is a lower backlift with autologous gluteal augmentation. (Reprinted from Shermak MA, Mallalieu J, Chang D. Does thighplasty for upper thigh laxity after massive weight loss require a vertical incision? *Aesthet Surg J*. 2009;29:513-522.)

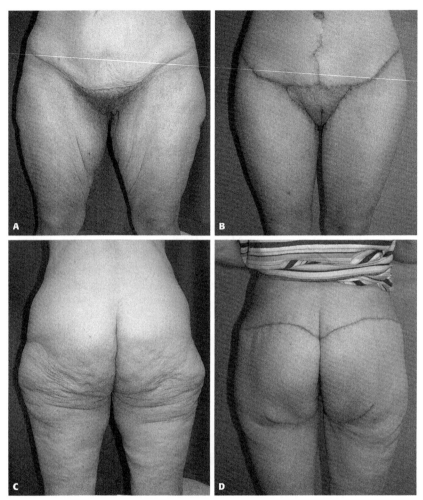

FIGURE 3.—A, C, Preoperative views of a 41-year-old woman who lost 167 lb after laparoscopic gastric bypass surgery, reaching a body mass index of 22.6. She desired a lower body lift. This same patient is featured in Figures 1 and 2. B, D, Two months after thighlift with the anterior proximal extended thigh-lift (APEX) technique. (Reprinted from Shermak MA, Mallalieu J, Chang D. Does thighplasty for upper thigh laxity after massive weight loss require a vertical incision? *Aesthet Surg J*. 2009;29:513-522.)

performed. The outcomes that were assessed included wound healing and lymphedema. Extended vertical thighlift was performed in 11 patients and anterior superior thighlift in 86 patients.

Results.—Complications of thighlift included wound healing problems (n = 18; 18.6%); lymphedema (n = 8; 8.3%); cellulitis (n = 7; 7.2%); seroma (n = 3; 3.1%); and bleeding (n = 1; 1%). On multivariate statistical analysis, age and BMI were found to impair healing in the entire thighlift group. For patients with a BMI greater than or equal to 35, the odds ratio (OR) for a wound healing complication was 13.7 ($P = .03$). Hypothyroidism was strongly associated with lymphedema, with an OR of 23 ($P = .06$). Extended thighlift trended toward lymphedema (OR = 16.7; $P = .08$).

Conclusions.—Thighlift can be a satisfying procedure for both the patient and surgeon because it provides aesthetic improvement in terms of skin excess and laxity. The APEX thighlift is a new technique that expands upon those previously described in the literature to effectively treat upper thigh laxity with a hidden scar after MWL (Figs 2 and 3).

▶ The described anterior proximal extended (APEX) thighlift technique offers greater improvement in thigh contouring in massive weight loss (MWL) patients than does a classic Lockwood "crescent excision" thighlift without the long incisions associated with the vertical thighlift typically done for these patients. The preoperative markings are easy to perform (Fig 2A & B), the results are good (Fig 3A, B, C & D), and a change from the prone position to the supine position is required. However, some MWL may not be candidates for the APEX thighlift as it does not seem to address the redundant tissue in the lower thigh and medial knee regions. For patients agreeable to the longer scars, a vertical thighlift will offer better results when there is moderate or severe tissue excess distal to the mid thigh. This technique stresses the importance of deep ischial periosteal suspension of the elevated thigh tissue to minimize scar spreading and vulvar distortion. The authors recommend large interrupted braided sutures for the tissue suspension, but I stopped using such sutures due to late suture abscess formation (even up to 6 years postoperatively) and occasional patient discomfort. Instead, long-lasting absorbable monofilament sutures seem to provide similar results without the problems associated with permanent sutures.

K. A. Gutowski, MD

Implications of Weight Loss Method in Body Contouring Outcomes
Gusenoff JA, Coon D, Rubin JP (Univ of Pittsburgh Med Ctr, PA)
Plast Reconstr Surg 123:373-376, 2009

Background.—Patients frequently present for body contouring after massive weight loss resulting from bariatric procedures or diet and exercise. The authors investigated whether body contouring complications vary by weight loss method.

Methods.—Four hundred forty-nine patients (511 cases) were entered into a prospective registry. Diet and exercise patients were matched to bariatric patients based on identical procedures performed. Conditional logistic regression was used to test for differences between groups. One-to-one matching was then performed by nearest neighbor matching to the most similar patient who underwent bariatric procedures based on sex, age, and body mass index. The t test was used to compare matched patients.

Results.—Twenty-nine patients (6.5 percent) lost weight exclusively through diet and exercise. They had significantly higher preoperative hematocrit ($p = 0.02$) and hemoglobin ($p = 0.05$), and tended to have multiple procedures performed at the same time, higher absolute complication rates, and significantly higher infection rates ($p = 0.03$). When matched to 191 bariatric patients based on procedures performed, diet and exercise patients had a higher complication rate that did not reach significance (odds ratio, 1.5; $p = 0.28$). One-to-one matching resulted in 34 procedure-matched pairs with nonsignificant trends toward better nutrition and more complications in diet and exercise patients.

Conclusions.—Infection rates were higher in patients who had body contouring after massive weight loss from diet and exercise versus bariatric procedures. When matched, despite lower nutrition markers, patients treated with bariatric procedures had outcomes similar to those of diet and exercise patients. We did not find evidence for an association between weight loss method and risk in the body contouring patient.

▶ Since the population of patients who have body contouring procedures after massive weight loss following diet and exercise is small compared with the number of those who had bariatric surgery, this and previous studies have been unable to show a difference in complication rates between the 2 groups. Intuitively, one would expect the bariatric surgery group to have more complications, presumably due to underlying metabolic deficiencies. The higher infection rate in patients who lost weight by diet and exercise is difficult to explain; however, postbariatric surgery patients may be more likely to be followed by dedicated physicians who monitor and manage these patients' nutritional status. Surprisingly, the bariatric surgery group had poorer nutritional markers but did not have a higher complication rate compared with the diet and exercise group. Clearly, more research needs to be done to better define nutritional and other risk factors for these patients.

K. A. Gutowski, MD

Management of the Mons Pubis and Labia Majora in the Massive Weight Loss Patient
Alter GJ (Univ of California, Los Angeles)
Aesthet Surg J 29:432-442, 2009

The high incidence of female obesity and weight loss has resulted in common complaints of a large, protuberant mons pubis and labia majora (outer labial lips) related to unsightly fat deposits and skin ptosis. The author presents a technique to correct the protuberant mons and pubic descent by performing a pubic lift, fat excision, and liposuction, and then tacking the superficial fibrofatty tissue to the rectus fascia. The labia majora enlargement is treated by fat excision and/or liposuction and skin excision. These techniques eliminate difficulties with sexual intercourse, poor hygiene, and discomfort, while also improving self-esteem.

▶ Female external genitalia procedures are becoming more common, particularly to achieve an improved aesthetic appearance. In female massive weight loss patients, functional and hygiene problems can also be addressed by elevating the mons and reducing the labia majora and minora as needed. The techniques described are well suited for this patient population and can easily be incorporated into abdominoplasty and body lift procedures, or they can be done separately. When elevating the mons, care should be taken to avoid distortion of the clitoral hood, which can lead to an abnormal appearance and patient discomfort. Similarly, overaggressive debulking of the mons may result in not only an unnatural flat shape but also complaints of patient discomfort due to loss of the normal protective padding over the symphysis pubis.

K. A. Gutowski, MD

The Effect of Weight Loss Surgery and Body Mass Index on Wound Complications After Abdominal Contouring Operations
Greco JA III, Castaldo ET, Nanney LB, et al (Vanderbilt Univ, Nashville, TN)
Ann Plast Surg 61:235-242, 2008

Abdominal contouring operations are in high demand after massive weight loss. Anecdotally, wound problems seemed to occur frequently in this patient population. Our study was designed to delineate risk factors for wound complications after body contouring. Our retrospective institutional analysis was assembled from 222 patients between 2001 and 2006 who underwent either abdominoplasty (N = 89) or panniculectomy (N = 133). Weight loss surgery (WLS) before body contouring occurred in 63% of our patients. Overall the wound complication rate in these patients was 34%: healing-disturbance 11%, wound infection 12%, hematoma 6%, and seroma 14%. WLS patients had an increase in wound complications overall (41% vs. 22%; $P < 0.01$) and in all categories of wound complications compared with non-WLS-patients by univariate methods of analysis. In a multivariate regression model, only American Society of Anesthesiologists Physical Status Classification was a significant independent risk factor for wound complications. In conclusion, WLS patients are at increased risk for wound complications and American Society of Anesthesiologists Physical Status Classification is the most predictive of risk.

▶ Studies of metabolic profile changes after liposuction have shown mixed results. It has been reported that after liposuction, a compensatory increase in the size of the remaining fat deposits, mainly in the visceral cavity, occurs if the weight lost after surgery is regained. Such body fat redistribution is associated with an increase in the metabolic complications of obesity and with the risk of experiencing cardiovascular disease. It appears reasonable to minimize the recurrence and unfavorable storage of fat after liposuction. Orlistat (a pancreatic lipase inhibitor) is effective in achieving weight loss and weight management while selectively reducing visceral fat and improving insulin sensitivity. Unfortunately, orlistat did not produce significant protection against visceral fat accumulation after liposuction, but it did result in a significant lowering of low-density lipoprotein (LDL) cholesterol levels. The favorable and unfavorable metabolic profile changes after liposuction need further study.

K. A. Gutowski, MD

Composite Body Contouring
Pereira LH, Sterodimas A (LH Clinic, Rio de Janeiro, Brazil)
Aesthetic Plast Surg 33:616-624, 2009

Background.—Aesthetic surgery of the thoracoabdominal region is one of the most frequently performed surgical procedures in plastic surgery. The combination of circumferential liposuction, autologous fat grafting of the buttocks and/or lower limbs, and the modified transverse abdominoplasty as an adjuvant procedure all done in a single surgical procedure is not very common. The authors present a prospective study of the surgical technique of composite body contouring, emphasizing the low rate of complications and the high overall patient satisfaction.

Methods.—A total of 64 consecutive female patients were operated on between January 2004 and January 2007. All the patients who were included in the study were candidates for a classical abdominoplasty. Posterior and lateral syringe-assisted liposuction combined with fat insertion into the buttocks and/or lower limbs was performed. Autologous fat grafting was done in the gluteal area for buttocks enhancement and in the lower limbs to correct contour deformities. Anterolateral liposuction with modified transverse abdominoplasty was done as an adjuvant procedure. Overall satisfaction with body appearance after composite body contouring was rated on a scale of 1–5.

Results.—From 1,500 to 4,600 ml of fat was obtained with liposuction (mean = 2,478 ml). Forty-five patients had fat grafting only to the buttocks area. Six patients had fat insertion into the lower limbs and 13 had fat injection into the buttocks and lower limbs. The amount of fat transplanted to the buttocks varied from 165 to 625 ml (mean = 346 ml) and to the lower limbs it varied from 75 to 270 ml (mean = 195 ml). Three patients (5%) suffered from early complications, including infection (3%) and hematoma formation (2%). Nine patients (14%) had late complications, including hypertophic scars (7.5%), dog ears (4.5%), and localized fat excess (2%). Nine patients (14%) underwent revision surgery. Sixty-three percent reported that their appearance after composite body contouring was "very good" (42%) or "excellent" (21%) and 27% responded that their appearance was "good." Only 10% thought their appearance was less than good, (7% "fair" and 3% "poor"). The average follow-up time has been 3.2 years (range = 2–5 years).

Conclusion.—Composite body contouring combines circumferential liposuction, fat grafting of the buttocks and lower limbs, and modified transverse abdominoplasty to accomplish very good aesthetic results in a single surgical procedure with a low rate of complications and high patient satisfaction.

▶ This article extends the lipoabdominoplasty concept[1] of extensive anterior abdominal liposuction with concurrent lower abdominal tissue excision and limited abdominal flap undermining to achieve an anterior trunk contour that would not be possible with abdominoplasty alone. The results are acceptable and confirm that lipoabdominoplasty is safe when properly performed. The composite component adds buttock fat grafting to improve the overall shape of the trunk. The grafting technique described is simple and uses syringe aspiration and saline irrigation of the harvested fat grafts. Although patient satisfaction was reported as being favorable, specific evaluation of the fat graft results was not done.

K. A. Gutowski, MD

Reference

1. Saldanha OR, Federico R, Daher PF, et al. Lipoabdominoplasty. *Plast Reconstr Surg.* 2009;124:934.

Maximizing Aesthetics and Safety in Circumferential-Incision Lower Body Lift With Selective Undermining and Liposuction
Kolker AR, Lampert JA (Mount Sinai School of Medicine, New York)
Ann Plast Surg 62:544-548, 2009

Circumferential dermolipectomy has been an effective means of reducing excess skin and fat after massive weight loss, however, regions of residual midabdominal and epigastric fat frequently confer a suboptimal contour, and often mediocre cosmetic results. Liposuction in association with lower body lift surgery has been regarded with caution, for fear of ischemia or necrosis of the undermined flaps as potential dire consequences. In this study, a theoretical and technical approach that maximizes safety and aesthetics in circumferential lower body lift after massive weight loss with contouring using liposuction is described and evaluated. Twenty-four patients were treated with follow-up ranging from 6 to 40 months (mean follow-up 17 months). All patients were treated with the resection of circumferential skin and fat maintaining a low-lying transverse suture line with a prone-to-supine approach. Dorsally, liberal liposuction is performed after the instillation of lidocaine-free wetting solution above and below the resection lines. Ventrally, the upper flap is elevated widely to the umbilical horizontal. The umbilicus is circumcised, and the dissection then progresses in a narrow column above the rectus sheaths to the xiphoid. Judicious subcostal undermining is performed, maintaining an intact bilateral subcostal "perforator zone" of 4 to 6 cm. Diastasis repair and anterior sheath plication are performed, and the umbilicus is anchored to the fascia. Wetting solution is instilled, and suction-assisted lipoplasty of the entire flap, particularly in the midline and in the region of the neo-umbilicus, is performed, removing excess fat and providing discontinuous lateral flap "undermining." There was 1 hematoma (4%) requiring re-exploration and 4 seromas (17%) treated with percutaneous aspiration. There was no infection, skin loss, or wound dehiscence. Unlike standard dermolipectomy procedures with wide undermining, the maintenance of a broad subcostal blood supply with selective direct undermining allows for liberal flap contouring with suction and the establishment of lower suture-line position. With this technique, liposuction can be safely used during lower body lift to maximize aesthetic outcomes.

▶ The lipoabdominoplasty concept can be used safely in body lift procedures for massive weight loss patients. The demonstrated enhanced results from more liberal liposuction of the truck, particularly in epigastric area, are possible when the blood supply is respected and preserved. The described technique to maximize flap vascularity, and consequently safety, is similar to other lipoabdominoplasty procedures. Particular attention should be paid to the selective direct midline undermining of the anterior abdominal flap and discontinuous lateral undermining, which preserves perforator blood vessels.

K. A. Gutowski, MD

Circumference reduction and cellulite treatment with a TriPollar radiofrequency device: a pilot study

Manuskiatti W, Wachirakaphan C, Lektrakul N, et al (Mahidol Univ, Bangkok, Thailand)
J Eur Acad Dermatol Venereol 23:820-827, 2009

Background.—A wide variety of treatments for circumference reduction and cellulite are available, but most procedures offer suboptimal clinical effect and/or delayed therapeutic outcome.

Objective.—To determine the safety and efficacy of the TriPollar radiofrequency device for cellulite treatment and circumference reduction.

Methods.—Thirty-nine females with cellulite received eight weekly TriPollar treatments. Treatment areas included the abdomen, thighs, buttocks and arms. Subjects were evaluated using standardized photographs and measurements of body weight, circumference, subcutaneous thickness, and skin elasticity of the treatment sites at baseline, immediately after and 4 weeks after the final treatment. Physicians' evaluation of clinical improvement scores using a quartile grading scale was recorded.

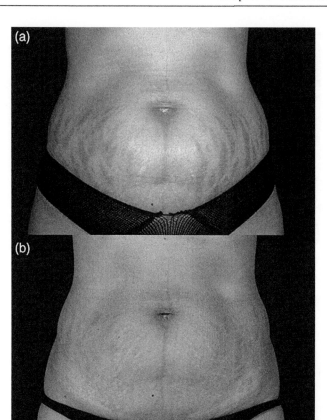

FIGURE 2.—Abdomen region, before treatment (a), Clinical appearance at 4 weeks after eight treatments (b). Note the appearance of stretch marks, before and after the series of treatment. (Reprinted from Manuskiatti W, Wachirakaphan C, Lektrakul N, et al. Circumference reduction and cellulite treatment with a TriPollar radiofrequency device: a pilot study. *J Eur Acad Dermatol Venereol*. 2009;23:820-827.)

Results.—Thirty-seven patients (95%) completed the treatment protocol. There was significant circumference reduction of 3.5 and 1.7 cm at the abdomen ($P = 0.002$) and thigh ($P = 0.002$) regions, respectively. At 4 weeks after the last treatment, the average circumferential reductions of the abdomen and thighs were sustained. No significant circumferential reductions of the buttocks and arms at the last treatment visit compared to baseline were demonstrated ($P = 0.138$ and 0.152, respectively). Quartile grading scores correlating to approximately 50% improvement in cellulite appearance were noted.

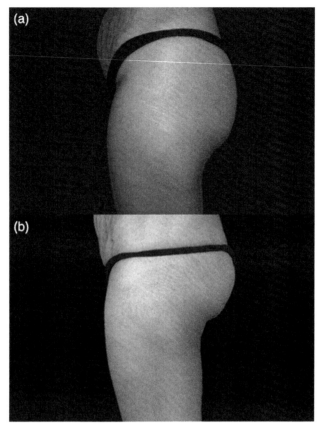

FIGURE 3.—Thigh region, before treatment (a). Clinical appearance at 4 weeks after eight treatments (b). (Reprinted from Manuskiatti W, Wachirakaphan C, Lektrakul N, et al. Circumference reduction and cellulite treatment with a TriPollar radiofrequency device: a pilot study. *J Eur Acad Dermatol Venereol.* 2009;23:820-827.)

Conclusions.—Tripollar radiofrequency provided beneficial effects on the reduction of abdomen and thigh circumference and cellulite appearance (Figs 2 and 3).

▶ Noninvasive external radiofrequency (RF) and light technologies are showing promise in skin tightening and body contouring by volumetric heating of tissues. RF devices have shown beneficial effects in both monopolar and bipolar mode, but pain is associated with the treatment. TriPollar RF combines monopolar and bipolar modalities and produces heating of deep subcutaneous tissue with significantly less patient discomfort. This well-designed study demonstrated significant improvement in abdominal and thigh contouring (Figs 2 and 3), but not in the arms or buttock. The improvement was sustained 4 weeks after cessation of treatment, but no further follow-up was done. While this technology has potential for tissue tightening and contouring, longer follow-up is needed. As with other noninvasive methods of adipose tissue reduction (mesotherapy), it will be important to know what happens metabolically to the affected fat. While the improvements are significant, based on body region circumference measurements and tissue thickness, they need to be compared with what can be achieved with other modalities (eg, liposuction) that are more likely to produce greater improvement and higher patient satisfaction.

K. A. Gutowski, MD

Liposuction

Liposuction: 25 Years of Experience in 26,259 Patients Using Different Devices

Triana L, Triana C, Barbato C, et al (Colombian Society of Plastic, Aesthetic, Maxillofacial, and Hand Surgery)
Aesthet Surg J 29:509-512, 2009

Background.—The development of liposuction provided plastic surgeons with a safe and effective way to sculpt the human figure. The techniques and instrumentation used in the performance of liposuction have evolved significantly since its introduction.

Objective.—The authors review their experience with different liposuction techniques over the past 25 years.

Methods.—Data from patients who had undergone liposuction were collected from the personal databases of four different surgeons and from the database at the Corpus and Rostrum Plastic Surgery Clinic in Cali, Colombia. A retrospective review was conducted and the results from different liposuction techniques were compared.

Results.—A total of 26,259 patient charts were reviewed. The results showed that 5% of patients experienced a postsurgical seroma. Postsurgical fibrosis developed to some degree in 2.3% of patients. Anemia was present in 18% of all patients and in 60% of those patients who underwent dry liposuction. Ninety percent of patients reported postoperative pain. The incidence of deep vein thrombosis was 0.03%, as was the incidence of pulmonary embolism. Mortality was 0.01% and was mainly caused by pulmonary embolism. Patient satisfaction was similar for all of the described techniques.

Conclusions.—The incidence of anemia was reduced significantly in patients undergoing tumescent liposuction versus dry liposuction. However, the occurrence of seroma increased with the introduction of tumescent liposuction. The incidence of postoperative pain and fibrosis was similar for all liposuction techniques reviewed. The aesthetic results obtained using ultrasound- or laser-assisted liposuction were similar to those obtaining using other techniques.

▶ While it may be hard to draw conclusions regarding outcomes of different liposuction techniques from a retrospective review of cases done over a 25-year period, some observations can be made. The authors used dry liposuction, tumescent liposuction, tumescent ultrasound-assisted liposuction (UAL), and tumescent laser-assisted liposuction (LAL). Better improvement in skin retraction in the front part of the axillae, submental area, and inner thighs was seen with LAL when compared with tumescent liposuction alone, but no difference was observed in these regions between LAL and UAL. These findings support other observations that UAL and LAL may offer better results in certain body regions, particularly where skin laxity is common. Patient satisfaction with results averaged 82% and was similar for all 4 liposuction techniques. Furthermore, LAL was associated with less inflammation and ecchymosis compared with tumescent liposuction alone. From a safety perspective, the incidence of deep vein thrombosis (DVT) and of pulmonary embolism (PE) was 0.03% while mortality was 0.01%, mainly due to PE. Surprisingly, of the patients who died all had a low surgical risk and did not undergo any associated procedures. Since 2004, enoxaheparine (Enoxaparin) was administered to all liposuction patients 1 day before and for 1 to 4 days after surgery. However, the complications (if any) of adding anticoagulation were not discussed.

K. A. Gutowski, MD

Assessing the Long-Term Viability of Facial Fat Grafts: An Objective Measure Using Computed Tomography

Fontdevila J, Serra-Renom JM, Raigosa M, et al (Univ of Barcelona, Spain)
Aesthetic Surg J 28:380-386, 2008

Background.—Autologous fat transplantation for soft tissue augmentation is a commonly used technique without a universally accepted approach. The literature includes a variety of reports describing varying degrees of success or failure.

Objective.—To evaluate the behavior of facial fat grafts in humans with the use of an objective measuring tool.

Methods.—A prospective randomized study, comparing patients pre- and postoperatively, was designed to evaluate the long-term viability of fat grafting. Participants were 18 men and 8 women between 34 and 59 years of age (mean, 45.07 yrs; standard deviation, 6.54 yrs). A total of 52 hemifaces in 26 patients diagnosed with HIV and demonstrating facial lipoatrophy were treated with fat transplantation using Coleman's technique. HIV-positive patients were chosen as study participants because their nearly total lack of subcutaneous fat diminishes the bias in the evaluation of fat volume. Fat graft viability was evaluated by measuring the volume of adipose tissue evolution via computed tomography scan before fat grafting, at the second month after fat grafting, and 1 year after fat grafting. Descriptive statistical analysis was performed.

Results.—The mean volume on the right and left cheeks before fat grafting was 1.57 cc. The mean volume 2 months after the procedure was 2.93 cc with a statistically significant mean increase of 1.36 cc ($P < .001$) between baseline and the second month after the procedure. The mean

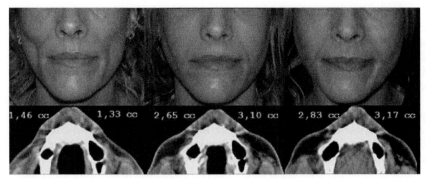

FIGURE 5.—This 40-year-old woman demonstrates grade 3 facial lipoatrophy. In each side of her face, 14 cc of fatty tissue was injected. The numbers indicate the volume of fat detected by CT scan in a fixed cheek area before treatment and 2 and 12 months postinjection. (Reprinted from Fontdevila J, Serra-Renom JM, Raigosa M, et al. Assessing the long-term viability of facial fat grafts: an objective measure using computed tomography. *Aesthetic Surg J.* 2008;28:380-386.)

volume after 12 months was 3.29 cc ($P < .001$), with a mean increase compared with the baseline of 1.72 cc, and of 0.36 cc between months 2 and 12. The statistically significant posttreatment improvement ($P < .001$) was maintained until month 12 of the follow-up period.

Conclusions.—Using objective measurement, this study demonstrates that with one fat grafting procedure a durable result can be achieved, persisting for a minimum of 12 months without any trend towards reabsorption (Fig 5).

▶ The powerful results seen with fat grafts are well demonstrated. Because fat grafting appears to be technique dependant (and the optimal technique has not yet been described) and possibly recipient-site dependent, care should be used when applying these results to regions outside the midface. The CT findings demonstrate that the soft-tissue augmentation is due to viable fat and not fibrosis or fat necrosis. The dramatic results are seen in Fig 5 where a patient is seen before 2 months and 12 months after 14 cc of fat was injected into each side of the face.

K. A. Gutowski, MD

Analysis of a Series of Autologous Fat Tissue Transfer for Lower Limb Atrophies
Mojallal A, Veber M, Shipkov C, et al (Edouard Herriot Hosp, Lyon, France; et al)
Ann Plast Surg 61:537-543, 2008

Localized and circumferential atrophies of the lower extremities have been difficult to treat with few simple autologous solutions available. The aim of this study was to analyze the efficacy of fat grafting in lower limb atrophies.

There were 20 patients (17 females and 3 males) at an average age of 33 years. Twelve patients had localized and 8 patients circumferential atrophies of various etiologies: traumatic (60%), congenital (25%), and iatrogenic (15%). The average number of fat injections was 1.1 per patient (range 1–2) for localized atrophies and 2.2 per patient (range 1–3) for circumferential atrophies. The average follow-up period was 2 years.

The average volume injected at each stage was 79 mL for localized atrophies and 137 mL for circumferential atrophies. In the cases of circumferential atrophies, an average augmentation of 1.9 cm (range 1–6 cm) of the limb perimeter per injection was achieved. The overall satisfaction of the patients was high.

Autologous fat grafting is a reliable technique for lower limb atrophies.

▶ This article provides a relatively simple and safe solution to a somewhat challenging problem. Previous methods for correcting contour deformities of the extremities usually involved placement of implants that were usually made of silicone. Standardized implants are available but usually require some form of customization to achieve symmetric extremity contours. Placement of the implant requires an incision, although some patients already have scars from previous trauma or surgery. The complication rate of implants, especially in the lower extremity, is high. The authors' use of fat injection eliminates the need for any new incisions, minimizes the risk of infection, and maximizes the potential for effective recontouring. The only downside is the need to repeat injections one or more times in many patients. The authors chose to keep their patients hospitalized for 48 hours, but there is no evidence that this is necessary. This is a procedure in which the sculpturing skill of the plastic surgeon can truly be demonstrated.

R. L. Ruberg, MD

Evaluation of Skin Tightening After Laser-Assisted Liposuction
DiBernardo BE, Reyes J (Univ of Medicine and Dentistry of New Jersey)
Aesthet Surg J 29:400-407, 2009

Background.—Lasers have been used to enhance the emulsification of fat and coagulation of small blood vessels in conjunction with lipoaspiration. Although seen anecdotally, documented skin tightening has not been established.

Objective.—The authors sought to establish a model and a quantifiable method for documenting changes in skin tightening and skin shrinkage after laser lypolysis.

Methods.—Five female patients with focal abdominal adiposity were treated in a prospective evaluation with a sequentially firing 1064-/1320-nm laser. Skin shrinkage was measured from four quadrants of tattoo skin markings and evaluated using a three-dimensional camera.

Skin tightening was measured with a skin elasticity device. Measurements were taken at baseline and at one and three months postoperatively.

Results.—At three months postoperatively, the average skin tightening index (elasticity) increase indicating skin elasticity improvement was 26%; the average reduction in area or skin shrinkage was 17%. Both the skin tightening index and skin shrinkage at three months postoperatively (P < .01) were higher than baseline.

Conclusions.—Our findings represent the first documentation of quantifiable evidence of positive skin changes resulting from the addition of laser treatment to liposuction.

▶ This report serves as a pilot study to conduct a larger scale evaluation of skin tightening following liposuction. Only the SmartLipo MPX laser (Cynosure) was tested and there was no control group. However, favorable improvements in tissue endpoints were demonstrated. Future studies will hopefully address any differences in tissue changes using the various liposuction modalities available, and will offer insight as to which patients can benefit most from these more expensive technologies.

K. A. Gutowski, MD

Effects of Orlistat on Visceral Fat After Liposuction

Montoya T, Monereo S, Olivar J, et al (Getafe Univ Hosp, Madrid, Spain)
Dermatol Surg 35:469-474, 2009

Background.—Liposuction can aggravate metabolic complications associated with obesity. It has been shown that the recovery of weight lost through these interventions is associated with body fat redistribution toward the visceral cavity, increasing metabolic risk factors for coronary heart disease such as insulin resistance and high triglyceride levels.

Objectives.—The aim of this study was to evaluate the consequences of liposuction on body mass redistribution and metabolic parameters 6 months after surgery and to evaluate the use of orlistat treatment (tetrahydrolipstatin) in controlling these parameters.

Methods.—A population of 31 women with a mean body mass index of 26.17 ± 3.9 kg/m^2 and undergoing liposuction of more than 1,000 cm^3, was studied. Twelve of them were treated postsurgery with 120 mg of orlistat every 8 hours for the following 6 months. Anthropometric, analytical, and radiological (computed tomography) tests were performed to quantify visceral fat area before surgery and 6 months after surgery.

Results.—Despite weight loss after liposuction, visceral fat was not modified. Patients treated with orlistat showed a greater reduction in visceral fat, although not statistically significant. Orlistat use induced a reduction in low-density lipoprotein cholesterol values of 20.0 ± 22.5 mg/dL, compared with an increase of 8.46 ± 20.1 mg/dL in controls ($p = .07$).

Conclusions.—Visceral fat does not decrease despite weight loss after liposuction. Orlistat use post-liposuction might be a useful tool because it shows a tendency to reduce visceral fat and improve blood lipids profile.

▶ Studies of metabolic profile changes after liposuction have shown mixed results. It has been reported that after liposuction, a compensatory increase in the size of the remaining fat deposits, mainly in the visceral cavity, occurs if the weight lost after surgery is regained. Such body fat redistribution is associated with an increase in the metabolic complications of obesity and with the risk of experiencing cardiovascular disease. It appears reasonable to minimize the recurrence and unfavorable storage of fat after liposuction. Orlistat (a pancreatic lipase inhibitor) is effective in achieving weight loss and weight management while selectively reducing visceral fat and improving insulin sensitivity. Unfortunately, orlistat did not produce significant protection against visceral fat accumulation after liposuction, but did result in a significant lowering of low-density lipoprotein (LDL) cholesterol levels. The favorable and unfavorable metabolic profile changes after liposuction need further study.

K. A. Gutowski, MD

A New Approach for Adipose Tissue Treatment and Body Contouring Using Radiofrequency-Assisted Liposuction

Paul M, Mulholland RS (Univ of California, Irvine; Private Aesthetic Plastic Surgery Practice, Toronto)
Aesthetic Plast Surg 33:687-694, 2009

A new liposuction technology for adipocyte lipolysis and uniform three-dimensional tissue heating and contraction is presented. The technology is based on bipolar radiofrequency energy applied to the subcutaneous adipose tissue and subdermal skin surface. Preliminary clinical results, thermal monitoring, and histologic biopsies of the treated tissue demonstrate rapid preaspiration liquefaction of adipose tissue, coagulation of subcutaneous blood vessels, and uniform sustained heating of tissue.

▶ New technologies continue to offer variants on traditional liposuction but do not always lead to proven clinical advantages, particularly in patient outcome. The radiofrequency-assisted liposuction (RFAL) technique using the BodyTite system (Invasix Ltd) claims to offer faster treatment times, reduced tissue trauma, improved safety, uniform heating of the skin and the subcutaneous layer, and the potential skin contraction. This device uses an internal RF emitting electrode, which is inserted into the adipose tissue at the desired depth for adipose and blood vessel coagulation. An external electrode with a larger contact area is applied to the skin surface, creating a lower power density in the skin than in the adipose tissue. The RF current creates heat and coagulates the adipose, vascular, and fibrous tissue in the operative area. Histological analysis of treated tissue suggested less trauma and bleeding compared with traditional liposuction. However, the time of treatment is somewhat longer, and despite pictures of good postoperative results there is no proof of improved safety or superior skin retraction. The cost of the device and associated operating expenses is not provided. While this technology may offer some advantages, it is yet to be determined what role, if any, it will have in body contouring.

K. A. Gutowski, MD

6 Breast

General

Use of the microdebrider for treatment of fibrous gynaecomastia
Goh T, Tan BK, Song C (Singapore General Hosp)
J Plast Reconstr Aesthet Surg 63:506-510, 2010

Background.—In the quest for reduced scars and better aesthetic outcomes in minimally invasive surgical techniques for gynaecomastia, suction-assisted lipoplasty and ultrasound-assisted lipoplasty are now considered accepted recent advancements. Nevertheless, the fibrous glandular breast disc encountered in young, thin patients requires a separate peri-areolar incision as the disc cannot be removed with suction lipoplasty. The use of a microdebrider (powered shaving rotary device) is a potential solution to this problem.

We present a series of eight patients with fibrous gynaecomastia that was successfully treated in this way.

Method.—The surgery is performed under general anaesthesia. The microdebrider cannula is used to remove the fibrous glandular breast tissue. Drains are inserted and fibrin glue is sprayed subcutaneously. Patients are discharged on the next day. Drains are removed on the 5th postoperative day. A compressive vest is worn for 6 weeks. (A video of the procedure can be seen on http://www.microflap.com/video3.asp).

Results.—The eight patients were successfully treated. No bleeding, haematoma or seroma was encountered. All patients were satisfied with the results of the surgery.

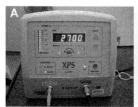 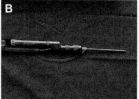 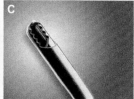

FIGURE 1.—A. Microdebrider machine. B. Microdebrider cannula. C. Close-up of cannula tip showing cutting trough. (Reprinted from Goh T, Tan BK, Song C. Use of the microdebrider for treatment of fibrous gynaecomastia. *J Plast Reconstr Aesthet Surg.* 2010;63:506-510, with permission from British Association of Plastic, Reconstructive and Aesthetic Surgeons.)

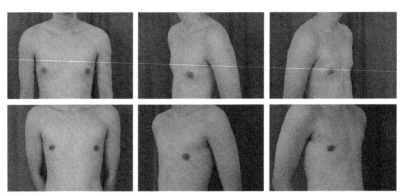

FIGURE 4.—A 20-year-old male with bilateral gynaecomastia treated with the microdebrider technique. (Above) Preoperative views. (Below) postoperative views at 6 months. (Reprinted from Goh T, Tan BK, Song C. Use of the microdebrider for treatment of fibrous gynaecomastia. *J Plast Reconstr Aesthet Surg.* 2010;63:506-510, with permission from British Association of Plastic, Reconstructive and Aesthetic Surgeons.)

Conclusion.—The microdebrider is a viable solution in the treatment of gynaecomastia with a fibrous breast disc. Excellent aesthetic results can be achieved with a single 3-mm incision (Figs 1 and 4).

▶ This is an interesting technique using a microdebrider originally developed for the excision of nasal polyps via endoscopic sinus surgery. I think most of us have had little success in removing the fibrous component of gynecomastia with liposuction with or without ultrasound. As a consequence, we often have to extend the incision and remove the tissue by direct excision. Rarely has this approach required much more than a 1.5 to 2 cm periareolar incision allowing one to directly and safely excise the fibrous tissue. The authors in a very small number of cases suggest that the microdebrider can safely and efficiently remove the fibrous tissue without injury to the overlying skin or development of postoperative hematoma. Although promising, further studies are warranted and the surgeon attempting this for the first time should practice being cautious to avoid damage to the vasculature or overlying areolar.

S. H. Miller, MD, MPH

Development of a New Patient-Reported Outcome Measure for Breast Surgery: The BREAST-Q

Pusic AL, Klassen AF, Scott AM, et al (Memorial Sloan-Kettering Cancer Ctr, NY; McMaster Univ, Hamilton, Canada; Univ of British Columbia, Vancouver, Canada; et al)

Plast Reconstr Surg 124:345-353, 2009

Background.—Measuring patient-reported outcomes has become increasingly important in cosmetic and reconstructive breast surgery.

The objective of this study was to develop a new patient-reported outcome measure to assess the unique outcomes of breast surgery patients.

Methods.—Patient interviews, focus groups, expert panels, and a literature review were used to develop a conceptual framework and a list of questionnaire items. Three procedure-specific questionnaires (augmentation, reduction, and reconstruction) were developed and cognitive debriefing interviews used to pilot each questionnaire. Revised questionnaires were field tested with 1950 women at five centers in the United States and Canada (response rate, 72 percent); 491 patients also completed a test-retest questionnaire. Rasch measurement methods were used to construct scales, and traditional psychometric analyses, following currently recommended procedures and criteria, were performed to allow for comparison with existing measures.

Results.—The conceptual framework included six domains: satisfaction with breasts, overall outcome, and process of care, and psychosocial, physical, and sexual well-being. Independent scales were constructed for these domains. This new patient-reported outcome measure "system" (the BREAST-Q) contains three modules (augmentation, reconstruction, and reduction), each with a preoperative and postoperative version. Each scale fulfilled Rasch and traditional psychometric criteria (including person separation index 0.76 to 0.95; Cronbach's alpha 0.81 to 0.96; and test-retest reproducibility 0.73 to 0.96).

Conclusions.—The BREAST-Q can be used to study the impact and effectiveness of breast surgery from the patient's perspective. By quantifying satisfaction and important aspects of health-related quality of life, the BREAST-Q has the potential to support advocacy, quality metrics, and an evidence-based approach to surgical practice.

▶ The development of the BREAST-Q constitutes a very important advance in Plastic Surgery. A validated tool that allows surgeons to assess the effectiveness of cosmetic and reconstructive procedures involving the breast will contribute enormously to our ability to make evidence-based judgments about new and existing procedures. It is important to note that there are commercial implications of the development of this assessment tool. A visit to the web site cited in the article will allow the potential user to fully understand the conditions for use of this device for different purposes. But most important in the various restrictions for use of the BREAST-Q is its availability free of charge for "nonfunded academic research and nonfunded clinical purposes." This and other evaluation tools currently in use, or perhaps still to be developed, will help plastic surgeons to make rational decisions about treatment of a variety of different breast problems in the not-too-distant future.

R. L. Ruberg, MD

Improved Postoperative Pain Control using Thoracic Paravertebral Block for Breast Operations

Boughey JC, Goravanchi F, Parris RN, et al (Mayo Clinic, Rochester, MN; The Univ of Texas M. D. Anderson Cancer Ctr, Houston)
Breast J 15:483-488, 2009

Thoracic paravertebral block (PVB) in breast surgery can provide regional anesthesia during and after surgery with the potential advantage of decreasing postoperative pain. We report our institutional experience with PVB over the initial 8 months of use. All patients undergoing breast operations at the ambulatory care building from September 09, 2005 to June 28, 2005 were reviewed. Comparison was performed between patients receiving PVB and those who did not. Pain scores were assessed immediately, 4 hours, 8 hours and the morning after surgery. 178 patients received PVB and 135 patients did not. Patients were subdivided into three groups: Group A–segmental mastectomy only ($n = 89$), Group B–segmental mastectomy and sentinel node surgery ($n = 111$) and Group C–more extensive breast surgery ($n = 113$). Immediately after surgery there was a statistically significant difference in the number of patients reporting pain between PVB patients and those without PVB. At all time points up until the morning after surgery PVB patients were significantly less likely to report pain than controls. Patients in Group C who received PVB were significantly less likely to require overnight stay. The average immediate pain scores were significantly lower in PVB patients than controls in both Group B and Group C and approached significance in Group A. PVB in breast surgical patients provided improved postoperative pain control. Pain relief was improved immediately postoperatively and this effect continued to the next day after surgery. PVB significantly decreased the proportion of patients that required overnight hospitalization after major breast operations and therefore may decrease cost associated with breast surgery.

▶ This is a very worthwhile article to bring to the attention of plastic surgeons, and their anesthesiologists who are performing outpatient augmentation and reduction breast surgery. While the study was not randomized, the data certainly suggest that thoracic paravertebral blocks can reduce postoperative pain and hospitalization rates at relatively low costs, economically and in terms of complications. One caveat is to be aware that the complication rate initially may be higher than after a greater degree of experience of the anesthesiologist. Similar material was published from Duke University in 2000 and included patients who underwent plastic surgical breast operations.[1] I believe this type of anesthetic might prove especially beneficial for submuscular augmentations and extensive breast reductions. Needless to say, randomized studies, in both general and plastic surgery, should be performed to document its value and potential for cost savings.

S. H. Miller, MD, MPH

Reference

1. Klein SM, Bergh A, Stelle SM, Georgiade GS, Greengrass RA. Thoracic paravertebral blocks for breast surgery. *Anesth Analg.* 2000;90:402-405.

The Serial Free Fat Transfer in Irradiated Prosthetic Breast Reconstructions

Panettiere P, Marchetti L, Accorsi D (Università degli Studi di Bologna, Italy; Ospedale Privato Accreditato "Villa Chiara", Casalecchio di Reno (Bo), Italy)
Aesthetic Plast Surg 33:695-700, 2009

Background.—This study investigated the effects of lipofilling on both the functional and the aesthetic aspects of breast reconstruction.

Methods.—Sixty-one consecutive patients with irradiated reconstructed breasts (62 breasts) were offered free fat transfer to enhance the results and correct the defects. Twenty patients were enrolled (active branch) and underwent multiple sessions of lipofilling, while the others were considered controls. The fat was harvested by syringe and processed by saline washing only (no centrifugation). Three months after the last session the functional outcome was evaluated using the LENT-SOMA scoring system and the aesthetic outcome was evaluated using a visual 5-point scale.

Results.—A significant improvement in all the LENT-SOMA scores after free fat grafting was observed; the scores after treatment were all significantly lower than those before it and were also significantly lower than those of untreated breasts. These results also were confirmed by comparing homogeneous subgroups of breasts with similar LENT-SOMA ranks before treatment. Similarly, the cosmetic outcomes were significantly enhanced after serial lipofilling. The four cases in the active branch with severe flap thinning resolved with no implant exposure (mean follow-up = 17.6 months), while implant exposure occurred in the two cases with the same problem in the control group. In one case, a Baker 3-4 capsular contracture was downgraded to Baker 1 after only one session of lipofilling. No complications occurred in the treated cases.

Conclusion.—Free fat transfer is a safe and reliable technique in improving the outcomes of irradiated reconstructed breasts with implants.

▶ Individual anecdotal studies—including this one, which involved consecutive irradiated patients—fail to randomize patients, fail to match patients, and also fail to provide readers with an adequate follow-up to allow one to assess the long-term risks and benefits. There is little question, in my mind, that the technique is being widely used, but evidence for its efficacy is lacking.[1] Haven't we reached the stage where this issue needs to be studied collaboratively? The American Society of Plastic Surgeons (ASPS) and American Society for Aesthetic Plastic Surgery (ASAPS) and their educational foundations really do need to come up with a reliable evidence-based study. For those unfamiliar with the scoring system used in this study—it is an international system for evaluating the effects of radiation therapy on normal tissues. In the United

States it has been incorporated by the National Cancer Institute (NCI) into a Common Terminology Criteria for Adverse Events (CTCAE) rating system to look at both the early and late-term effects of radiation therapy.

S. H. Miller, MD, MPH

Reference

1. Coleman SR, Saboeiro AP. Fat grafting to the breast revisited: safety and efficacy. *Plast Reconstr Surg.* 2007;119:775-785.

Autologous Fat Transplantation to the Breast: A Personal Technique with 25 Years of Experience
Illouz YG, Sterodimas A (Saint Louis Hosp, Paris, France; 4224 Av Epitacio Pessoa, Brazil)
Aesthetic Plast Surg 33:706-715, 2009

Background.—Over the last 30 years there has been interest in the use of autologous fat transplantation for breast reconstructive and cosmetic purposes. Up until now injection of adipose tissue into the breast has been subject to two limiting factors. First, fat injection into the breast could result in fat necrosis, cyst formation, and indurations that could be mistaken as cancerous calcifications. Second, the degree of reabsorption of the injected adipose tissue is unpredictable.

Methods.—Patients included in the study were candidates for either breast reconstruction after tumor resection or breast augmentation and were divided into three groups. Group I included patients with asymmetry after mastectomy and breast reconstruction; Group II consisted of patients with congenital breast asymmetry; and Group III included patients requesting bilateral breast augmentation. All patients signed a consent form acknowledging potential complications of infiltrating fat into the breast.

Results.—A total of 820 consecutive female patients were operated on between 1983 and 2007. The age distribution of the patients ranged from 19 to 78 years, with a mean of 45.6 years. There were 381 patients in Group I, 54 in Group II, and 385 in Group III. Complications included ecchymosis in 76 patients, striae in 36 patients, 12 hematomas, and 5 infections. Long-term breast asymmetry was observed in 34 cases. Six hundred seventy patients have undergone mammography and ultrasonography 6 months and 1 year after their first intervention under our care. The majority of complications resulting from lipofilling of the breast have been seen in this series during the first 6 months after each session. Breast lesions, including calcifications, cysts, and cancer, that are not apparent in the first year after the final procedure of lipofilling we believe may not be directly associated with the autologous fat grafting to the breast. This has been confirmed by the long-term follow-up of 230 patients (range = 2–25 years, mean = 11.3 years) who have been followed up yearly with mammographic examination.

Conclusion.—In the last 25 years the results of autologous fat transplantation have been predictable and satisfying on the condition that the treatment is performed in stages with small quantities of adipose tissue fat injected in each treatment session. To prevent major complications the final expected result should not be the aim of a single procedure. Mammary lipografting is a procedure that can be offered to patients for breast reconstructive and cosmetic purposes.

▶ There have been a number of recent articles documenting the safety and efficacy of fat injection for contour restoration or augmentation of the breast. This article stands out for several reasons: (1) It probably represents the largest series of cases published so far. The authors report a single-surgeon series of 820 patients. Based on an average of approximately 3 procedures per patient, their experience would represent more than 2000 operations, and the experience extends over 25 years. (2) The technique described by the authors is as simple as any method recommended to date. Ordinary syringe liposuction is used for fat harvest. No centrifugation of fat is required. Larger droplets of fat are injected than suggested by some authors, and 10 mL syringes (as opposed to 1 mL as recommended by some authors) are used. (3) Relatively long-term follow-up shows a low complication rate and a high success rate. It is important to note, however, that no matter how simple this method of fat injection to the breast (mammary lipografting) appears, it still must be performed with great caution in order to achieve consistently good results.

R. L. Ruberg, MD

Complications after Autologous Fat Injection to the Breast
Hyakusoku H, Ogawa R, Ono S, et al (Nippon Med School, Tokyo, Japan)
Plast Reconstr Surg 123:360-370, 2009

Background.—Although autologous fat injection (fat grafting) to the breast was performed widely throughout the twentieth century, the authors at their hospital have recently had to repair the damage suffered by a number of patients subjected to this procedure. The authors are concerned that this procedure is being performed incorrectly by untrained and untutored individuals, especially in Japan. The authors report several cases of complications after this procedure. Several related issues are discussed.

Methods.—The authors retrospectively reviewed 12 patients who had received autologous fat grafts to the breast and required breast surgery and/or reconstruction to repair the damage presenting between 2001 and 2007. The symptoms are described and the fat grafting procedures that were used are analyzed.

Results.—All 12 patients (mean age, 39.3 years) had received fat injections to the breast for augmentation mammaplasty for cosmetic purposes.

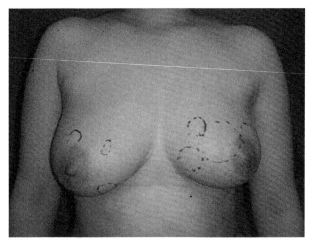

FIGURE 6.—Preoperative view of the 41-year-old woman in case 7. After fat grafting, many small indurations developed. (Reprinted from Hyakusoku H, Ogawa R, Ono S, et al. Complications after autologous fat injection to the breast. *Plast Reconstr Surg.* 2009;123:360-370.)

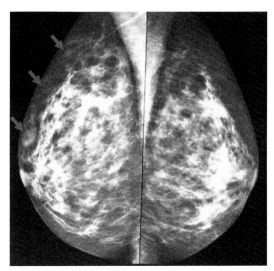

FIGURE 7.—Mammography of the patient in case 7. Multiple round permeates with fibrous capsules, oil cysts, and eggshell-like calcifications were detected in the subcutaneous tissue (*red arrows*). For interpretation of the references to color in this figure legend, the reader is referred to web version of this article. (Reprinted from Hyakusoku H, Ogawa R, Ono S, et al. Complications after autologous fat injection to the breast. *Plast Reconstr Surg.* 2009;123:360-370.)

They presented with palpable indurations, three with pain, one with infection, one with abnormal breast discharge, and one with lymphadenopathy. Four cases had abnormalities on breast cancer screening. All patients underwent mammography, computed tomography, and magnetic resonance imaging to evaluate the injected fats.

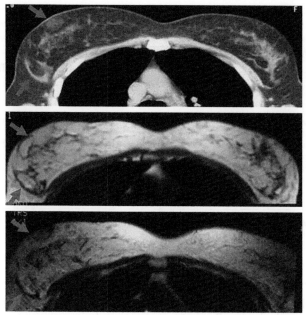

FIGURE 8.—Computed tomographic and T1- and T2-weighted magnetic resonance imaging scans of the patient in case 7. Multiple low-density areas encapsulated with high-density areas (degenerated fat) in the subdermis were observed (*red arrows*). It appears that multiple fat injections were performed but the volume per injection was large and/or the injected layer was too shallow. For interpretation of the references to color in this figure legend, the reader is referred to web version of this article. (Reprinted from Hyakusoku H, Ogawa R, Ono S, et al. Complications after autologous fat injection to the breast. *Plast Reconstr Surg.* 2009;123:360-370.)

Conclusions.—Autologous fat grafting to the breast is not a simple procedure and should be performed by well-trained and skilled surgeons. Patients should be informed that it is associated with a risk of calcification, multiple cyst formation, and indurations, and that breast cancer screens will always detect abnormalities. Patients should also be followed up over the long-term and imaging analyses (e.g., mammography, echography, computed tomography, and magnetic resonance imaging) should be performed (Figs 6-8).

▶ The authors describe their experience with 12 patients having complications after autologous fat injections into the breast in Japanese women (Figs 6-8 and Fig 9 in the original article). All of the procedures were performed for cosmetic indications. The concerns expressed by these authors are that untrained individuals are performing these procedures in Asia generally and Japan specifically, and that the procedure is not without risks. It should only be performed by well-trained surgeons who understand and have been fully trained in the technique, and who inform patients of the potential risks of the procedure. Certainly, their admonition of limiting the volume of injection and avoidance of placing the fat too superficially in the breast is wise counsel. While the authors suggest that all patients undergo a battery of expensive follow-up studies, it is not very likely that these suggestions will or should be universally adopted. However, I believe the surgeon who performs these injections must follow his/her patients clinically for a long period of time, just as they do when using prosthetic implants.[1,2]

S. H. Miller, MD, MPH

References

1. Coleman SR, Saboeiro AP. Fat Grafting to the breast revisited: safety and efficacy. *Plast Reconstr Surg.* 2007;119:775-785.
2. Missana MG, Laurent I, Barreau I, Balleyguier C. Autologous fat transfer in reconstructive breast surgery: indications, technique and results. *Eur J. Surg. Oncol.* 2007;33:685-690.

Mastopexy and Reduction

Rotation Mastopexy: An Anatomical Approach
Corduff N, Taylor GI (Aesthetic Breast Surgery Centre, Australia; Royal Melbourne Hosp, Australia)
Aesthetic Plast Surg 33:377-385, 2009

The goal of a mastopexy is to restore the shape and volume of the breast after ptosis of the breast. Ptosis occurs commonly in response to aging and breastfeeding. A low nipple position on the breast mound can be corrected by addressing the skin envelope, but maintenance of upper pole fullness and a youthful shape of the breast is the challenge to surgeons. To address this, techniques using local glandular flaps and implants have been suggested. A new technique has been created with regard to a detailed knowledge of the breast gland's vascular anatomy. The lower breast gland is raised as a large vascularized flap and rotated into a pocket beneath the upper pole. The operative procedure is presented together with the experience of the first author with a consecutive series of 25 patients.

▶ After years of experience performing mastopexy, I have concluded that the procedure is least successful when the technique focuses principally on lifting the existing breast tissue (despite the fact that the term "pexy" implies lifting) without altering the actual shape of that tissue. Many techniques have been developed over the years to assist in holding up the breast tissue on the chest wall once the "lifting" has taken place. These methods include different types of artificial material used as kind of a hammock to support the lifted tissue, or various autogenous slings using local muscle or fascia. The optimal lifting technique really requires some anatomic alteration of the tissue itself to achieve a more long-lasting result. For many years I elevated the lower half of the breast, split it vertically, and overlapped the 2 resulting segments to achieve a sling for support. More important, by overlapping the tissues, I increased the thickness (projection) of the existing breast tissue. But this increase was mostly in the lower pole of the breast. The authors of this article have described a technique that allows rotation of existing breast tissue into the mid and upper portion of the breast, where it really is needed to achieve a more aesthetically pleasing shape (in addition to a lift). The effect of stacking the pieces of breast tissue permits increased projection of the existing tissue (without implant augmentation) where it is needed. I think that this technique merits serious consideration.

R. L. Ruberg, MD

Dermal Suspension and Parenchymal Reshaping Mastopexy after Massive Weight Loss: Statistical Analysis with Concomitant Procedures from a Prospective Registry
Rubin JP, Gusenoff JA, Coon D (Univ of Pittsburgh Med Ctr, Life after Weight Loss Ctr)
Plast Reconstr Surg 123:782-789, 2009

Background.—An increasing number of women are presenting for mastopexy after massive weight loss. The authors analyzed data from a prospective registry of massive weight loss patients who underwent the dermal suspension and parenchymal reshaping mastopexy alone or with concomitant operations to assess safety and efficacy.

Methods.—One hundred eight female massive weight loss patients underwent mastopexy. Variables included operative time; time since gastric bypass; body mass index; revision; and complications such as seroma, dehiscence, hematoma, and infection. Univariate analyses were performed to assess outcome measures.

Results.—Ninety-one patients underwent mastopexy without implant [mean age, 43.7 ± 9 years; mean intraoperative time, 8.5 ± 3 hours (mastopexy plus concomitant procedures), mean body mass index, 28.3 ± 3.9; mean time since gastric bypass, 27.5 ± 13.4 months; mean follow-up, 7.3 months], whereas 17 had augmentation/mastopexy. Eighty-five of 91 patients (93.4 percent) had multiple procedures performed. Wound dehiscence was the most common complication in 26 patients (29.2 percent); however, breast-specific complications overall occurred in only eight patients (8.8 percent). Body mass index and operative time did not predict an increase in complication rates. Patients who underwent augmentation/mastopexy had a lower current body mass index than those who had mastopexy alone ($p = 0.01$).

Conclusions.—Dermal suspension, parenchymal reshaping mastopexy is a safe, effective, and durable method of treating the deflated breast after massive weight loss. Although patients with massive weight loss are likely to present for longer procedures and have a higher rate of wound-healing complications, these complications occur most frequently in areas other than the breast.

▶ This article demonstrates an effective way to restructure the breast after massive weight loss, and also provides valuable insights into other aspects of this potentially complicated problem. 1) The authors achieved a very satisfactory and relatively long-standing lifting of the breast using various autogenous tissues to achieve suspension of the very ptotic, deflated breast. There are other methods that other authors have espoused (including use of various artificial materials) to lift and hold the tissues, but the techniques described in this article certainly seem to work. 2) In addition to lifting the breast, the authors also describe effective ways of reshaping the existing structures to achieve a very aesthetically pleasing, projecting breast. The plication methods are carefully documented in the article. 3) The authors successfully combined the mastopexy with other body contouring procedures (particularly for the abdomen, which from a logistic standpoint can be done easily). Although many of the combined procedure patients experienced complications, only a few of the problems were related to the breast portion of the procedure. 4) Recognizing that adding a breast implant to the procedure adds significant additional risk, the authors note that an implant can be placed later, allowing their various suspensions of the breast to be carried out for maximum benefit without the need to leave extra room for a prosthesis.

R. L. Ruberg, MD

Augmentation and Silicone

Breast Augmentation Under General Anesthesia Versus Monitored Anesthesia Care: A Retrospective Comparative Study
Eldor L, Weissman A, Fodor L, et al (Technion-Israel Inst of Technology, Haifa; et al)
Ann Plast Surg 61:243-246, 2008

Breast augmentation is one of the leading esthetic surgeries, enjoying high satisfaction rates. Pain, nausea, and vomiting are frequent shortcomings of the immediate postoperative period. The aim of this study was to compare breast augmentation from the anesthetic point of view: general anesthesia (GA) versus monitored anesthesia care (MAC). The charts of 115 patients were reviewed in this retrospective study performed over a period of 2 years. Sixty-nine women chose to have the surgery done under MAC, and 46 under GA. Statistically significant differences were noted in both postoperative hospital stay (16.1 ± 6.78 hours vs. 11.7 ± 6.10 hours) and frequency of vomiting (mean, 0.5 vs. 0.22 times per patient) after GA and MAC, respectively (Mann-Whitney, $P < 0.01$). Postoperative pain, assessed using the visual analog scale, was significantly higher (mean visual analog scale, 5 vs. 3.27) when the prosthesis was placed in the submuscular plane compared with the subglandular plane (Mann-Whitney, $P = 0.043$). When offered a choice, more women preferred MAC over GA for their breast augmentation procedure. Less vomiting and shorter postoperative hospitalization were prominent in the MAC group.

▶ This article provides some useful information regarding anesthetic techniques for breast augmentation, but still leaves some questions unanswered. The useful information includes: the shorter length-of-stay in the hospital and the reduced rate of vomiting in patients who had managed anesthesia care (MAC) as opposed to general anesthesia, and the increased pain of submuscular implant placement compared with subglandular. None of these conclusions is particularly surprising. Maybe what is surprising is the fact that these patients stayed at the hospital for many hours after their surgery. I think many surgeons send their augmentation mammaplasty patients home much earlier than these surgeons do (usually in a few hours, as opposed to 16 hours for the general anesthesia patients, and 11 hours for the MAC patients in this study), and the patients do perfectly well if provided with appropriate postoperative medicines. The authors note that more of their patients chose MAC than general, but this piece of information really represents the limitation of the study—ie, the unanswered question. The anesthetic choice was based on preoperative expressed preference, not upon objective data. To really determine which approach patients prefer, one would have to do a prospective study in which the patients were not given a choice, but were randomized to the different anesthetic techniques. Then, after the procure was concluded and the patient had recovered, a more accurate evaluation of patient preference could be determined.

R. L. Ruberg, MD

Breast Augmentation, Antibiotic Prophylaxis, and Infection: Comparative Analysis of 1,628 Primary Augmentation Mammoplasties Assessing the Role and Efficacy of Antibiotics Prophylaxis Duration
Khan UD (Re-shape House, West Malling, Kent, UK)
Aesth Plast Surg 34:42-47, 2010

Background.—Infections after augmentation mammoplasty are not uncommon, and prophylactic antibiotics are routinely administered to minimize infection. However, there is paucity of information on the relationship between the length of prophylaxis cover and its benefits in primary augmentation mammoplasty. A retrospective analysis of different antibiotic cover regimens, their effectiveness in preventing infections, and the management of infection in established cases is reviewed.

Methods.—A retrospective chart analysis of periprosthetic infections in primary augmentation mammoplasties performed over the past 10 years was conducted. Periprosthetic infection was determined by the presence of pain, swelling, redness, and discharge. Each breast was taken as an individual unit in 1,628 patients, and data for 3,256 breasts were analyzed. The patients had their augmentation in the partial submuscular plane (214 breasts in 107 patients), the subglandular plane (1,548 breasts in 774 patients), and the muscle-splitting biplane (1,494 breasts in 747 patients). All the patients had soft round cohesive gel silicone implants. Of the 3,256 implants, 3,218 were textured, and 38 were smooth surfaced. The patients received antibiotics as a single intravenous dose of cephalosporin (474 breasts in 237 patients), a single intravenous dose plus an oral dose for 24 h (344 breasts in 172 patients), or a single intravenous dose plus an oral course for 5 days (2,438 breasts in 1,219 patients). Infection was recorded as superficial (e.g., wound breakdown, stitch extrusion, stitch abscess) or deep (periprosthetic). The patients with established periprosthetic infections, determined clinically by the presence of pain, discharge, swelling, and redness of the breasts, were managed either conservatively using antibiotics, passive wound drainage, and healing of the wound with secondary intention or by explantation and replacement after 3 to 4 months. In selected cases of periprosthetic infection, the implants were removed after a course of antibiotics and negative swab cultures. The cavity was washed thoroughly with betadine and saline, and new implants were simultaneously reimplanted.

Results.—The incidence of infection was lowest with a single perioperative dose of intravenous antibiotic compared with a combination of intravenous and oral antibiotics. Superficial infection was seen in 38 breasts (all unilateral), with an incidence of 1.2%, and periprosthetic infection was observed in 17 breasts (13 unilateral and 2 bilateral), giving an infection incidence of 0.52% ($p = 0.002$). In patients with a single intravenous dose of antibiotic, superficial and periprosthetic infection was seen in four breasts (0.8%) and no breasts, respectively. The difference was not significant ($p = 0.13$). The patients receiving a single intravenous antibiotic and a 24-h oral antibiotic had superficial and periprosthetic infection rates of 2.3% (8 breasts) and 0.3% (1 breast), respectively, and the difference between the two sub-groups was significantly higher ($p = 0.04$). The patients receiving an intravenous antibiotic and 5 days of oral antibiotics had superficial and periprosthetic infection rates of 1.1% (26 breasts) and 0.65% (14 breasts), respectively. The difference between the two subgroups was not significant ($p = 0.09$). Of the 17 periprosthetic infections in 15 patients (13 unilateral and 2 bilateral), 11 breasts (1 bilateral and 9 unilateral) were treated conservatively using antibiotics, passive drainage, and wound healing with secondary intention. Capsular contracture developed in two of the conservatively treated breasts, requiring capsulotomies with change of implants. Of the six periprosthetic infections in six patients, requiring surgical intervention, two implants were treated using explantation with immediate replacement after a course of antibiotics and a negative culture, and two implants were explanted followed by reimplantation later. One patient had both implants removed after unilateral infection, and no reimplantation was performed. One patient had a bilateral infection. In this case, one implant was explanted and the other was treated conservatively. The patient had bilateral reimplantion 6 months later, and bilateral Baker 4 capsular contracture developed in both breasts within 6 months. No other complications were seen in the patients who underwent surgery.

Conclusion.—A single dose of intravenous antibiotic is adequate for prophylaxis in breast augmentation surgery, and the extra duration of antibiotic cover does not result in reduced superficial or periprosthetic infections. Infection can be managed in more than one way depending on the nature, degree, and extent of infection.

▶ This article provides us with 1 important piece of information regarding the use of antibiotics to prevent infection after augmentation mammoplasty: A single dose of antibiotic is just as good as an initial dose at the time of surgery followed by oral antibiotics for a defined period of time thereafter—probably. In fact, the lowest infection rate was in the group of patients who received only the single dose administration of antibiotic when compared with those receiving an initial dose followed by postoperative oral administration, although the difference between the groups was not statistically significant. I added the term "probably" because there are a number of uncontrolled variables in the study that make it a less-than-optimal scientific exercise and they are as follows: (1) this is a retrospective study, not a prospective study; (2) the patients are not randomized to one or another antibiotic regimen—in fact, we have no way of knowing why a particular regimen was selected for a particular patient; (3) the implants were not all placed in the same location (some were submuscular, some were subglandular, etc); (4) not all the same type of implant was used—most were textured, but a few were smooth-walled; and (5) not all of the implants were made by the same manufacturer. Some more important questions were not even addressed: (1) is antibiotic even necessary? and (2) could the antibiotic be used as wound irrigation instead of systemic administration? However, despite these many concerns, based on this study, I would conclude that oral antibiotic administration in the postoperative period does not enhance the success of augmentation mammoplasty and is therefore not needed.

R. L. Ruberg, MD

Pilot Study of Association of Bacteria on Breast Implants with Capsular Contracture
Del Pozo JL, Tran NV, Petty PM, et al (Mayo Clinic College of Medicine, Rochester, MN)
J Clin Microbiol 47:1333-1337, 2009

Capsular contracture is the most common and frustrating complication in women who have undergone breast implantation. Its cause and, accordingly, treatment and prevention remain to be elucidated fully. The aim of this prospective observational pilot study was to test the hypothesis that the presence of bacteria on breast implants is associated with capsular contracture. We prospectively studied consecutive patients who underwent breast implant removal for reasons other than overt infection at the Mayo Clinic from February through September 2008. Removed breast implants were processed using a vortexing/sonication procedure and then subjected to semiquantitative culture. Twenty-seven of the 45 implants collected were removed due to significant capsular contracture, among which

9 (33%) had ≥20 CFU bacteria/10 ml sonicate fluid; 18 were removed for reasons other than significant capsular contracture, among which 1 (5%) had ≥20 CFU/10 ml sonicate fluid $(P = 0.034)$. *Propionibacterium* species, coagulase-negative staphylococci, and *Corynebacterium* species were the microorganisms isolated. The results of this study demonstrate that there is a significant association between capsular contracture and the presence of bacteria on the implant. The role of these bacteria in the pathogenesis of capsular contracture deserves further study.

▶ The quest to determine the cause (or causes) of capsular contracture around breast implants continues. This article provides us with some preliminary, but revealing, information regarding the currently popular culprit in capsular contracture – biofilms. For years surgeons have clung to the belief that infection must play a significant role in capsular contracture. Unfortunately, most efforts to verify this association have been less than convincing, with data that support the hypothesis only in indirect fashion. Now, use of more sophisticated techniques of collecting bacteria from implants with contracture (eg, sonication, as opposed to simple swabbing) have yielded more useful and more strongly supportive data. Still, the results must be considered preliminary, and only suggestive of, but not definitive for, the role of bacteria in capsular contracture. One would have preferred to find that 100% of the implants from patients with contracture grew bacteria, and 100% of implants without contracture were "sterile." However, only about one-third of the implants with contracture had significant growth. Is this because our methods of documenting infection are still not adequate, or because something else besides, or in addition to, infection is the cause of contracture? More studies are needed, but at least it appears as though we are moving in the right direction on this issue.

R. L. Ruberg, MD

Breastfeeding After Augmentation Mammaplasty with Saline Implants
Cruz NI, Korchin L (Univ of Puerto Rico, San Juan)
Ann Plast Surg 64:530-533, 2010

It has been reported that breastfeeding problems occur in women who have breast implants.

The breastfeeding success of women who had augmentation with saline implants and subsequently had a live birth (n = 107) was compared with that of women of similar age who had hypoplastic breasts and had children before their consultation (n = 105). A self-administered 11-item questionnaire was used to collect data on demographics and breastfeeding success. The information requested included age, weight, height, whether breastfeeding was attempted, if it was successful, and the need to supplement. Additional information requested from the study group included position of breast scar, implant volume, and whether loss of nipple sensation had occurred after the surgery (as judged by the patient).

The groups were not significantly different in age (22 ± 7 vs. 23 ± 5). There was, however, a significant difference ($P < 0.05$) in the breastfeeding success and need to supplement feedings. Successful breastfeeding occurred in 88% of the control and 63% of the study group. A need to supplement breastfeeding occurred in 27% of the control group but increased to 46% in the study group. No significant difference ($P > 0.05$) was found in the breastfeeding experience between periareolar and inframammary approaches. Loss of nipple sensation after augmentation mammaplasty was reported by 2% of both the periareolar and inframammary subgroups.

The success rate of breastfeeding decreases ~25% and the need to supplement breastfeeding increases 19% in young women with hypoplastic breasts after augmentation mammaplasty, irrespective of whether a periareolar or inframammary approach is used.

▶ This study confirms some of the findings, but contradicts others, of previous investigators regarding breastfeeding after augmentation mammoplasty. A common conclusion of a number of studies, including this one, is that women experience less success with breastfeeding after breast augmentation with either saline implants (in this study) or silicone gel implants (several other studies). This study differs from others by concluding that the location of the incision on the breast for implant placement has no influence on the success or failure of postoperative breastfeeding. The authors speculate about factors that may be contributing to their findings, not the least of which may be the conscious decision on the part of postimplant patients to avoid or limit breastfeeding for fear that they will alter the quality of their cosmetic result. These findings reinforce the need to discuss potential postoperative adverse effects on breastfeeding with patients contemplating augmentation mammoplasty.

R. L. Ruberg, MD

A Prospective, Multi-Center Study of Psychosocial Outcomes After Augmentation With Natrelle Silicone-Filled Breast Implants

Murphy DK, Beckstrand M, Sarwer DB (Allergan, Santa Barbara, CA; Univ of Pennsylvania School of Medicine, Philadelphia)
Ann Plast Surg 62:118-121, 2009

Psychosocial outcomes are believed to be a critical factor in determining the success of cosmetic surgery, but little research has focused on measuring these factors in breast augmentation patients. In the multicenter study for FDA approval of Natrelle silicone-filled breast implants, 455 augmentation patients completed paper and pencil measures of body image, self-esteem, and quality of life before implantation and at 1, 2, 4, and 6 years postimplantation. Subjects' satisfaction with their implants was uniformly high throughout the follow-up period, from 99% in the month after implantation to 95% at 6 years. Satisfaction with breast size, shape, and feel improved significantly postimplantation and continued through 6 years. Significant improvements in body image were found postoperatively and remained throughout the study. Improvements in health-related quality of life, however, were not observed. Results provide additional information on patient satisfaction and improvement in body image that typically occur after breast augmentation.

▶ Does breast augmentation work? The answer to this question depends on how one defines success in breast augmentation. Certainly the operation works to increase the size of the breast. But what else does the operation accomplish? This article provides answers to this question with reliable data, and with unique long-term (6-year) follow-up. The patients are overwhelmingly satisfied with the physical aspects of the procedure, with only minimal decline in satisfaction over time. They (not surprisingly) experience long-term improvement in body image. However, patients who expected the procedure to improve their health-related quality of life will be disappointed in the results. Is this operation worth the operative risk? The answer depends on what the patient hopes to accomplish.

R. L. Ruberg, MD

Breast Implant Stability in the Subfascial Plane and the New Shaped Silicone Gel Breast Implants
Sampaio Góes JC (Rua Campos Bicudo, São Paulo, Brazil)
Aesth Plast Surg 34:23-28, 2010

The author presents his experience with breast augmentation using a next-generation, form-stable, anatomically shaped silicone gel breast implant. Rotation is a potential complication for anatomically shaped breast implants. Anatomically shaped saline implants have been reported to have a rotation rate as high as 14%, while lower rotation rates of 1–2.6% for anatomic cohesive gel silicone implants have been reported. Currently, these implants are limited in the United States to US FDA-approved clinical trials. The author reviews the appropriate surgical techniques to prevent rotation when using these devices. A recent innovation, placement of the superior pole of the implant underneath the superficial fascia of the pectoralis major muscle, is described. Primary and secondary breast augmentations in 241 procedures using the Allergan Style 410 implant resulted in a 0.0% rotation rate. Overall, the anatomic form-stable silicone gel breast implants, when placed subfascially, improve common complications such as capsular contracture and implant rupture with improved aesthetic outcomes and patient satisfaction.

▶ Over the past several years there have been a number of reports (mostly from outside of the United States) on breast augmentation with implants placed under the pectoral fascia. The authors of these articles make the case that this implant location combines some of the favorable aspects of both subglandular and submuscular implant placement, while eliminating the disadvantages of each method. The technique in this particular article might be called a dual plane partially subfascial approach. It appears as though the subfascial pocket is not closed at the end of the procedure, making this a fairly simple and quick operation to do. The author claims that implant rotation and skin/muscle rippling, somewhat common problems with submuscular placement, are eliminated entirely. This particular series is done using only the new form-stable type of implant but could conceivably apply to softer implants as well. An important advantage claimed by the author is camouflage of the upper pole of the form-stable implant by something more than just skin and a thin layer of breast tissue, although I am not sure how much extra coverage is really afforded by the pectoral fascia. In this series, the author advocates use of a suction drain for 5 days, but other authors do not find a drain to be needed with this approach, even if the fascial pocket is closed. As with all other new approaches to breast augmentation, long-term studies of this anatomic location and this style of implant are not yet available.

R. L. Ruberg, MD

Long-Term Safety and Effectiveness of Style 410 Highly Cohesive Silicone Breast Implants

Hedén P, Bronz G, Elberg JJ, et al (Akademikliniken, Stockholm, Sweden; Bronz Clinic, Lugano, Switzerland; Rigshospitalet, Copenhagen, Denmark)
Aesthetic Plast Surg 33:430-436, 2009

Background.—In 2006, a single-center Swedish study demonstrated a low rupture rate and high patient satisfaction with the Style 410 shaped, form-stable gel implant. The current study aimed to validate the accuracy of the previously published results across multiple European sites.

Methods.—A total of 163 subjects (~70% had augmentation [$n = 112$], 15% had reconstruction [$n = 25$], and 15% had revision [$n = 26$]) underwent a physical examination followed by breast magnetic resonance imaging (MRI) for rupture detection. These subjects had been implanted for 5 to 11 years with at least one Style 410 shaped gel breast implant before examination. The secondary end points included lactation, reproductive and breast disease history before and after implantation, and quality-of-life measurements and complications after implantation.

Results.—The implant rupture rate was 1.7% a median of 8 years after implantation. Capsular contracture was the most common complication noted at the physical examination, occurring for 5.3% of implants, and there were no cases of grade 4 capsular contracture. The postimplantation rates for lactation and reproductive problems and breast disease were lower than the preimplantation rates. Breast implantation surgery was considered advantageous by 91% of the subjects, demonstrating high patient satisfaction.

Conclusions.—The Style 410 anatomically shaped, form-stable gel breast implants demonstrated long-term safety and effectiveness.

▶ We now have available the data on long-term safety and effectiveness of round silicone gel implants from several different manufacturers used in the United States. These devices have been made available for use by all surgeons in the United States after extensive premarket testing. What we do not have available for general use in the United States is the so-called form-stable implant, which has a highly cohesive gel and is offered in an "anatomic" shape. This study reports the results of a multicenter European study, with long-term follow-up, of this type of implant. The results are consistent with earlier preliminary studies, and confirm the safety, effectiveness, and use of these devices in the hands of many different surgeons. However, it is difficult to compare these results with those of surgeons in the United States, especially with regard to breast augmentation. These European devices are textured surface implants, and most used in the United States are smooth-walled. For reasons that are not completely clear, most European surgeons continue to favor a subglandular position for their implants, whereas most American surgeons use a submuscular (or at least partially submuscular) implant placement. Ultimately, before the form-stable implants are accepted for use in the United States, data relating to the American way of placing implants will probably be necessary, although the likelihood of any significant difference in outcome seems small.

R. L. Ruberg, MD

Capsular Flaps for the Management of Malpositioned Implants After Augmentation Mammoplasty
Yoo G, Lee P-K (The Catholic Univ of Korea, Yeoungdeungpo-gu, Seoul; Apgugeong Avenue Plastic Surgery Clinic, Gangnam-gu, Seoul, Korea)
Aesth Plast Surg 34:111-115, 2010

Among the reasons for reoperation after augmentation mammaplasty is the malpositioned implant, especially a lowered inframammary fold or symmastia, which is difficult to repair. The peri-implant capsule, a physiologic response to a foreign body, is naturally formed and suitable for use as a flap because of its high vascularity. In addition, it is sufficiently tough for suspension of the implant. The authors introduce the idea that the capsular flap is very useful for the correction of symmastia or a lowered inframammary fold. In such situations, the capsular flaps are used to prevent migration of the implant after raising of the inframammary fold or defining of the midline with capsulorrhaphy. This technique successfully corrected the malpositioned implants in this study, and all the patients were satisfied. There was no recurrence of a lowered inframammary fold or symmastia.

These findings suggest that the capsular flap should be considered a safe and effective option for the management of malpositioned implants.

▶ The use of a capsular flap to reinforce capsulorrhaphy appears to be a valuable addition to techniques for correcting implant malposition. I have used capsulorrhaphy combined with appropriate capsulotomy (when needed) to achieve successful implant repositioning in most instances. I initially used absorbable sutures for the capsule closure but had to later reinforce the closure with permanent sutures in a few instances. I think the area that requires the strongest capsule closure is at the inframammary fold area. The weight of the implant in this location will contribute to the re-establishment of the deformity unless the closure of the capsule is completely secure. Others have suggested reinforcing this closure with material such as acellular dermis. But the technique espoused by these authors eliminates the expense for biomaterials and offers an autogenous vascularized source of reinforcement. Development of the flap will potentially increase the time needed to perform the procedure compared with the use of acellular dermis or similar material. But I would expect that the slight increase in operating time would still result in a much lower cost than the use of the biomaterial patch.

R. L. Ruberg, MD

Dynamic Breasts: A Common Complication Following Partial Submuscular Augmentation and its Correction Using the Muscle-Splitting Biplane Technique
Khan UD (Belvedere Private Hospital, London SE2 0GD)
Aesth Plast Surg 33:353-360, 2009

Background.—Dynamic breast deformity following partial submuscular augmentation is not uncommon. The complication is due primarily to the release of the pectoralis and the true incidence of this complication is not known. The submuscular biplane pocket is a new pocket and is used to correct dynamic breasts following augmentation mammaplasty in the partial submuscular plane.

Methods.—After the first submuscular biplane muscle-splitting augmentation mammaplasty in October 2005, the author has performed 58 secondary augmentation mammaplasties for various reasons. Of these, nine patients showed marked dynamic breast deformity following partial submuscular augmentation and the submuscular muscle-splitting biplane was used to correct this complication.

Results.—Good to excellent results were achieved in all patients with complete elimination of the dynamic breast deformity.

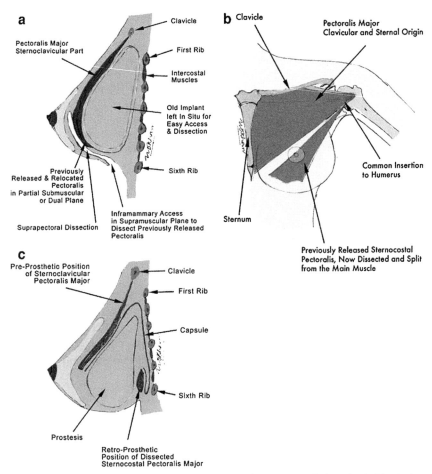

FIGURE 3.—a, Illustration showing supramuscular plane dissection up to the lower level of the nipple-areola complex to free up previously released muscle from the breast parenchyma and skin. At this stage the old implant is left undisturbed to facilitate this maneuver. b, Illustration showing extent of dissected and split muscle in a medial to lateral direction. Muscle remains attached laterally to the rest of the pectoralis at the anterior axillary fold. c, Implant replacement is done in the submuscular biplane and released split muscle has acquired its new retroprosthetic position once the procedure is complete. (Reprinted from Khan UD, Dynamic breasts: a common complication following partial submuscular augmentation and its correction using the muscle-splitting biplane technique. *Aesthetic Plast Surg.* 2009;33:353-360, with permission from Springer Science+Business Media.)

Conclusion.—The submuscular biplane is a new and versatile pocket and is used to correct dynamic breast deformity seen following partial submuscular augmentation mammaplasty (Fig 3 a to c).

▶ Superior displacement of a breast implant (dynamic breast) may occur after release of the pectoralis major muscle in partial submuscular breast augmentation. One option for correction is to replace the implant in a subglandular pocket. However, in patients with saline implants and thin soft tissue coverage in the superior pole, this may not be a good option.

In the previously described submuscular biplane technique,[1] the pectoralis major muscle lies in front of the implant in the upper part of the pocket and behind the implant in the lower part of the pocket. The sternocostal pectoralis fibers, responsible for implant displacement and deformity, are left attached and kept behind the prosthesis in the lower part of the pocket. This submuscular biplane technique prevents dynamic breast deformity.

The use of this technique (Fig 3) adds another option in correcting dynamic breasts in patients where replacement to a subglandular position is not possible.

K. A. Gutowski, MD

Reference

1. Khan UD. Muscle splitting biplane breast augmentation. *Aesthetic Plast Surg.* 2007;31:353-358.

Multisite Analysis of 177 Consecutive Primary Breast Augmentations: Predictors for Reoperation

McCafferty LR, Casas LA, Stinnett SS, et al (Univ of Pittsburgh School of Medicine, Pittsburgh, PA; Northwestern Univ Feinberg School of Medicine, Evanston, IL; Duke Univ School of Medicine, Durham, NC; et al)
Aesthetic Surg J 29:213-220, 2009

Background.—Plastic surgeons and manufacturers of breast implants have been examining the complication and reoperation rates of primary breast augmentations for more than 18 years. The seemingly high rates reported by the manufacturers to the United States Food and Drug Administration (FDA) were the impetus for this multicenter study.

Objective.—This paper reports on data pooled from three plastic surgery practices that were geographically distributed across the United States and examines the reoperation rate, time to reoperation, the reason for reoperation, and specific complications in 177 consecutive primary breast augmentation patients. These data are statistically compared to the manufacturers' 2005 and 2008 FDA data. In addition, the significance of selected variables from our data are examined as predictors for reoperation.

Methods.—Data were retrospectively collected from 177 consecutive primary breast augmentations performed between 2001 and 2004 from three surgical practices. Direct physician-to-patient follow-up periods ranged from 12 to 58 months, with 100% of patients having at least one year of follow-up. Each practice extracted chart data on variables and complications, including reoperations. These data were independently collated and sent to an independent biostatistician for analysis.

Results.—Our three year Kaplan–Meier (KM) reoperation rate (8%) and capsular contracture rate (2%) were both lower than the manufacturers' KM 3-year rates for reoperation (13%-21%) and capsular contracture (8.2%-9%). Logistic regression identified only simultaneous mastopexy and preexisting ptosis as predictors of reoperation.

▶ This study is valuable for a number of reasons. First of all, it reaffirms several important pieces of information about breast augmentation: (1) the likelihood of reoperation is significantly higher when breast augmentation is combined with mastopexy, and (2) the presence of ptosis raises the reoperation rate—and the greater the degree of ptosis, the higher the chances of reoperation. Secondly, it provides us with some hope that the implant manufacturer's previously reported reoperation rate of 13% to 21% for breast augmentation can be reduced in the hands of experienced surgeons. The authors also report a reduction in capsular contracture, but one has to have some degree of skepticism about this claim because of the great variability and inconsistency in interpretation of the degree of capsular contracture. Finally, the fact that a significant number of patients still request surgical size changes within the first year after operation, despite careful preoperative evaluation and counseling, is disturbing. It is important to note that this is a relatively small series of patients, and more data, including rates of specific complications, could be gleaned from a much larger study.

R. L. Ruberg, MD

Psychological Characteristics of Danish Women with Cosmetic Breast Implants
Lipworth L, Kjøller K, Hölmich LR, et al (International Epidemiology Inst, Rockville, MD; Inst of Cancer Epidemiology, Denmark; et al)
Ann Plast Surg 63:11-14, 2009

An excess of suicide among women with cosmetic breast implants compared with controls has consistently been reported in epidemiologic studies. We have evaluated psychological characteristics among 423 Danish women with cosmetic breast implants, compared with 414 controls. Odds ratios (OR) with 95% confidence intervals (CI) for self-reported psychological symptoms were calculated using multiple logistic regression. Substantial excesses of all studied symptoms before implant surgery were reported among women with breast implants compared with women with other cosmetic surgery, whereas ORs for virtually all symptoms occurring after surgery were close to or below 1.0. In particular, ORs for treatment for depression, cognitive/depressive symptoms, and depression/low spirit before surgery were 4.6 (95% CI = 2.1–10.0), 3.9 (95% CI = 1.9–7.8), and 2.5 (95% CI = 1.1–5.5), respectively. In contrast, the corresponding ORs for these 3 psychological symptoms after surgery were 0.9 (95% CI = 0.6–1.4), 1.0 (95% CI = 0.7–1.5), and 1.0 (95% CI = 0.6–1.5), respectively. In conclusion, women with cosmetic breast implants reported preoperative psychological symptoms indicative of depressive disorders substantially more frequently than women with other cosmetic surgery. Future studies using standardized, validated psychiatric assessment tools are needed to determine whether this can explain the higher risk for suicide among a subset of women seeking cosmetic breast implants.

▶ The observation that women who undergo augmentation mammaplasty have a higher rate of suicide than both the normal population and women undergoing other types of cosmetic surgery is consistent and troubling. Therefore, plastic surgeons are motivated to prevent the conclusion (not in the plastic surgical literature, but in lay publications and discussions) that something in the implant, or some aspect of the operation itself, is the cause of this suicide risk. The more information we know about the psychologic characteristics of the patients undergoing breast augmentation, the more we can counter this conclusion and understand more fully the various factors which may contribute to this disturbing finding. This article contributes useful data about the presurgical psychological characteristics of these patients. As surgeons, we must understand that patients undergoing breast augmentation, as a group, are indeed different from other women having cosmetic surgery, and could therefore be expected to behave differently than others after surgery. The observation does not mean that the surgery shouldn't be done—it only suggests that surgeons be more cautious with individuals requesting this procedure. Exactly what to do to prevent the suicide problem is not addressed in this study, and clearly needs more investigation.

R. L. Ruberg, MD

Effect of Verapamil on Reduction of Peri-implant Capsular Thickness

Benlier E, Unal Y, Usta U, et al (Med Faculty of Trakya Univ, Edirne, Turkey)
Aesthetic Plast Surg 33:570-575, 2009

Silicone is a material commonly used in reconstructive and aesthetic surgery, but capsular formation is a very frequent complication of silicone implants. This study aimed to investigate whether verapamil, a calcium-channel blocker, can reduce the thickness of the peri-implant capsule in rats when it is instilled into the subcutaneous pockets. For this study, 60 female Wistar albino rats were used, and cubes of silicone blocks (10 × 10 × 5 mm) were crafted. The rats were divided into five groups of 12 each, and the groups were distinguished according to the use of silicone and artificially created hematoma relevant to administration of a single dose of 5 mg verapamil (Isoptin). The control group was left without silicone. In two of the four silicone groups, hematoma was artificially created around the silicone by a 1-ml injection of blood. The implants were removed 6 months later, and capsulectomy was performed. Under light microscopic examination, no severe inflammation was observed in any of the capsule tissues. Additionally, the thickness of the capsule was measured and found to be significantly reduced statistically in all the verapamil-treated groups, including the groups with the artificially created hematoma. In conclusion, based on the statistically significant data obtained in this study, subcutaneous verapamil administration may be a useful adjunct for preventing formation of capsular contracture after silicone implantations. This preliminary work in rats should be confirmed with larger mammals before carefully controlled clinical trials are considered.

▶ Verapamil, a calcium channel blocker, has been used to dissolve plaques in Peyronie's disease[1] as well as to alter the shape of fibroblasts and increase the production of collagenase in burn patients.[2] Use of verapamil to reduce/ ameliorate capsular contracture caused by silicone implantation is intriguing, and in this well-conducted study in a rat model the authors have demonstrated that instillation of 5 mg of verapamil at the time of silicone implantation does significantly reduce the thickness of the capsule 6 months after implantation, even when an artificial hematoma has been created in the pocket. Obviously, further studies will be necessary to confirm that calcium channel blockers do actually reduce the incidence of capsular contracture as opposed to just reducing capsular thickness. Also, it will be necessary to document these changes in larger mammals and ultimately in human beings.

S. H. Miller, MD, MPH

References

1. Rehman J, Benet A, Medman A. Use of intralesional verapamil to dissolve Peyronie's disease plaque: a long term single-blind study. *Urology.* 1998;51: 620-626.
2. Doong H, Dissanayake S, Gowrishanker TR, LaBabera MC, Lee RC. Calcium antagonists alter cell shape and induce protocollagenase synthesis in keloid and normal human fibroblasts. *J Burn Care Rehbil.* 1996;17:497-514.

Capsular Contracture and Possible Implant Rupture: Is Magnetic Resonance Imaging Useful?
Paetau AA, McLaughlin SA, McNeil RB, et al (Mayo Clinic, Jacksonville, FL; Vanderbilt Med Ctr, Nashville, TN)
Plast Reconstr Surg 125:830-835, 2010

Background.—Currently, magnetic resonance imaging is considered the accepted standard to evaluate breast implant integrity.

Methods.—To evaluate its utility in diagnosing ruptured silicone implants in the setting of capsular contracture and to correlate the preoperative assessment of implant integrity with or without magnetic resonance imaging with operative findings, 319 capsulectomies (171 patients with capsular contractures) were retrospectively reviewed. Preoperative magnetic resonance imaging was done on 160 implants, whereas the remaining 159 were evaluated using only physical examination and/or mammography. Postoperative results were analyzed to determine the sensitivity, specificity, and accuracy of preoperative magnetic resonance imaging in comparison with clinical and/or mammography evaluation alone.

Results.—Although occasionally valuable, overall, preoperative magnetic resonance imaging was no more accurate than clinical evaluation with or without mammography in predicting implant status: magnetic resonance imaging 124 of 160 (78 percent) and clinical 121 of 159 (76 percent; $p = 0.77$).

Conclusions.—In the setting of capsular contracture, physical examination with or without mammogram is as accurate as magnetic resonance imaging in determining implant integrity. Although magnetic resonance imaging is a sensitive diagnostic tool, in symptomatic patients with capsular contracture, it cannot be viewed as infallible.

▶ At first glance this article would appear to say that MRI works for, but is not needed for, the diagnosis of ruptured silicone gel breast implants. But it is important to focus on the specific context in which this principle can be applied. The data are in reference only to the situation in which the patient has established capsular contracture, especially with symptoms. The study concludes that the MRI, in that circumstance, is not of any real benefit. And the patient probably already has requested surgery (although the study does not provide us with that information), so performance of an MRI just to confirm the diagnosis is indeed a waste of both time and money. However, a number of questions still remain. Some of the patients in this study had no capsular contracture at all (12%-14%). Did these women simply want surgery to change the size of their implants? In that case, the presence or absence of rupture is irrelevant, and an MRI would again be superfluous. And what about asymptomatic patients who are just having MRI in accordance with the current Food and Drug Administration (FDA) recommendations? How many of those women will be found to have occult rupture (ie, no symptoms and no physical findings)? It would seem as though this is indeed the place where MRI would be of great value, but the study is not designed to address this important question.

R. L. Ruberg, MD

Intrapulmonary and Cutaneous Siliconomas after Silent Silicone Breast Implant Failure
Dragu A, Theegarten D, Bach AD, et al (Univ of Erlangen-Nürnberg, Germany; Univ of Duisburg-Essen, Germany; et al)
Breast J 15:496-499, 2009

Since the implementation and use of silicone implants in breast surgery the risks are published and discussed. Especially, the incidence of late silicone implant rupture and its potential risk to induce local siliconomas are still under discussion and not sufficiently evaluated. So far literature data offer no information of intrapulmonal or peripheral located cutaneous siliconomas because of systemic migration of silicone after breast augmentation. In light of silicones checkered history, and given the large and growing number of women who choose to undergo breast augmentation surgery each year, the presented clinical findings in our study are likely to be of interest to medical professionals, producers, and consumers alike. We present six female patients with an average age of 55 (±5) years with bilateral rupture of silicone implants after breast augmentation for aesthetic reasons. The average time after operation was 18 (±6) years. In five patients, we identified peripheral located cutaneous siliconomas and one patient suffered from an intrapulmonal siliconoma. The diagnosis of bilateral rupture of the silicone implants was performed preoperatively by MRI-scans. All five peripheral cutaneous siliconomas and the intrapulmonal siliconoma were validated by histopathologic analysis. Six female patients suffered from bilateral rupture of silicone implants after breast augmentation. In five patients, we identified peripheral located cutaneous siliconomas which were surgically excised. One patient suffered from an intrapulmonal siliconoma. In this unique case a lobectomy with resection of the pulmonal segment 10 had to be performed. Clinical findings of peripheral cutaneous and even intrapulmonary siliconomas after bilateral rupture of silicone breast implants indicate a systemic hematogen or lymphatic pathway of silicone. These findings suggest that it is mandatory to inform the patient about the potential risk of local siliconomas, but also about the potential risk of peripheral cutaneous or even intrapulmonary siliconomas caused by systemic hematogen or lymphatic pathways of silicone after silent implant failure.

▶ This article is important because it is published in a journal which will likely reach far beyond the plastic surgery community and could have widespread repercussions for those of us who regularly use silicone gel breast implants for either cosmetic or reconstructive purposes. Certainly this phenomenon has been reported before, but this review shows perhaps the largest number of collected cases with careful documentation of history, physical findings, and pathology. Therefore, we must acknowledge to our patients that implant rupture has the potential to result not only in local siliconomas (which I have seen), but also in distant lesions (which I personally have never seen). And we must be prepared to face criticism once again from the opponents of the use of silicone gel breast implants as a result of this study and its attendant publicity. However, besides the useful information that is in the article, there is a great deal of potentially useful information which is not. We can't know for sure which types and which manufacturers' implants may be predisposed to this phenomenon. We don't know the denominator—that is, the total number of women who received implants. This probably is a very rare phenomenon, but we can't give any statistics which show exactly how rare it is. We can't state unequivocally that old implants need to be removed and possibly replaced, although some have certainly suggested this approach. What we do know, and perhaps the real bottom line in this discussion, is that we now can offer the latest generation of silicone implants (the form stable type), which probably have a much lower possibility of rupture with distant migration of silicone. But can we be sure? Time will tell.

R. L. Ruberg, MD

Efficacy of Neopectoral Pocket in Revisionary Breast Surgery
Maxwell GP, Birchenough SA, Gabriel A (Loma Linda Univ Med Ctr, CA; Greenville, SC)
Aesthet Surg J 29:379-385, 2009

Background.—An increasing number of patients present today with volume-depleted breasts from large saline or silicone gel–filled implants most commonly placed under the pectoral muscle. Revisionary (secondary or tertiary) surgeries are performed for late complications of breast augmentation, such as implant extrusion, gel bleed, rupture with extravasation of the gel, saline implant deflation, capsular contracture, palpability, rippling, "double- bubble," "Snoopy breast," symmastia, and implant malposition. Because most patients undergoing revisionary surgery in the past decade presented with subglandular implants, little has been published regarding the treatment of revisionary surgery in patients with subpectoral implants.

Objective.—The authors describe the efficacy of a new technique for the management of late breast augmentation (augmentation mastopexy) complications.

Methods.—A retrospective chart review was conducted of all consecutive patients who underwent revisionary breast surgery with the creation of a neopectoral pocket. Data were collected regarding the presenting complaints, original augmentation date, original implant location, revision date, type of implant used for revision, incision used in revision, length of follow-up, and any ensuing complications.

Results.—There were 198 patients who underwent revisionary surgery with the creation of a neopectoral pocket over a four-year period. Patients' presenting complaints involved concerns related to either capsular contractures or implant malposition. Only three of 198 patients required reoperation for complications.

Conclusions.—The neopectoral pocket is a new type of site change operation. This procedure will address many of the issues seen today in revisionary aesthetic breast surgery for subpectoral implants that are already in place. These are frequently large implants that have displaced medially, inferomedially, inferiorly, or are encapsulated.

▶ Correction of deformities associated with breast implants frequently requires a pocket change procedure of some sort in order to find a location for the implant that has not been previously used in order to get a fresh start on healing around the implant. When the implant is in a subglandular position, the logical step is to relocate the implant under the pectoralis major muscle. But when the implant is already under the muscle (as in the cases presented in this series), a new position for the implant is harder to achieve. These authors solve this problem not by changing the position, but simply by making a new pocket in the same location. An important component of their approach is the preservation of the old capsule, which is managed simply by pocket obliteration. This innovation obviates the need to remove the old capsule, a step that can entail a risk of thoracic injury when the posterior portion of the capsule is dissected away from the chest wall. The authors attribute their successful reduction in capsular contracture in part to the neopectoral pocket and in part to the use of textured surface implants. Unfortunately, they cannot confirm the validity of the latter observation because of insufficient numbers of cases. Future studies should address this issue.

R. L. Ruberg, MD

Difficulties with Subpectoral Augmentation Mammaplasty and Its Correction: The Role of Subglandular Site Change in Revision Aesthetic Breast Surgery
Lesavoy MA, Trussler AP, Dickinson BP (Univ of California, Los Angeles; Univ of Texas Southwestern Med Ctr, Dallas)
Plast Reconstr Surg 125:363-371, 2010

Background.—Difficulties that arise with subpectoral breast implant placement include the following: malpositioning of the implant; improper superior contouring; and unnatural movement with chest muscle contraction. Correction of these deformities is easily achieved by removal of the subpectoral implant, resuspension of the pectoralis major muscle to the chest wall, and reaugmentation with a new implant in the subglandular plane. This study defines a correction modality for the adverse results of subpectoral implant placement in augmentation mammaplasty.

Methods.—Pectoralis major resuspension was performed in 36 patients undergoing revision aesthetic breast surgery from 1995 to 2006. All patients had previously placed subpectoral breast implants performed elsewhere with unwanted movement, malposition, and/or capsular contracture. All patients underwent explantation of the breast implant, modified capsulectomy, pectoralis major resuspension, and reaugmentation of the breast in the subglandular position. In cases of symmastia, medial capsulodesis and sternal bolster sutures were used. Patients were evaluated for resolution of symptoms, satisfaction, and complications.

Results.—Malposition (62 percent), capsular contracture (53 percent), and symmastia (10 percent) were the most common indications for revision, but 100 percent of patients were dissatisfied with abnormal breast movement. The average follow-up time was 20 months. The silicone implants were commonly used, with an average volume change decrease of 27 cc. Unwanted implant movement was eliminated completely (100 percent), symmastia was corrected (100 percent), and capsular contraction was significantly decreased in each respective group. Patient satisfaction with this procedure was high, with a low complication rate.

Conclusions.—Pectoralis major resuspension can be performed successfully in aesthetic breast surgery. It can be applied safely to correct problems of unwanted implant movement, symmastia implant malposition, and capsular contraction. The use of silicone gel implants in a novel tissue plane may be beneficial in this diverse, reoperative patient population.

▶ The authors describe a successful approach to a somewhat unusual breast augmentation complication: unwanted implant movement. To solve this problem, they apply a somewhat unusual solution–conversion of the implant position from a subpectoral to a subglandular location. What makes this solution unusual is that most of the problems that have been reported after breast augmentation are treated by converting from a subglandular to a subpectoral location. In this series, the approach is reversed. The authors identify the muscle (and its previous extent of dissection) as the source of abnormal implant position and movement. Instead of trying to repair the muscle or alter its influence on the implant, they essentially take the muscle out of the equation by restoring the pectoralis to its presurgical location. Some might find the use of a smooth silicone implant in a subglandular location to be problematic, particularly with regard to future capsular contracture. The authors report that this is only a minor problem, but their duration of follow-up is rather limited.

R. L. Ruberg, MD

Augmentation Mammaplasty by Reverse Abdominoplasty (AMBRA)

Zienowicz RJ, Karacaoglu E (Brown Univ School of Medicine, Providence, RI)
Plast Reconstr Surg 124:1662-1672, 2009

Background.—The purpose of this article is to describe a novel technique of providing autologous tissues for breast augmentation and simultaneously rejuvenating the abdomen.

Methods.—Thirty-seven patients underwent augmentation mammaplasty by reverse abdominoplasty (AMBRA) between 1997 and 2006. The upper abdominal pannus present in women whose lower abdomen was typically less aesthetically compromised was harvested as deepithelialized adipofascial flaps, maintaining their connection to and thus blood supply from the attached breast parenchyma. These flaps are transposed subglandularly, creating autologous tissue breast implants, and reverse abdominoplasty accomplishes donor-site closure and aesthetic improvement. If previous surgery or inadequate inframammary fold tissue thickness renders the superior circulation unfavorable, the upper abdominal tissues can be used as advancement flaps vascularly supplied by their attachment to the abdominal skin apron.

Results.—Twenty-three patients (62 percent) had simultaneous mastopexy and 16 (43 percent) had simultaneous panniculectomy. Complications in the superior pedicle group were minimal. In the inferior pedicle group, complications were more extensive because of the premorbidity of this group of patients and the limitations of this technique, where the resuspension of the abdominal wall apron is less facile and generally weaker than closure with superiorly based flaps.

Conclusions.—Augmentation mammaplasty by reverse abdominoplasty is a versatile procedure that in the carefully selected patient can successfully address two aesthetic concerns simultaneously, providing durable autologous tissue that can obviate or enhance the outcome provided by prosthetic implants and rejuvenating the abdomen. It also shows promise as a significant adjunct to the techniques available to the breast reconstructive surgeon.

▶ The authors present a valuable technique for using tissue that would, under other circumstances, be discarded. Although the degree of augmentation achieved in these cases would probably be judged as only moderate, the breast change combined with the abdominal rejuvenation makes the overall result more impressive. Clearly, there are significant forces pulling on the tissues at the upper abdominal site of closure; the authors' carefully detailed closure technique helps to minimize the potential problems of this tight closure. It is important to note that this technique is *not* applicable to most patients seeking abdominoplasty and simultaneous breast augmentation—only those with clearly defined upper abdominal excess tissue and those willing to accept a long upper abdominal scar. In some cases, the authors used both an upper abdominal and a lower abdominal transverse incision. I would worry about tissue viability between these incisions, but the authors assure us that preservation of periumbilical perforators obviates this problem. This same principle of use of ordinarily discarded tissue has been applied on the other side of the body, and going in the opposite direction, when simultaneous belt lipectomy and autologous buttock augmentation are done!

R. L. Ruberg, MD

The influence of cosmetic breast augmentation on the stage distribution and prognosis of women subsequently diagnosed with breast cancer
Xie L, Brisson J, Holowaty EJ, et al (Public Health Agency of Canada, Ottawa, Ontario; Laval Univ, Quebec, Canada; Cancer Care Ontario, Toronto, Canada; et al)
Int J Cancer 126:2182-2190, 2010

This study aimed to determine whether cosmetic breast implants impair the early detection of breast cancer, and adversely influence survival. This analysis derives from a cohort of 24,558 women who received bilateral cosmetic breast implants, and 15,893 women who underwent other plastic surgery procedures at the same practices in Ontario and Quebec, Canada, between 1974 and 1989. Incident cancers and vital status through 1997 were determined by record linkage to the Canadian Cancer Registry and Canadian Mortality Database. The Analyses are based on a total of 182 and 202 incident cases of breast cancer identified among the implant and control groups, respectively. Contingency table analyses were performed to test for differences in the stage distribution of breast cancers between the 2 groups. Potential differences in survival were evaluated using the Kaplan–Meier estimates and Cox proportional hazards models. Women who received breast implants were more likely to have advanced stage breast carcinoma relative to the other plastic surgery patients (crude and adjusted $ps < 0.01$). No statistically significant differences in distributions between the implant and control patients were found for age at diagnosis, tumor size, histological type, period of diagnosis or length of follow-up. The delayed diagnosis in augmented women did not appear to influence the overall prognosis. Breast cancer-specific survival was similar in both groups (hazard ratio $= 1.06$; 95% confidence interval $= 0.65$–1.74). In conclusion, this study suggests that breast implants delay the detection of breast cancer, but there was no statistically significant difference in survival between the breast implant and other plastic surgery groups.

▶ This article does not change what we know about cosmetic breast implants and early detection of breast cancer, but it provides very important reinforcement for previous reports. The specific value is the large number of women included in this study. Previous reports appeared to have statistical validity, but the small number of cancers that were detected led some to question whether there really was a slight difference in survival, which might become evident with larger cohorts of women. Now we can have even more confidence in telling women that cosmetic breast implants do not appear to alter their prognosis if they develop breast cancer. Nevertheless, I think we are also obligated to tell our patients that studies show that if they develop breast cancer, it is likely to be at a more advanced stage than had they not had the implants. Will this deter patients from undergoing the surgery? Based on the popularity of this operation, probably not.

R. L. Ruberg, MD

Cancer and Reconstruction

Private insurance is the strongest predictor of women receiving breast conservation surgery for breast cancer
Moreland A, Zhang Y, Dissanaike S, et al (Texas Tech Univ Health Sciences Ctr, Lubbock)
Am J Surg 198:787-791, 2009

Background.—It is widely accepted that mastectomy and breast-conserving surgery (BCS) with irradiation yield similar results, yet many women continue to receive mastectomy. This study evaluates factors contributing to surgical decision-making in breast cancer. Registry data were obtained on all patients treated at the Southwest Cancer Treatment and Research Center (SWCTRC) between 2002 and 2006. Patient demographics, including age and race, and insurance type, tumor characteristics, surgical procedure performed, lymph node status, stage, adjuvant therapy, and outcome were analyzed against mastectomy versus BCS using bivariate and multivariate analysis.

Results.—There was a higher proportion of uninsured patients in the mastectomy cohort, which also included more patients with later stage disease, larger tumor size, and a higher number of lymph node metastases. The only independent predictors of BCS were fewer lymph node metastases and having insurance. Patients with private insurance were almost 4 times more likely to receive BCS (odds ratio 3.90, 95% confidence interval 1.20–12.67).

Conclusions.—Insurance status is an important predictor determining whether a patient receives BCS or mastectomy for breast cancer.

▶ The study purports to show that an important predictor of whether or not a patient in the cancer registry of the Southwest Cancer Treatment and Research Center undergoes breast conservation surgery versus mastectomy is their insurance status. It was of interest that the data were significant for those with private insurance and tended toward but did not reach significance for those with government-sponsored insurance when compared with those with no insurance. Of course, the patients without insurance had larger tumors, higher numbers of lymph node metastasis, and generally worse prognosis for survival. The limits of this study are fairly obvious in so far as the data from the registry did not capture information about socioeconomic status, education, patient income levels, or the characteristics or preferences of the operating surgeon. Finally, this is a report from a single cancer center with a high proportion of uninsured Hispanic patients. Is it possible that we are seeing not only an effect related to economics but also one due to culture? I am concerned that many of the uninsured suffer from lack of availability of early screening and diagnosis and then face limited choices for therapy. Will these factors change should health care reform become a reality?

S. H. Miller, MD, MPH

Immediate Postmastectomy Reconstruction Is Associated With Improved Breast Cancer-Specific Survival: Evidence and New Challenges From the Surveillance, Epidemiology, and End Results Database
Bezuhly M, Temple C, Sigurdson LJ, et al (Dalhousie Univ, Halifax, Nova Scotia; Univ of Western Ontario, London; Univ of Manitoba, Winnipeg; et al)
Cancer 115:4648-4654, 2009

Background.—Although immediate breast reconstruction is increasingly offered as part of postmastectomy psychosocial rehabilitation, concerns remain that it may delay adjuvant therapy or impair detection of local recurrence. No single population-based study has examined the relationship between immediate breast reconstruction and breast cancer-specific survival.

Methods.—By using data from the US National Cancer Institute's Surveillance, Epidemiology, and End Results (SEER) registries, breast cancer-specific survival was compared for female unilateral mastectomy patients who did or did not undergo immediate breast reconstruction. Cox proportional hazards models were fitted, adjusting for known demographic and disease severity variables and stratifying on reconstruction type (implant or autologous) and age.

Results.—Improved breast cancer-specific survival was observed among all immediate breast reconstruction patients compared with patients who underwent mastectomy alone (hazard ratio [HR] = 0.74; 95% confidence interval [CI], 0.68 to 0.80). Implant reconstruction patients below 50 years of age demonstrated the greatest apparent survival benefit (HR = 0.47; 95% CI 0.28 to 0.80). Similarly, autologous reconstruction was associated with improved cancer-specific survival among patients below the age of 50 (HR = 0.58; 95% CI, 0.42 to 0.80) and between ages 50 to 69 (HR = 0.61; 95% CI, 0.43 to 0.85).

Conclusions.—Immediate breast reconstruction is associated with decreased breast cancer-specific mortality, particularly among younger women. We believe this association is more likely attributable to imbalances in socioeconomic factors and access to care than to inadequate adjustment for tumor characteristics and disease severity. Further research is needed to identify additional prognostic factors responsible for the improved cancer survival among women undergoing immediate postmastectomy reconstruction.

▶ This is a very important population-based study, not because it confirms what most of us would like to believe, which is that breast reconstruction, be it in the form of implant or autologous reconstruction, seems to improve survival, but because evaluated appropriately, it points to issues difficult to control; that socioeconomic and cultural factors[1] are very likely to affect patient outcomes. The authors appropriately point to factors other than socioeconomic/cultural ones which might have produced some of the results they reported, including relatively short median follow-up of only 59 months, comorbidities, and lack of data about patients who did or did not receive adjuvant hormonal or chemotherapy. That being said, it seems clear that limitations in the type of data archived in the Surveillance, Epidemiology, and End Results (SEER) registries, upon which this report is based, suggest that further study, using different techniques such as qualitative structured interviews, might help dissect out some of these socioeconomic/cultural issues. On a more global view, it also points to the potential effects of socioeconomic and cultural issues on access to equivalent health care and patient outcomes.

S. H. Miller, MD, MPH

Reference

1. Maly RC, Liu Y, Kwong E, et al. Breast reconstructive surgery in medically under-served women with breast cancer: the role of physician communication. *Cancer.* 2009;115:4819-4827.

Computer-Based Learning Module Increases Shared Decision Making in Breast Reconstruction

Lee BT, Chen C, Yueh JH, et al (Beth Israel Deaconess Med Ctr, Boston, MA)
Ann Surg Oncol 17:738-743, 2010

Background.—Shared decision making (SDM) combines evidence-based medicine with individual patient preferences. Patients who are actively engaged in their own health care management with their physicians have been shown to experience not only increased compliance, but also higher satisfaction and better outcomes. We hypothesize that a computer-based learning module for breast reconstruction increases patient involvement in the decision-making process.

Materials and Methods.—Women who underwent either immediate or delayed breast reconstruction at an academic teaching hospital from 2004 to 2007 were identified. Patients meeting inclusion criteria were mailed questionnaires on demographics, informational resources, and decision-making processes. Questionnaire results were divided into 2 groups for analysis: patients who received a standard surgeon consultation and patients who were shown a computer-based decision aid in addition to the standard consultation.

Results.—There were 358 women eligible for our study. A total of 255 patients (75.9%) responded to the survey; 168 patients were shown the computer-based decision aid and 87 patients were not. Patients who used the computer-based learning module reported a greater role in choosing the type of reconstruction ($P < .001$). Additionally, these patients reported a greater number of reconstructive options offered to them ($P < .001$) and were more satisfied with the amount of information provided by their reconstructive surgeon ($P = .049$).

Conclusions.—A computer-based learning module allows patients to assimilate information and actively participate in choosing type of breast reconstruction. Use of this educational modality represents a simple and effective way to improve the shared decision-making process.

▶ I applaud the authors for developing a computer-based, patient-oriented model to educate patients about breast reconstruction with the goal of increasing shared decision making and for reporting the results of this preliminary study. The results indicate that the use of the computer program increased shared decision making and led to greater patient satisfaction with the amount of information provided. Still, patients who had the benefit of this educational tool were no more satisfied with their reconstructions than those who were not provided with the learning module, due, no doubt, to the many other factors involved that determine patient satisfaction. It would be very useful to know if the authors had a priori input from patients into the development and design of the educational module. Other issues to consider in future studies include lack of randomization of patients and surgeons; the use of 5 different surgeons (based on preassigned roles), potentially giving different spins on reconstruction during the face to face surgical consultations; and the fact that some patients had an opportunity to use the learning module at home prior to the office visit and others just prior to the surgical consultation.

S. H. Miller, MD, MPH

Video-Assisted Skin-Sparing Breast-Conserving Surgery for Breast Cancer and Immediate Reconstruction with Autologous Tissue
Nakajima H, Fujiwara I, Mizuta N, et al (Kyoto Prefectural Univ of Medicine, Japan)
Ann Surg 249:91-96, 2009

Objective.—To analyze therapeutic results of video-assisted breast-conserving surgery (VA-BCS) for early stage breast cancer.

Background.—VA-BCS for breast cancer has been developed in Japan, and is indicated for breast cancer unaccompanied by skin involvement. The surgical incision is made at an inconspicuous site, followed by skin-sparing partial mastectomy (SSPM) and immediate reconstruction of the breast. This technique affords good cosmetic results. The long-term results are reported herein.

Methods.—VA-BCS was performed on 551 patients. The skin incision was made as a peri-areolar incision or at the midaxillary line. Skin-sparing partial mastectomy was performed using an endoscope and the lifting and tunneling method. Morbidity, curability, and degree of satisfaction with regard to cosmesis were analyzed.

Results.—Skin necrosis in 22 patients (4.0%) and necrosis of fatty tissue-muscle flap in 17 patients (3.1%) were recorded as postoperative complications. No other serious complications were encountered. Local recurrence occurred in 23 patients (4.2%) after a mean follow-up of 38.4 months. Distant-metastasis-free survival rate at 66 months was 100% for Tis, 95.5% for T1, and 90.7% for T2. Overall survival rate was 100% for Tis, 97.3% for T1, and 95.7% for T2. Degree of satisfaction with surgery as investigated by questionnaire was "good" for 76.1% of patients.

Conclusion.—VA-BCS for early stage breast cancer showed no association with increases in local or distant organ recurrence. The technique yielded improved cosmesis and a high degree of patient satisfaction.

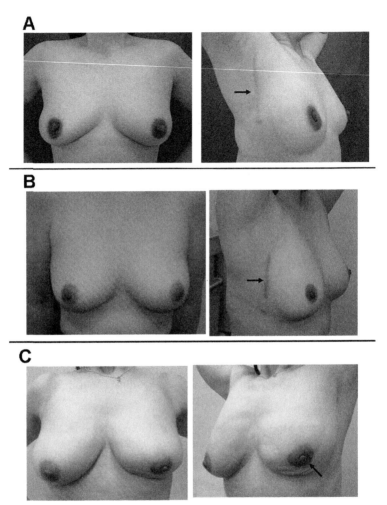

FIGURE 4.—Esthetic results of video-assisted breast-conserving surgery. A, A 44-year-old woman who had right breast cancer (diameter, 3.9 cm) in the upper-outer area and received VA-BCS and reconstruction with LDMF via a midaxillary line incision. Skin incision was invisible from the frontal view as of 3 years after operation. B, A 35-year-old woman who had right breast cancer (diameter, 1.9 cm) in upper-outer area and received VA-BCS and reconstruction with LTF via a midaxillary line incision. Skin incision was invisible from the frontal view as of 2.5 years after operation. C, A 48-year-old woman who had left breast cancer (diameter, 2.2 cm) in the lower-outer area and received VA-BCS and reconstruction with mobilization of the remnant breast gland and fat tissue via peri-areolar incision. Skin incision was inconspicuous as of 1 year after operation. Arrows show skin incision. (Reprinted from Nakajima H, Fujiwara I, Mizuta N, et al. Video-assisted skin-sparing breast-conserving surgery for breast cancer and immediate reconstruction with autologous tissue. *Ann Surg.* 2009;249:91-96.)

Follow-up observation of patients for a longer period is necessary, but VA-BCS seems useful for local treatment of breast cancer (Fig 4).

▶ This is a very large series of endoscopically aided partial breast excisions and reconstructive surgery for early stage breast cancer. The primary goal was to improve cosmesis of skin-sparing mastectomy procedures by making the incision site inconspicuous. Skin incisions for the procedure were either periareolar or axillary. Reconstruction was performed through the same incision by rearranging the local breast tissues or in instances of large tissue resections through the use of a lateral tissue flap or a latissimus dorsi muscle flap. Axillary dissection or sentinel node biopsies were performed through either the axillary incision or a small midaxillary incision when the periareolar incision was chosen for the original resection. The local recurrence and metastasis rates were comparable with those reported for skin-sparing partial mastectomy. Of concern was the relatively large number (20%) of the resections that had tumor demonstrated at the margins of the specimens, but no further resections were performed. Will the low incidence of local recurrence and distant metastasis in this series hold up after a longer, 5-year follow-up? There are a significant number of patients (almost 25% to 30%) who report fair to poor overall cosmetic results. It is not clear whether these resulted from the choice of the incision, the degree of extirpation, the tissues used, or the technique of reconstruction. The one photo of a patient in whom the periareolar approach was used has a good deal of wrinkled skin, and the breast is retracted superiorly when compared with the opposite side. It would be of interest to know if there were differences in patient satisfaction based on the siting of the incision.

S. H. Miller, MD, MPH

Implant Breast Reconstruction After Salvage Mastectomy in Previously Irradiated Patients

Persichetti P, Cagli B, Simone P, et al (Univ of Rome, Italy; et al)
Ann Plast Surg 62:350-354, 2009

The most common surgical approach in case of local tumor recurrence after quadrantectomy and radiotherapy is salvage mastectomy. Breast reconstruction is the subsequent phase of the treatment and the plastic surgeon has to operate on previously irradiated and manipulated tissues. The medical literature highlights that breast reconstruction with tissue expanders is not a pursuable option, considering previous radiotherapy a contraindication. The purpose of this retrospective study is to evaluate the influence of previous radiotherapy on 2-stage breast reconstruction (tissue expander/implant). Only patients with analogous timing of radiation therapy and the same demolitive and reconstructive procedures were recruited. The results of this study prove that, after salvage mastectomy in previously irradiated patients, implant reconstruction is still possible. Further comparative studies are, of course, advisable to draw any conclusion on the possibility to perform implant reconstruction in previously irradiated patients.

▶ This article is selected because of the raw data brought to us by the authors, but not because of their conclusions. In fact, in spite of their statistical analysis, I would come to a different conclusion. The study compares 2 groups of patients with breast cancer who undergo mastectomy followed by tissue expander reconstruction. One group (A) had previous lumpectomy and radiation therapy followed by tumor recurrence; the second group (B) had mastectomy without previous radiation therapy. The incidence of minor complications in both groups was about the same (group B was slightly, but not significantly, higher). The incidence of major complications was 50% in the radiation group and only 16% in the other group. The authors' statistical analysis does not demonstrate significance between these 2 groups. They conclude that there is "no difference," and tissue expander reconstruction is perfectly acceptable in the face of previous radiation. I conclude that they simply didn't have enough patients to show that there really is a striking increase of major complications of tissue expander reconstruction after previous radiation. I still think there is a place for tissue expanders after radiation, but only in very special circumstances: (1) patients who have too many risk factors, preventing more complex (autogenous) reconstruction, and (2) patients who could have more complex surgery but simply refuse. I tell those patients undergoing implant reconstruction after failed lumpectomy and radiation that they should expect a 50% chance of having a major complication. Finally, the article really doesn't address the issue of the quality of the reconstruction after previous radiation. In my experience, I would rate the completed reconstructions as "acceptable" at best. In spite of the conclusions offered by these authors, I would strongly discourage surgeons from performing implant reconstruction after radiation therapy except in the rare circumstances outlined above.

R. L. Ruberg, MD

Transposition of the Malpositioned Nipple-Areola Complex in Breast Reconstruction with Implants
Takayanagi S (Mega Clinic, Higashiyodogawa-ku, Osaka, Japan)
Aesth Plast Surg 34:52-58, 2010

Background.—The goal of breast reconstruction after breast cancer is to obtain symmetrical breasts, including the nipple-areola complex. However, in some cases the nipple-areola complex may not be symmetrical even though a symmetrical breast shape has been created. In such cases the nipple-areola complex has been transpositioned, leaving a scar to close the wound or skin graft in the original position.

Methods.—To treat this problem, skin surrounding the areola is removed and two pedicles are created to bear the nipple-areola complex.

The nipple-areola complex is then moved to the proposed position and the surrounding circular edge of the skin is closed using a purse-string suture.

Results.—The author performed this technique in three nipple-areolae of two patients. All the nipple-areolae were transposed to the proposed position to create symmetrical breasts without any complications.

Conclusion.—This technique can be used when the malpositioned nipple-areola complex is not too far from the proposed position. The nipple-areola complex can be moved without leaving any scar at the original position of the complex.

▶ Moving a malpositioned nipple is often a challenge. The difficulty involves performance of the procedure without leaving a significant scar at the original location of the structure. The problem is most challenging when the nipple needs to be moved down. A scar superior to the nipple is almost always unsightly. The author combines several well-established plastic surgical techniques (subcutaneous pedicle flaps and circumareolar purse-string sutures) to achieve the result. An important adjunct to the procedure is the excision of a crescent of tissue at the new position and grafting of this tissue to fill out a potential indentation at the original site. An alternative to this tissue transplantation might be fat injection to achieve the same purpose. The author cautions that the procedure can be used only when the distance between the old and the proposed new location is not too great—which is defined as 3.5 cm. Even this distance might be too great in some cases. The results shown in 3 cases (2 patients, 3 nipples) are really quite good.

R. L. Ruberg, MD

Evolution of the Pedicled TRAM Flap: A Prospective Study of 500 Consecutive Cases by a Single Surgeon in Asian Patients
Kim EK, Eom JS, Ahn SH, et al (Univ of Ulsan College of Medicine, Seoul, Korea)
Ann Plast Surg 63:378-382, 2009

Although free flap has largely replaced pedicled transverse rectus abdominis musculocutaneous (TRAM) flap, the latter has also evolved by increased understanding of anatomy and physiology. We report the outcomes in 500 consecutive pedicled TRAM in Asian patients performed by a single surgeon, providing incidences of complications and ideas of prevention. Fascia was minimally harvested with full width of muscle. The eighth intercostals nerve was severed and back-cut was made at the lateral belly. Anterior rectus sheath was directly repaired. Breast complication occurred in 24.6% with the most common being skin envelope necrosis. Major flap loss occurred in 1 (0.2%), and the incidence of fat necrosis was 14.2%. Abdominal complication rate was 16.4%, and bulging occurred in 3%. Exercise performance was almost completely restored after 1 year. Pedicled TRAM is still a competitive procedure with overall flap survival rate of 99.8%, yielding consistent results with acceptable complication rates for most patients under experienced hands.

▶ This is a very interesting report of a large series of pedicle transverse rectus abdominis musculocutaneous (TRAM) breast reconstructions in Asian patients performed by a single surgeon at a large university based medical center in Korea. The results described by the author are quite good. While recognizing the benefits of free TRAM flap breast reconstruction, the authors make the point that in their hands and patient population the results are equivalent. Some of the reasons may relate to their patient population and the fact that tissue requirements for breast reconstruction are less than in nonAsian patients. The latter might also account for why they seemed to have fewer abdominal wall complications. They state that they transfer less abdominal fascia than others performing this surgery and postulate that Asian women have thicker and tougher abdominal fascia than do nonAsian women. No evidence is offered to support this contention. It is difficult to be certain whether their good results are based on uncontrollable differences in patient population, which are based on controllable technical factors. Nonetheless the technical suggestions made by these authors are worthy of study by all surgeons performing TRAM flap breast reconstruction.

S. H. Miller, MD, MPH

Upper Cervicothoracic Sympathetic Block Increases Blood Supply of Unipedicled TRAM Flap

Tsoutsos D, Kakagia D, Gravvanis A, et al (Athens General State Hosp "G. Gennimatas", Greece; et al)
Ann Plast Surg 61:247-251, 2008

A prospective clinical study was conducted to evaluate the impact of upper cervicothoracic sympathetic block (CTGB) on blood supply of the unipedicled transverse rectus abdominis musculocutaneous (TRAM) flap. The use of the technique is first reported herein, as a manipulation improving arterial blood flow within the flap in high-risk patients, thus reducing postoperative morbidity. From March 2003 to September 2006, 28 heavy smokers, who underwent delayed breast reconstruction with unipedicled TRAM flap, were included in the study. Intraoperative upper cervicothoracic block (ganglia C5,6,7 and T1,2) was performed in 16 patients (group A), while 12 patients, who did not consent to have the blockade (group B), were the control. Clinical evaluation and thermographic monitoring of skin temperature, using the Thermacam A40 (FLIR systems, Wilsonville, OR), was used in all patients and determined the blood flow within the flap. All patients were monitored for early and late complications. In all group A patients, CTGB resulted in TRAM flap temperature increase within 9.5 to 16 min. Flap temperature elevation was found to be significantly higher ($P < 0.001$) and hospital stay was significantly shorter ($P = 0.004$) in group A patients. No CTGB or TRAM flap complications were recorded in group A patients. However, in group B, major fat necrosis occurred in 2 patients and partial (1/3) flap necrosis in 1 patient. Upper cervicothoracic sympathetic block is a reliable, safe, and useful technique for increasing blood flow within TRAM flaps in high-risk patients, like heavy smokers, and it minimizes postoperative morbidity.

▶ This is an intriguing study using a well-published technique to improve blood flow. While the results do suggest that the adjunctive cervical sympathetic blockade is effective in increasing blood flow to transverse rectus abdominis musculocutaneous (TRAM) pedicle flap reconstructions and reducing ischemic complications in smokers, the control group was self selected by their refusal to accept the adjunctive therapy. However, the 2 groups were similar demographically and with regards to comorbidity. Another limitation to this study was the relatively short follow-up evaluation of those with negative outcomes. Most studies of breast reconstruction in the United States recommend not operating on smokers until they have ceased smoking for at least 3 to 4 weeks before surgery, a few suggest delaying the TRAM flap or supercharging it, or performing a deep inferior epigastric pedicle (DIEP) TRAM reconstruction. The potential benefits of adjunctive cervical sympathetic blockade include: its relative simplicity, low cost, and usefulness in other types of flap reconstructive surgery. It would be very interesting to see this study repeated in a randomized fashion. It would also be of interest to see if an equally effective blockade could be performed by placement of a catheter (for the instillation of local anesthesia bath) directly around the vascular anastomosis. Finally, could a local or cervical sympathetic blockade improve blood flow and reduce complications in free TRAM flaps more effectively and efficiently than supercharging or delaying the flap?

S. H. Miller, MD, MPH

Postoperative analgesia and flap perfusion after pedicled TRAM flap reconstruction – continuous wound instillation with ropivacaine 0.2%. A pilot study
Dagtekin O, Hotz A, Kampe S, et al (Univ of Cologne, Germany)
J Plast Reconstr Aesthet Surg 62:618-625, 2009

Transverse rectus abdominis musculocutaneous (TRAM) flap surgery is a complex procedure characterised by an extensive wound site. We present a pilot study with 17 patients receiving continuous wound instillation with ropivacaine or isotonic saline.

Patients undergoing TRAM flap surgery were included in the study and randomised to the ropi group or the control group. Two catheters were placed subcutaneously before wound site closure. At the end of surgery patients received a single shot dose of 20 ml ropivacaine 0.2% or isotonic saline. After surgery the continuous instillation of ropivacaine or isotonic saline was commenced at an infusion rate of 10 ml/h per catheter. The perfusion of the TRAM flap was measured intraoperatively and postoperatively over 48 h. Pain scores, patient satisfaction, and the quality of recovery score were also assessed postoperatively over 48 h. Ropivacaine plasma levels were quantified 24 and 48 h after start of infusion.

Pain scores at rest and on coughing were lower for the ropi group and reached significance in the first 8 h at rest ($P = 0.007$). Patient satisfaction, quality of recovery score, and adverse events were also comparable between the groups. Patients of the ropi group had bowel movement earlier than the control group ($P = 0.003$). No differences were seen in the flap perfusion. Ropivacaine plasma levels were within therapeutic range.

Our data show a trend that continuous wound instillation of ropivacaine 0.2% increases pain relief after TRAM flap surgery with earlier bowel movement than intravenous opioid patient controlled analgesia (IV-PCA) alone. A dose of 960 mg of ropivacaine daily did not result in toxic plasma concentrations. Ropivacaine 0.2% did not show a vasoconstrictor effect.

▶ Perfusion of continuous long-acting local anesthetics, with either bupivacaine or ropivacaine into the abdomen after complex procedures, transverse rectus abdominis musculocutaneous (TRAM) flaps, abdominoplasties, and component surgery for large ventral hernias can reduce the need for postoperative systemic narcotics and obviate the increased risk, cost, and discomfort attendant on placement of an epidural catheter. I have been quite impressed having had the opportunity recently to see the technique using bupivacaine. Is the dosage and time of treatment reported in this study optimal? Would a larger group of patients demonstrate that patients treated with ropivacaine had in fact a lower consumption of postoperative narcotics?

S. H. Miller, MD, MPH

Perforator Flaps: Recent Experience, Current Trends, and Future Directions Based on 3974 Microsurgical Breast Reconstructions
Massey MF, for the Group for the Advancement of Breast Reconstruction (Med Univ of South Carolina and The Dr. Marga Practice Group, Chicago, IL; et al)
Plast Reconstr Surg 124:737-751, 2009

Perforator flap breast reconstruction is an accepted surgical option for breast cancer patients electing to restore their body image after mastectomy. Since the introduction of the deep inferior epigastric perforator flap, microsurgical techniques have evolved to support a 99 percent success rate for a variety of flaps with donor sites that include the abdomen, buttock, thigh, and trunk. Recent experience highlights the perforator flap as a proven solution for patients who have experienced failed breast implant–based reconstructions or those requiring irradiation. Current trends suggest an application of these techniques in patients previously felt to be unacceptable surgical candidates with a focus on safety, aesthetics, and increased sensitization. Future challenges include the propagation of these reconstructive techniques into the hands of future plastic surgeons with a focus on the development of septocutaneous flaps and vascularized lymph node transfers for the treatment of lymphedema.

▶ This is a very large and quite successful series of microsurgical perforator flap breast reconstructions. The procedures reported in this article were performed in a 12-month period at several community hospital centers in diverse geographic areas. The authors freely admit to a bias for autologous breast reconstruction with perforator flaps. Nonetheless, they do provide a great deal of useful information. Especially interesting was the reliance on and the rationale provided for preoperative MRI or CT assessments or, in at least the case of 1 coauthor, both CT and MRI assessments in all candidates for this type of surgery. Equally valuable is the authors' call for centers of excellence such as the one they have established to recognize their potential adjunctive role in educating future plastic surgeons. I have always believed that all of us who have had the privilege to learn plastic surgery also incur a responsibility to teach future generations and to do so in conjunction with established residency and fellowship training programs.

S. H. Miller, MD, MPH

A new classification system for muscle and nerve preservation in DIEP flap breast reconstruction

Lee BT, Chen C, Nguyen M-D, et al (Beth Israel Deaconess Med Ctr, Boston, MA)
Microsurgery 30:85-90, 2010

The main advantage of deep inferior epigastric perforator (DIEP) flap breast reconstruction is muscle preservation. Perforating vessels, however, display anatomic variability and intraoperative decisions must balance flap perfusion with muscle or nerve sacrifice. Studies that aggregate DIEP flap reconstruction may not accurately reflect the degree of rectus preservation. At Beth Israel Deaconess Medical Center from 2004–2009, 446 DIEP flaps were performed for breast reconstruction. Flaps were divided into three categories: DIEP-1, no muscle or nerve sacrifice (126 flaps); DIEP-2, segmental nerve sacrifice and minimal muscle sacrifice (244 flaps); DIEP-3, perforator harvest from both the medial and lateral row, segmental nerve sacrifice and central muscle sacrifice (76 flaps). Although the rate of abdominal bulge was similar among groups, fat necrosis was significantly higher in DIEP-1 when compared with DIEP-3 flaps (19.8% vs. 9.2%,

$P = 0.049$). We describe a DIEP flap classification system and operative techniques to minimize muscle and nerve sacrifice.

▶ This is a very large retrospective study describing and classifying types of vascular and nerve anatomy found by the authors in their deep inferior epigastric perforator flap (DIEP) breast reconstructions. The key point of the article is that the authors consider nerve preservation important to maintain integrity of the rectus, which remains within the abdominal wall. There was no difference in flap loss, abdominal hernia, or abdominal bulging in the 3 types of DIEP flaps studies. Does that suggest that sacrifice of segmental nerve and some central muscle is not of major importance? The finding of more frequent fat necrosis in single perforator DIEP reconstructions in this study than in reconstructions which contained more perforating vessels is not surprising. What is not clear is whether they correlated fat necrosis with the diameter of the perforating vessel(s) used for the flap. In addition, the authors neither delineate the degree of necrosis nor its effect on the ultimate outcome. Their classification system should prove useful to other breast reconstructive surgeons. As the authors state, it would be very useful to evaluate and to develop a classification system that can document the functional outcome results for their patients. Those interested in keeping abreast of new findings will discover some important new information about the vascular perfusion zones based on work by Rozen et al.[1]

S. H. Miller, MD, MPH

Reference

1. Rozen WM, Ashton MW, LeRoux CM, Wei-Ren P, Corlett RJ. The perforator angiosome: a new concept in the design of deep inferior epigastric artery perforator flaps for breast reconstruction. *Microsurgery.* 2010;30:1-7.

Fat Necrosis in Deep Inferior Epigastric Perforator Flaps: An Ultrasound-Based Review of 202 Cases

Peeters WJ, Nanhekhan L, Van Ongeval C, et al (Univ Hosp Leuven, Belgium; H. Hart Roeselare, Belgium)

Plast Reconstr Surg 124:1754-1758, 2009

Background.—In autologous breast reconstruction after mastectomy, fat necrosis is a rather common complication that may lead to secondary corrective surgery. The understanding of fat necrosis until now has been limited because previous studies were based exclusively on physical examination and used diverse definitions.

Methods.—The authors retrospectively reviewed the incidence of fat necrosis and the correlation of several risk factors in 202 deep inferior epigastric perforator (DIEP) flaps for breast reconstruction. The incidence of fat necrosis was based on both physical examination and ultrasound imaging. The following risk factors were studied: age, smoking, body mass index, timing of reconstruction, and timing and extent of radiation therapy fields.

Results.—Physical examination revealed a palpable mass or nodule in 14 percent of the DIEP flaps (28 of 202). Ultrasound examination added another 21 percent of DIEP flaps (42 of 202) with a firm area of scar tissue (diameter ≥5 mm). The overall ultrasound incidence of fat necrosis in this study was 35 percent (71 of 202). Although the overall ultrasound incidence of fat necrosis was very high, only 7 percent of the DIEP flaps (15 of 202) needed to undergo an extra surgical procedure for removal of this area. In contrast to previous studies, none of the risk factors studied was statistically significant for the occurrence of fat necrosis.

Conclusions.—These results suggest that there is no significant association between previously suspected risk factors and fat necrosis. The overall incidence of fat necrosis, however, is much higher than previously accepted, even though the need for corrective surgery is limited.

▶ This study adds new information to the current debate in breast reconstruction regarding whether the new techniques in breast reconstruction (such as deep inferior epigastric perforator (DIEP) flaps) have a higher incidence of complications (such as fat necrosis or failure) than the older techniques. Unfortunately, while the absence of a control group makes definitive conclusions impossible, the data from a major DIEP center demonstrating a 14% clinically evident presence of fat necrosis with another 21% demonstrable by ultrasound give one pause. Although the authors note that only 7% of the patients needed to have a surgical revision because of this, it is not clear how the other 50% of the patients felt about the palpable nodules remaining in their reconstructed breast and whether they would have preferred a surgical revision. The growth in DIEP flaps has been driven by marketing until now, and further scientific evidence comparing it with other techniques is sorely needed. This article begins this process and hopefully will be followed by further more rigorous studies.

G. C. Gurtner, MD

The value of multidetector-row CT angiography for pre-operative planning of breast reconstruction with deep inferior epigastric arterial perforator flaps
Minqiang X, Lanhua M, Jie L, et al (Plastic Surgery Hosp, Beijing, China; et al)
Br J Radiol 83:40-43, 2010

The deep inferior epigastric artery perforator (DIEP) flap has recently become the first option for breast reconstruction. However, the anatomy of the deep inferior epigastric artery varies greatly from one individual to another and even from one hemiabdomen to the other. An optimal pre-operative evaluation method that adequately maps the underlying vasculature has been lacking. The advent of multidetector-row CT

(MDCT) angiography has proven highly accurate at detailing the vasculature, but no reports have documented its value during pre-operative planning. From December 2006 to May 2008, 22 consecutive patients who underwent MDCT angiography before breast reconstruction using DIEP flaps were selected as the test group, and 22 former patients who did not undergo MDCT before the same procedure were selected as the control group. The two groups were evaluated for the ratio of pre-operative redesign, intra-operative method changes, time spent on flap harvest and the ratio of flap-associated complications. The pre-operative redesign ratio was 22.7% in the test group and 0% in the control group. The intra-operative method change ratio was 0% in the test group and 13.6% in the control group. The mean time spent on flap harvest was 2.8 ± 0.2 h in the test group and 4.4 ± 0.2 h in the control group ($p < 0.05$). The flap complication rate was 1/22 in the test group and 3/22 in the control group ($p = 0.04$). In conclusion, use of MDCT angiography during pre-operative planning promotes a significant reduction in operating time and complication rate.

▶ There are an increasing number of reports promoting the use of various types of radiological preoperative planning for all patients before undergoing breast reconstruction using deep inferior epigastric artery perforator (DIEP) flaps.[1,2] Apparently at this time the gold standard is the CT scan because it is said to be more accurate. It is very difficult to truly evaluate which of these techniques, if any, are really invaluable to the clinical surgeon. All of them require exposure to radiation, all likely increase the global costs involved in breast reconstruction, but the net cost in saved operating room (OR) time complications has not really been studied or reported. While the initial studies have established that the techniques are capable of providing a great deal of anatomic information about the vasculature of the abdominal wall, they have not really been subjected to a random study to establish a cost-benefit analysis of the different radiological techniques. Moreover, this study should also include an arm wherein experienced DIEP surgeons use only Doppler and intraoperative direct evaluation to determine how best to design the DIEP flap.

S. H. Miller, MD, MPH

References

1. Masia J, Larrañaga J, Clavero JA, Vives L, Pons G, Pons JM. The value of the multidetector row congenital tomography for the preoperative planning of deep inferior epigastric artery perforator flap: our experience in 162 cases. *Ann Plast Surg.* 2008;60:29-36.
2. Rozen WM, Stella DC, Bowdoin J, Taylor GI, Ashton MW. Advances in the preoperative planning of deep inferior epigastric artery perforator flaps: magnetic resonance angiography. *Microsurgery.* 2009;29:119-123.

The Pedicled Descending Branch Muscle-Sparing Latissimus Dorsi Flap for Breast Reconstruction

Saint-Cyr M, Nagarkar P, Schaverien M, et al (Univ of Texas Southwestern Med Ctr, Dallas)
Plast Reconstr Surg 123:13-24, 2009

Background.—The pedicled descending branch muscle-sparing latissimus dorsi flap with a transversely oriented skin paddle presents distinct advantages in breast reconstruction, including reduced donor-site morbidity and greater freedom of orientation of the skin paddle. This study reports the anatomical basis, surgical technique, complications, and aesthetic and functional outcomes following use of this flap for breast reconstruction.

Methods.—A retrospective study of 20 patients who underwent breast reconstruction with a pedicled muscle-sparing latissimus dorsi musculocutaneous flap was conducted. Indications for surgery included breast reconstruction following mastectomy, lumpectomy, and irradiation, and for correction of implant-related complications. Case-note review was performed, as was a functional evaluation consisting of a patient questionnaire, a Disabilities of the Arm, Shoulder, and Hand form, postoperative range-of-motion analysis, and instrumented strength testing comparing the operated and nonoperated sides. Aesthetic evaluation of the donor site was conducted by all patients. An anatomical study of 15 flaps harvested from fresh cadavers was performed to determine the location of the bifurcation of the thoracodorsal artery and the course of its descending branch.

Results.—Twenty-four descending branch muscle-sparing latissimus dorsi flaps were harvested. All donor sites were closed primarily, with skin paddle sizes ranging up to 25 × 12 cm. There was one case of minor flap tip necrosis and no instances of seroma. There was no statistically significant difference in strength or range of motion of the shoulder joint when comparing the operated to the nonoperated side. Two patients reported minor functional impact following surgery.

Conclusions.—The pedicled descending branch muscle-sparing latissimus dorsi flap with a transversely orientated skin paddle results in minimal functional deficit of the donor site, absence of seroma, large freedom of orientation of the skin paddle, low rate of flap complications, and a cosmetically acceptable scar.

▶ The authors use of the descending branch of the thoracodorsal artery to develop a muscle sparing transverse oriented flap taken from the region of the latissimus dorsi muscle has proven effective for a group of selected patients undergoing breast reconstruction in this retrospective report of 20 patients. The large majority of patients (16) underwent reconstruction using the flap plus a tissue expander after a skin-sparing mastectomy. The primary advantage of this technique is that sparing the latissimus muscle reduced the incidence of donor site morbidity, specifically, reduction of shoulder mobility and strength, the development of postoperative seroma, and presence of a long vertically oriented or oblique scarring. The major limitations in the use of this flap are its relatively small size, which often requires the use of an implant, and its reduced reliability in patients who have undergone postoperative radiation therapy. It would be of interest to see if the presence of this flap altered the incidence of capsular contracture in those patients who subsequently required radiation.

S. H. Miller, MD, MPH

Circumferential suction-assisted lipectomy for lymphoedema after surgery for breast cancer
Damstra RJ, Voesten HGJM, Klinkert P, et al (Nij Smellinghe Hosp, Drachten, The Netherlands; Tjongerschans Hosp, Heerenveen, The Netherlands; et al)
Br J Surg 96:859-864, 2009

Background.—The incidence of arm lymphoedema after treatment for breast cancer ranges from 1 to 49 per cent. Although most women can be treated by non-operative means with satisfying results, end-stage lymphoedema is often non-responsive to compression, where hypertrophy of adipose tissue limits the outcome value of compression or massage.

Methods.—This was a prospective study of 37 women with unilateral non-pitting lymphoedema. After initial conservative treatment for 2–4 days, circumferential suction-assisted lipectomy was used to remove excess volume. Limb compression was resumed after surgery with short-stretch bandages, followed by flat-knit compression garments.

Results.—The mean preoperative excess arm volume was 1399 ml. The total aspirate volume was 2124 ml with 93 per cent aspirate adipose tissue content. After 12 months, the mean reduction in excess volume was 118 per cent. The percentage reduction in excess volume after 12 months was linearly related to the preoperative excess volume but showed no linear relationship with the duration of lymphoedema or surgeon experience.

Conclusion.—Circumferential lipectomy combined with lifelong compression hose is an effective technique in end-stage lymphoedema after treatment for breast cancer.

▶ This is a small, nonrandomized study from the Netherlands that documents the beneficial effect of liposuction for reduction of lymphedema after surgery for breast cancer. In addition to liposuction, patients were required to wear flat-knit compression garments for 1 year. Those who would not or could not adhere to the latter requirement were not included in this study, thus there is an element of selection bias. Nonetheless, the results at 1 year are quite good (Fig 2 in the original article). Of interest, at 1 year the mean reduction in excess volume, measured using the a water displacement method, was greater than 100%. The authors use of a tourniquet on the upper arm to reduce blood loss during liposuction of the lower arm and hand, and tumescent technique for liposuction of the upper arm, was likely instrumental in resulting in a relatively small blood loss during the procedure. It would be of great interest to follow these patients for longer periods of time to be certain that the effect was long lasting in an effort to determine the differential benefits of liposuction and post-operative compression garment use, in addition to enlarging the numbers of patients studied.

S. H. Miller, MD, MPH

7 Scars and Wound Healing

Scars

Insights into Patient and Clinician Concerns about Scar Appearance: Semiquantitative Structured Surveys
Young VL, Hutchison J (BodyAesthetic Res Ctr, St Louis, MO; Renovo Ltd, Manchester, UK)
Plast Reconstr Surg 124:256-265, 2009

Background.—Few data are available regarding the psychological impact of scars arising from routine elective/aesthetic surgical procedures. To gain insight into both patients' and clinicians' concerns, the authors have undertaken structured semiquantitative surveys of (1) patients who had recently undergone a routine surgical procedure and (2) a cohort of plastic and aesthetic dermatological surgeons.

Methods.—All selected patients had undergone a surgical procedure within 6 to 24 months before survey and had a scar(s) that caused concern. Participants completed a previously validated Self Completion Form that aimed to investigate their concerns. Clinicians were surveyed via telephone interviews using a similar format of questionnaire but with questions tailored to clinicians.

Results.—Ninety-seven patients and 24 clinicians were interviewed. Patients were dissatisfied with scars resulting from surgery, irrespective of gender, age, ethnicity, or geographical location, and 91 percent would value even small improvements in scarring. Patients had scar(s) that they wished were less noticeable over a wide range of body sites (both "visible" and "nonvisible"). Male and female respondents had similar rates of dissatisfaction about their own scars. The survey revealed issues in the communication between patients and clinicians regarding scars; 71 percent of patients felt that they were more concerned than their surgeon about the scar resulting from a recent surgical procedure.

Conclusions.—This preliminary study indicates that patients are highly concerned about scarring following routine surgery, with most patients valuing any improvement in scarring. These data also show that there are disparities in patient-clinician communication regarding expectations following surgery.

▶ This is a very important and rigorously conducted survey of both patient and physician attitudes toward scar formation following elective surgical procedures. The patients underwent elective nonaesthetic procedures and represent a representative cross section across all demographic groups. Surprisingly, over 92 % of the respondents wished that their scars were less noticeable and smoother across all demographic groups. Over 60% of patients from this group were actively unhappy with the scar appearance and this dissatisfaction included both visible and hidden locations. Importantly, over 70 % felt that they were more concerned with their scars than were their surgeons. This study highlights the real unmet need of scar reduction in patients undergoing both aesthetic and nonaesthetic procedures in a variety of disciplines. Historically, the attitude of surgeons has been fatalistic toward scar prevention in the belief that nothing can be done to alter scar formation. However, exciting new approaches to scar reduction are being developed around the world, and it is important that plastic surgeons are leaders in the implementation of these new technologies if they prove to be efficacious. An active role in scar modulation is likely to benefit both practices and patients alike in the years ahead.

G. C. Gurtner, MD

Wound Healing

Serial surgical debridement: A retrospective study on clinical outcomes in chronic lower extremity wounds
Cardinal M, Eisenbud DE, Armstrong DG, et al (Advanced BioHealing, La Jolla, CA; Univ of Arizona College of Medicine, Tucson, et al)
Wound Repair Regen 17:306-311, 2009

This investigation was conducted to determine if a correlation exists between wound healing outcomes and serial debridement in chronic venous leg ulcers (VLUs) and diabetic foot ulcers (DFUs). We retrospectively analyzed the results from two controlled, prospective, randomized pivotal trials of topical wound treatments on 366 VLUs and 310 DFUs over 12 weeks. Weekly wound surface area changes following debridement and 12-week wound closure rates between centers and patients were evaluated. VLUs had a significantly higher median wound surface area reduction following clinical visits with surgical debridement as compared with clinical visits with no surgical debridement (34%, $p = 0.019$). Centers where patients were debrided more frequently were associated with higher rates of wound closure in both clinical studies ($p = 0.007$ VLU, $p = 0.015$ DFU). Debridement frequency per patient was not statistically correlated to higher rates of wound closure; however, there was some minor evidence of a positive benefit of serial debridement in DFUs (odds ratio—2.35, $p = 0.069$). Our results suggest that frequent debridement of DFUs and VLUs may increase wound healing rates and rates of closure, though there is not enough evidence to definitively conclude a significant effect. Future clinical research in wound care should focus on the relationship between serial surgical wound debridement and improved wound healing outcomes as demonstrated in this study.

▶ Most surgeons feel comfortable surgically debriding wounds that appear infected or have stalled in their healing, but many wounds are taken care of by health care professionals for whom debridement is approached with some anxiety. Certainly, we have all seen the chronic wound that has been limped along by another practitioner for months or even years without an adequate debridement, and that rapidly closes once this is done. This study attempts to answer the fundamental question of whether more debridement is better for both venous ulcers and diabetic foot ulcers. Although the study is not definitive, the answer appears to be yes. The study retrospectively analyzes data from 2 completed skin substitute studies and demonstrates that patients healed faster at centers that debrided more frequently and that individual wounds closed more rapidly following a debridement than a typical office visit. Thus, it appears likely that debridement in and of itself is able to accelerate wound closure, although a prospective randomized trial will be needed to definitively prove this. In the meantime, those of us with surgical skills and experience should not be shy about sharply debriding the wounds we see in the clinic or OR.

G. C. Gurtner, MD

Wounds and survival in cancer patients

Maida V, Ennis M, Kuziemsky C, et al (Univ of Toronto, Ontario, Canada; Applied Statistician, Markham, Ontario, Canada; Univ of Ottawa, Canada)
Eur J Cancer 45:3237-3244, 2009

A number of validated and objectively based prognostic models are available for use in cancer care. The quest for additional prognostic factors continues in order to increase their accuracy. To date, none has considered the effect that wounds may contribute to assessing survival. This study serves to demonstrate that certain wound classes affecting cancer patients carry associations with survival. As a prospective observational study, based on a sequential case series of 418 advanced cancer patients, all cutaneous and wound issues were documented and monitored. Three hundred and seventy seven patients were followed until their deaths. Univariate and multivariate survival analyses were performed using hazard ratios (HRs) derived from Cox-proportional hazard models. Forty-four percent of patients presented with at least one wound at referral. Patients with wounds displayed worse overall survival than those without wounds ($p \leq 0.0001$). A significant interaction was seen between pressure ulcers (PU's) and sex ($p = 0.0005$). After controlling for the co-occurrence of wounds, age, sex, Charlson comorbidity index and PPSv2, statistically significant increased risk of death was observed for female patients with

PU's (HR 2.00, $p = 0.0002$), but not for males with PU's (HR 0.83, $p = 0.328$). Malignant wounds were not associated with decreased survival (HR 1.17, $p = 0.285$). The presence of all other wounds was associated with decreased survival (HR 1.48, $p = 0.002$). In summary, the presence of PU's in female cancer patients and 'other' wounds in all cancer patients correlates with reduced survival. Therefore, this data should be incorporated into existing prognostic models or used in conjunction with them in order to enhance prognostic accuracy.

▶ This is an important article that demonstrates in a large series of patients (418 patients) the presence of wounds as a negative prognostic indicator for patients with cancer. In a large palliative care population at a single institution, patients with cancer who had open wounds had a much worse survival rate than patients without wounds and this difference was highly statistically significant ($P < .0001$). The authors' conclusion (which seems reasonable) is that the development of wounds is a sign of global deterioration within the patient, although the possibility exists that the presence of wounds hastens the patients' demise by diverting resources that hold the cancer in check. The only way to really find out whether the wounds are cause or effect is to randomize patients to either aggressive or nonaggressive wound care and see whether mortality is impacted. Subgroup analysis revealed some very interesting findings, including the fact that malignant wounds were the one type of wound that did *not* correlate with mortality, which again suggests that the other wounds are the end product of metabolic decline. Taken together, this work will be useful for those working in high acuity settings where frequent consults are obtained for cutaneous wounds. Although it remains unknown whether aggressive care would make any difference in mortality, at a minimum skin integrity appears to be a valuable metric to assess prognosis in patients with cancer and may be useful in determining when to convert from aggressive oncologic management to more palliative care.

G. C. Gurtner, MD

A randomized, prospective, controlled study of forearm donor site healing when using a vacuum dressing
Chio EG, Agrawal A (Ohio State Univ Med Ctr, Columbus, OH)
Otolaryngol Head Neck Surg 142:174-178, 2010

Objective.—1) Compare skin graft healing of the radial forearm free flap (RFFF) donor site when using a negative pressure dressing (NPD) versus a static pressure dressing (SPD). 2) Examine the association of graft size and medical comorbidities with healing of RFFF donor site.

Study Design.—Randomized, controlled trial.

Setting.—Tertiary care hospital.

Subjects and Methods.—After the study was approved, consenting adults undergoing RFFF for head and neck reconstructions were randomized into two arms: SPD and NPD groups. Fifty-four patients were enrolled from March 2007 to August 2009. Pre- and postoperative data were collected, including medical comorbidities, graft size, and area of graft failure/tendon exposure. Data were collected at two postoperative time points.

Results.—The overall wound complication rate was 38 percent (19/50). Wound complications at the first postoperative visit (44.4% [12/27] SPD and 30.4% [7/23] NPD) were not significantly different between groups ($P = 0.816$). Similarly, wound complications at the second visit (68.8% [11/16] SPD and 80% [12/15] NPD) were not significantly different ($P = 0.55$). Percentage of area of graft failure between the groups also showed no difference (4.5% SPD vs 7.2% NPD, $P = 0.361$). The association of graft size with wound complications was analyzed by dividing the data set into three groups ($<50 \, cm^2$, $51\text{-}100 \, cm^2$, and $>100 \, cm^2$). This difference was not found to be significant ($P = 0.428$). Finally, when evaluating comorbidities, 50 percent (8/16) of subjects with comorbidities experienced complications compared with 32.4 percent (11/34) without comorbidities, also not reaching significance ($P = 0.203$).

Conclusions.—Although an attractive option for wound care, the NPD does not appear to offer a significant improvement over an SPD in healing of the RFFF donor site.

▶ Negative pressure wound therapy (NPWT) has been rapidly adopted into plastic surgery practice. One of the areas that it has been felt to be most useful is in bolstering split thickness skin grafts. Here it is thought that the compressive effect of NPWT leads to better split thickness skin graft take when compared with standard tie-over bolster dressings. However, this belief has never been subjected to intense scrutiny in a controlled clinical trial. In this study, the authors examine the use of NPWT in grafting radial forearm free flap donor sites, certainly one of the most standardized skin graft sites available for this kind of comparison. This randomized controlled trial compared NPWT with petroleum gauze, adaptic and splinting with NPWT. Interestingly, this study showed no difference between the 2 groups, with similar numbers of graft complications in both groups. The high numbers of complications in both groups (30% to 40%) make the likelihood of type II error less likely, though still possible. In the absence of larger studies, the conventional wisdom is that NPWT increase skin grafts must be taken with a grain of salt, especially with the very high costs associated with this technology.

G. C. Gurtner, MD

Effect of Stitch Length on Wound Complications After Closure of Midline Incisions: A Randomized Controlled Trial

Millbourn D, Cengiz Y, Israelsson LA (Sundsvall Hosp, Sweden; Umeå Univ, Sweden)

Arch Surg 144:1056-1059, 2009

Hypothesis.—In midline incisions closed with a single-layer running suture, the rate of wound complications is lower when a suture length to wound length ratio of at least 4 is accomplished with a short stitch length rather than with a long one.

Design.—Prospective randomized controlled trial.

Setting.—Surgical department.

Patients.—Patients operated on through a midline incision.

Intervention.—Wound closure with a short stitch length (ie, placing stitches <10 mm from the wound edge) or a long stitch length.

Main Outcome Measures.—Wound dehiscence, surgical site infection, and incisional hernia.

Results.—In all, 737 patients were randomized: 381 were allocated to a long stitch length and 356, to a short stitch length. Wound dehiscence occurred in 1 patient whose wound was closed with a long stitch length. Surgical site infection occurred in 35 of 343 patients (10.2%) in the long stitch group and in 17 of 326 (5.2%) in the short stitch group ($P = .02$). Incisional hernia was present in 49 of 272 patients (18.0%) in the long stitch group and in 14 of 250 (5.6%) in the short stitch group ($P < .001$). In multivariate analysis, a long stitch length was an independent risk factor for both surgical site infection and incisional hernia.

Conclusion.—In midline incisions closed with a running suture and having a suture length to wound length ratio of at least 4, current recommendations of placing stitches at least 10 mm from the wound edge should be changed to avoid patient suffering and costly wound complications.

Trial Registration.—clinicaltrials.gov Identifier: NCT00508053.

▶ This is a very well-controlled study that could never be performed in the United States yet has substantial relevance for clinical practice in the United States. In this randomized controlled study, the authors demonstrate that taking smaller "bites" in abdominal closure results in lower rates of dehiscence, infection, and herniation than taking larger "bites" of the fascia. This contradicts many years of surgical training at some institutions where surgical trainees are admonished to get a good "bite" of the fascia during abdominal closure. There are several caveats to this study. The first is that the total length of the suture must exceed 4 times the length of the fascial closure. This means that more smaller "bites" need to be taken, which results in a 4-minute longer closure. The highly statistically significant results are likely due to the decreased tissue necrosis seen by taking small "bites." These findings are undoubtedly applicable to the plications commonly performed during abdominoplasty.

Thus, the debate is over. More frequently, smaller "bites" (5-8 mm from the fascial edge) under minimal tension are the right way to close an abdominal fascial incision.

G. C. Gurtner, MD

The Absorbable Dermal Staple Device: A Faster, More Cost-Effective Method for Incisional Closure
Cross KJ, Teo EH, Wong SL, et al (Weill Med College of Cornell Univ, NY; Columbia Univ Med Ctr and College of Physicians and Surgeons, NY)
Plast Reconstr Surg 124:156-162, 2009

Background.—Closure with dermal sutures is time consuming, may increase the risks of inflammation and infection secondary to foreign body reaction, exposes the surgeon to possible needlestick injuries, and has variable cosmetic outcomes depending on each surgeon's technique. The absorbable INSORB dermal stapler is hypothesized to be faster and more cost effective than sutures for dermal layer closures and provides a safer and more consistent result.

Methods.—This is a prospective, randomized, controlled study. Patients undergoing bilateral breast reconstruction with tissue expanders had one incision randomized to dermal closure with absorbable dermal staples. The contralateral side was closed with dermal sutures. During the expansion period, wounds were assessed by a blinded plastic surgeon using the 13-point Vancouver Scar Scale. At the time of implant exchange, both scars were excised and examined for histologic signs of inflammation.

Results.—Eleven patients (22 incisions) were enrolled in the study. The dermal stapler was four times faster than standard suture closure, reducing closure time by 10.5 minutes ($p \leq 0.001$). Overall cost savings with the dermal stapler was $220 per case. In the early postoperative period, the dermal stapler had a higher Vancouver Scar Scale score than sutures because of superior wound eversion, a beneficial characteristic for wound healing. By 4 months postoperatively, no significant difference in scar scores was found between interventions. At 6 months, histologic analysis suggested decreased inflammatory cell invasion of the dermal stapler–closed scar.

Conclusion.—Closure using the absorbable dermal stapler can be performed significantly faster than standard suture closure techniques, allowing for a more cost-effective incisional closure with equivalent cosmetic results.

▶ This is a small, protective, randomized study detailing some of the benefits of using absorbable dermal staples for wound closure in human beings. The authors make a good case for time and cost savings as compared with dermal sutures. Further studies will be needed to look at the effects of these closures in other sites of the body, rates of dehiscence, and rates of infection.

S. H. Miller, MD, MPH

8 Grafts, Flaps, and Microsurgery

Grafts

Resurfacing of colour-mismatched free flaps on the face with split-thickness skin grafts from the scalp
Lannon DA, Novak CB, Neligan PC (Univ of Toronto, Ontario, Canada)
J Plast Reconstr Aesthetic Surg 62:1363-1366, 2009

Free-tissue transfer is commonly used in micro-vascular head and neck reconstruction. In a significant proportion of cases, the reconstruction involves the placement of a conspicuous, colour-mismatched skin paddle on the face. This article presents our experience in resurfacing of free flaps on the face in seven patients, using split-thickness skin grafts harvested from the scalp. All patients had a noticeable improvement in colour

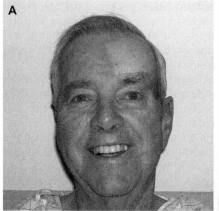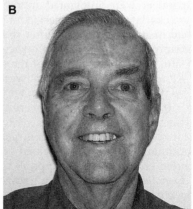

FIGURE 3.—(A) Pre- and (B) eight months post-resurfacing of a parascapular flap on the left forehead in a 72-year-old male. This patient had concomitant debulking of the parascapular flap. (Reprinted from Journal of Plastic, Reconstructive and Aesthetic Surgery, Lannon DA, Novak CB, Neligan PC. Resurfacing of colour-mismatched free flaps on the face with split-thickness skin grafts from the scalp. *J Plast Reconstr Aesthetic Surg*. 2009;62:1363-1366, with permission from British Association of Plastic, Reconstructive and Aesthetic Surgeons.)

match. This relatively minor procedure can significantly improve aesthetic outcome and merits consideration in appropriate patients (Fig 3).

▶ This is a useful bit of information on how to improve the color match of flaps placed on the face from distal donor sites that do not provide a good color match with the adjacent facial skin. I do think the results could be improved further by resurfacing according to the principles of replacing aesthethic facial units. Further improvement could also be gained by breaking up the straight lines, using z- or w-plasties, evident in the reconstructions of several of the patients demonstrated.

S. H. Miller, MD, MPH

Flaps, Experimental and Clinical

Application of Botulinum Toxin Type A in Myocutaneous Flap Expansion

Chenwang D, Shiwei B, Dashan Y, et al (Hebei Med Univ, People's Republic of China; Beijing Hosp, People's Republic of China; Plastic Surgery Hosp, People's Republic of China; et al)
Plast Reconstr Surg 124:1450-1457, 2009

Background.—Although the use of the expanded myocutaneous flap has many advantages, the time course is prolonged. The net gain in surface area during acute expansion is insufficient. In this study, botulinum toxin type A was applied to shorten the flap expansion period while obtaining an adequate surface area that would meet surgical requirements.

Methods.—Seven minipigs were used for the authors' experiments. Two sides of the dorsolumbar section in each pig were divided randomly into the botulinum toxin type A–treated and the saline-treated groups. Two 200-ml expanders were implanted in the submuscular pocket. Inflation began 2 weeks later, and the period of expansion was observed in a double-blind manner. Two weeks after the final inflation, the expansion area was measured, and a 10×6-cm myocutaneous flap was elevated and sutured in situ, and the contraction of the myocutaneous flap was observed.

Results.—Botulinum toxin type A shortened the expansion time by 17 days ($p < 0.001$). The average increment of effective expansion area ($p = 0.009$) and the average recruitment area ($p = 0.001$) in the botulinum toxin type A–treated group were significantly higher than in the saline-treated group. Moreover, contraction in axial length and width of the botulinum toxin type A–treated group was lower than that of the saline-treated group at each time point following transposition ($p < 0.001$).

Conclusions.—Botulinum toxin type A could decrease the resistance to myocutaneous flap expansion, speed up the inflation, increase the expansion area, and reduce the contraction of the myocutaneous flap. It is a safe and convenient method with which to assist myocutaneous flap expansion.

▶ This is an interesting use of botulinum toxin. Certainly, delay of myocutaneous flaps can be worthwhile but at the expense of considerable delay in accomplishing reconstruction. Attempts to speed up this process through the use of more rapid expansion can be painful, increase implant exposure, and result in significant contraction of the expanded tissues once the tissue has been placed in the recipient's site. These randomized, double-blinded studies are quite convincing as to the effects of the toxin versus the saline control. Expansion occurred more quickly and to a greater degree in both the effective and recruited areas and resulted in lesser amounts of postoperative contraction over several time periods in the botulinum-treated areas. I look forward to further reports about this technique and especially its use in human beings. I would also be interested to see whether these results actually hold up if the flap is actually transferred rather than merely inserted back into its original site.

S. H. Miller, MD, MPH

A method of controlled closure: the use of Ligaclips™ in the delayed primary closure of flaps

Hills AJ, Leo K-W, Tan B-K (Singapore General Hosp)
J Plast Reconstr Aesthet Surg 62:e322-e324, 2009

Background and Purposes of the Study.—Achieving primary closure of a flap may not always be possible initially. Current controlled closure techniques exert uniform pressure across a wound, which is unsuitable for a flap, as it can induce ischaemia in vulnerable areas. Using Ligaclips (Ethicon Inc., Somerville, NJ, USA) to secure tissue advancement along mattress sutures offers both the ease of expansion, like running sutures, and the ability to moderate tension in discrete areas, like interrupted sutures. The two cases here highlight variations of how this technique can be applied to close wounds boarded by vulnerable tissues such as flaps. We conclude that the use of Ligaclips in conjunction with mattress sutures in the controlled closure of defects around flaps is simple and fast, enabling greater control over the forces exerted over discrete areas, minimising the risk of compromising vulnerable tissues.

▶ Closure of a donor site can be a problem, particularly in the case of rotation flaps. As with fasciotomies, excessive tension on a donor site closure can lead to flap compromise, wound dehiscence, or in rare cases, ischemia in the distal upper or lower extremity. Leaving the wound open is not a panacea; either the open donor site can be painful or a portal for invasive infection. Moreover, in many cases delayed closure requires a return trip to the OR, which is inconvenient for both surgeon and patient, and leads to a prolonged hospital stay. Thus, there exists a need for a simple and reliable way to perform a delayed primary closure at the bedside. The present report describes a simple and inexpensive way to do this that would be applicable to nearly any clinical setting. The approach is similar to a ratchet mechanism that allows for a relentless slow advance of the sides of the defect to close the wound within 2 weeks. Large monofilament mattress sutures are placed but left untied. At 5 days postoperative these sutures are pulled tighter and ligaclips are placed flush with the skin surface to prevent the suture from sliding back. Over the next 7 to 10 days this process is repeated as the suture is gradually advanced until the wound is closed. The simplicity of this system makes it appealing in settings where expensive closure devices are unavailable.

G. C. Gurtner, MD

Attributes and Shortcomings of Acoustic Doppler Sonography in Identifying Perforators for Flaps from the Lower Extremity

Hallock GG (Sacred Heart Hosp and The Lehigh Valley Hosps, Allentown, PA)
J Reconstr Microsurg 25:377-382, 2009

The preoperative identification of perforators can facilitate the appropriate design of perforator flaps from the lower extremity. Although computed tomographic arteriography can now be considered the gold standard in this regard, this technology is not universally available or inexpensive, with a nonnegligible risk from radiation exposure. An old standby, the ubiquitous acoustic Doppler sonography, still has a role as an alternative, despite perhaps its too high sensitivity and low specificity. Regardless of the modality employed, the efficacious harvest of a perforator flap will still require constant vigilance during its dissection due to anatomic anomalies of the course of these perforators, which is the expected norm.

▶ This is a thoughtful and logical compendium of a single master surgeon's experience with different modalities commonly used to evaluate perforating vessels during microsurgical procedures. The perspective is from a private practice where the latest technology (as well as residents and fellows) is not readily available. The conclusion is that CT angiography (CTA) is probably the most useful because of its ability to evaluate the entire course of a perforator from source vessel to skin. This ability to provide a preoperative road map allows many decisions regarding number and location of perforators to be made preoperatively. Alternative technologies that have been proposed, such as ultrasound and MRI, suffer from either the need for specialized technicians (ultrasound) or poor spatial resolution (MRI) and have not been proved to be widely useful. However, even CTA suffers from requiring the patient to be exposed to ionizing radiation and can be difficult to obtain in the community hospital setting. For these reasons, the hand-held pencil doppler remains the workhorse for perforator flap surgery. Problems with hand-held doppler include the inability to provide anatomic detail and the lack of correlation between the amplitude of the sound and the size of the perforator. Newer technologies that are not covered in this overview but that might be important in the future include orthogonal polarization spectroscopy (OPS) and indocyanine green angiography (ICG), but their full utility remains to be determined.

G. C. Gurtner, MD

Depth of penetration of negative pressure wound therapy into underlying tissues

Murphey GC, Macias BR, Hargens AR (Univ of California, San Diego)
Wound Repair Regen 17:113-117, 2009

Negative pressure wound therapy has become ubiquitous in orthopedic surgery and it is therefore important to understand the physiologic conditions of this therapy. The purpose of this study was to determine the magnitude and depth of negative pressure transmission into underlying muscle tissue in a wound model. We hypothesized that the negative pressure is not transmitted beyond 2 mm into underlying muscle tissue. Using both an isolated muscle and a live animal wound model, we applied open cell foam dressing to the tissue. Using a series of vacuum-assisted closure negative pressure settings (0, -75, -125, -200 mmHg) interstitial fluid pressure was measured in the underlying tissue with a solid-state pressure transducer catheter at 1/10 mm depth intervals. In the ex vivo isolated-muscle model, the effect of negative pressure wound therapy on interstitial fluid pressure was extinguished and not significantly different than controls at a depth <2 mm. In the live animal wound model, the magnitude of interstitial fluid pressures corresponded directly with negative pressure settings ($p < 0.01$) and inversely with depth into muscle ($p < 0.01$). Interstitial fluid pressures were significantly ($p < 0.05$) less than control interstitial fluid pressures (0 mmHg setting) at depths of 0.5, 0.4, and 0.9 mm below the foam/muscle interface when the applied pressures were -75, -125, and -200 mmHg, respectively. Negative pressure wound therapy penetrates no more than 1 mm into rabbit wound tissue at the highest negative pressure setting (-200 mmHg) when using open-cell foam dressing.

▶ This study elegantly answers one of the many questions surrounding negative pressure wound therapy in the clinical setting. There have been concerns raised about the use of negative pressure wound therapy over exposed blood vessels (or other structures such as nerves or visceral structures) because of several case reports documenting near exsanguinating hemorrhage in this situation. The present report attempts to answer whether these incidents were due to transmission of negative pressure to underlying tissues leading to damage or disruption of blood vessels. This experimental study clearly demonstrates that the zone of negative pressure extends only about 1 mm even at the highest settings (-200 mm Hg). At the more commonly used pressures of -75 mm Hg this zone of negative pressure transmission was less than 0.4 mm. This should be reassuring to those who use a negative pressure dressing on a skin graft over a flap and worry about compromising the vascular supply. Whether or not this shallow rim of negative pressure is able to evacuate fluid in bulk from the wound bed is unanswered but is the obvious next step in this important work.

G. C. Gurtner, MD

Treatment of Recalcitrant Air Leaks: The Combined Latissimus Dorsi-Serratus Anterior Flap

Woo E, Tan B-K, Lim C-H (Singapore General Hosp)
Ann Plast Surg 63:188-192, 2009

Pleural space problems after lung resection and persistent air leaks are among the commonest challenges posed to thoracic surgeons. Surgical repair of air leaks are indicated when conventional tube thoracostomy has failed to solve the problem.

We would like to propose the novel application of the combined latissimus dorsi-serratus anterior transposition flap for selected cases of air leaks that are recalcitrant to conventional treatment. We discuss its indications and the surgical technique.

Five patients underwent the procedure between 2004 and 2007. They were male patients aged between 32 and 70 years. Four patients had alveolar-pleural fistulas resulting in persistent air leaks while the fifth patient had, in addition, a space problem following lung volume reduction surgery. All patients had prolonged treatment with chest drains without success.

With the patient in a lateral decubitus position, a lazy-S incision was used to expose the entire latissimus dorsi and the proximal slips of the serratus anterior muscles. They were raised as pedicled flaps and transferred in tandem. The latissimus dorsi was introduced into the pleural cavity via a thoracic window and used to reinforce the fistula repair. The serratus anterior muscle closed the rib window.

In all cases, the lungs reexpanded and chest drains were removed within 5 days post surgery. There were no recurrent air leaks at 1-year follow-up with all patients.

Conservative treatment in all our patients was unsuccessful. The dual flap technique has the advantage of allowing normal ventilation while providing a seal over the alveolar-pleural fistula. The muscle bulk of the latissimus dorsi fills the pleural dead space and the serratus anterior muscle seals the axilla preventing subcutaneous emphysema. There was minimal morbidity associated with the use of this dual muscle flap technique. This technique is an effective treatment option for recalcitrant air leaks.

▶ The authors of this article have described a comprehensive approach to a complicated problem. In effect, they are telling us that the technique they are using to repair one problem (the intrathoracic air leak), namely the transposition of a latissimus dorsi flap through a thoracic window to serve as an internal "patch," creates a second potential problem—the possibility of air leak through the chest wall. So to fix the second problem, a second flap is used immediately to reinforce the chest wall, prevent an external air leak, and permit immediate normal ventilation. The proximity of the 2 muscles used in this technique allows easy access through one incision. The successful outcome in 5 consecutive cases makes this aggressive approach appear to be very reasonable and appropriate.

R. L. Ruberg, MD

Microsurgery

"Lid technique": cyanoacrylate-assisted anastomosis of small-sized vessels
Gürhan Ulusoy M, Kankaya Y, Uysal A, et al (Ankara Training and Res Hosp, Turkey; et al)
J Plast Reconstr Aesthet Surg 62:1205-1209, 2009

This paper presents the details of an experimental study of arterial anastomosis, combining suture with the cyanoacrylate tissue adhesive. At the distal end of the vessel, two parallel incisions were made, 180° apart from each other, and two sutures were placed passing from the proximal end to exit from the most distal part of the longitudinal incisions. The tissue adhesive was then applied to the proximal vessel, and the full-thickness vascular 'lid' flap was closed over it on anterior and posterior surfaces. Eighty anastomoses were carried out at the left and the right femoral arteries of 40 Wistar rats. For all of the animals, conventional end-to-end anastomosis was carried out on the left side, and the lid technique was used on the right side. There was no statistically significant difference between the patency rates of the groups (two non-patent in control and two in the study group) ($P > 0.05$), whereas significantly reduced operation time (mean 16.2 and 10.7 min in control and study groups, respectively) ($P < 0.0001$) and bleeding time (median 1.5 and 0.5 min in control and study groups, respectively) ($P < 0.0001$) were documented in the study group. Histopathological evaluation of both the patent and non-patent vessels at day 21 revealed no signs of tissue toxicity or intraluminal adhesive leakage. In view of these data, it was concluded that the technique provides an effective and simple method for end-to-end anastomosis of small-calibre arteries.

▶ Vascular anastomosis has not changed since it was first described by Alexis Carrel over a hundred years ago. This technique (for which Carrel won the Nobel Prize in 1914) forms the basis for cardiac, vascular, transplant, and microsurgery, and has impacted millions of lives. However, the suture technique for vascular anastomosis has drawbacks, including the increasing technical challenges in smaller and diseased vessels, and the damage inflicted to the vascular wall by the passage of the needle itself. This trauma can lead to fibrosis, foreign body reaction, and late anastomotic failure. For these reasons, surgeons have been searching for an alternative to sutured techniques for several decades. This article describes one such attempt, using essentially a modified sleeve technique in which the outer sleeve is split longitudinally to allow the halves to be folded back and a cyanoacrylate adhesive used to approximate the vessel walls. This is a clever technique, but still requires 2 stay sutures (as opposed to the 6 in the controls) and according to the report elicits an intraluminal foreign body reaction, probably due to exposure of the adventitia to the blood flow. Thus, it is probably not the ultimate alternative to Alexis Carrel's technique, but may be one step on the pathway to a better anastomosis.

G. C. Gurtner, MD

The Use of Ultrasonic Shears for the Harvest of Perforator Free Flaps

Ahmed S, Sidell D, Blackwell KE, et al (Univ of California, Los Angeles; David Geffen School of Medicine, Los Angeles, CA)
Arch Facial Plast Surg 11:343-346, 2009

A retrospective chart review was performed at a university medical center to evaluate the use of ultrasonic shears for the harvest of perforator free flaps over an 18-month period. The anterolateral thigh (ALT) was the perforator free flap site selected for the study. The site of origin and the number of musculocutaneous perforator vessels that were dissected using ultrasonic shears were recorded, and ALT flap viability and wound-healing complications were evaluated to assess safety. Seventeen patients underwent harvest of ALT perforator free flaps. Successful dissection of musculocutaneous perforators was achieved in 96% (27 of 28) of the descending branch perforators and in 100% (9 of 9) of the transverse branch perforators. Flap viability was 100% (17 of 17). We found that ultrasonic shears were effective and safe to use for harvesting perforator free flaps. According to these preliminary findings, the use of ultrasonic shears appears promising, yet further prospective analysis is needed.

▶ Perforator flaps, although currently in vogue, in reconstructive microsurgery can be very tedious and time-consuming procedures. This is certainly the case for anterolateral thigh free flaps whose perforators can take an unpredictable intramuscular course, potentially for very long distances. The numerous muscular side branches of these perforators need to be either cauterized with bipolar electrocautery or clipped with fine microclips. Both of these maneuvers pose some peril to the flimsy and small caliber perforator and must be performed with caution—hence the tedium.

The authors (who disclose no financial conflicts) have provided an initial report of their experience with a tool that potentially can lessen this burden. Ultrasonic shears (Ethicon) function similarly to regular scissors but have high-frequency ultrasonic tips that are able to coagulate small vessels with a minimum of thermal damage. They used these shears to harvest 17 anterolateral thigh flaps and were impressed with the ease of use of the technology. All the flaps were successful but they were unable to determine whether there were time savings because of the small number of cases. One potential downside was the cost of the hand piece ($500), but this is undoubtedly a tool that many of us who do perforator flaps will explore to decrease the time commitment to these tedious cases.

G. C. Gurtner, MD

Early Experience with Fluorescent Angiography in Free-Tissue Transfer Reconstruction
Pestana IA, Coan B, Erdmann D, et al (Duke Univ Med Ctr, Durham, NC)
Plast Reconstr Surg 123:1239-1244, 2009

Background.—Soft-tissue and bony reconstruction with free-tissue transfer is one of the most versatile tools available to the reconstructive surgeon. Determination of flap perfusion and early detection of vascular compromise with prompt correction remain critical in free-tissue transfer success. The aim of this report is to describe the utility of laser-assisted indocyanine green fluorescent dye angiography in free-tissue transfer reconstruction.

Methods.—From October of 2007 to March of 2008, 27 nonrandomized, nonconsecutive patients underwent surgical free flaps in conjunction with intraoperative Novadaq SPY fluorescent angiography.

Results.—Twenty-seven patients underwent 29 free-tissue transfers. There was one partial flap loss in this group requiring operative revision. No complications attributable to indocyanine green fluorescent dye administration were noted. Imaging procedures (including dye administration) added minimal additional time to the operative time and anesthesia, and assisted in intraoperative decision-making.

Conclusions.—Novadaq's SPY fluorescent angiography system provides simple and efficient intraoperative real-time surface angiographic imaging. This technology places control of vascular anastomosis evaluation and flap perfusion in the hands of the surgeon intraoperatively in a visual manner that is easy to use and is helpful in surgical decision-making.

▶ Maintaining perfusion to the skin and soft tissues is central to nearly every plastic or aesthetic surgical procedure. The major complications that occur, such as retroauricular necrosis in a facelift or partial flap failure only in the place you need it, all relate to the failure of perfusion to maintain tissue viability. This article presents early experience with laser-assisted indocyanine imaging in the evaluation of both the microcirculation and macrocirculation in a wide variety of clinical settings. This technology allows real time assessment of vascular competency in the operating room where decisions can be made to correct problems before they lead to tissue necrosis. The authors found the technology to be simple, safe, and did not add to the overall operative time. Indocyanine green imaging was helpful in identifying perforators, determining the dimensions of a skin paddle supported by a vascular pedicle or perforator, and confirming the patency of microvascular anastomoses immediately. They conclude this new tool warrants further examination to confirm its ability to prevent postoperative complications in a variety of settings.

G. C. Gurtner, MD

Simultaneous Replantation of Both Lower Legs in a Child: 23 Years Later

Datiashvili RO (UMDNJ–New Jersey Med School, Newark)
J Reconstr Microsurg 25:323-329, 2009

Function is the single most important determinant in the assessment of the results of extremity replantations. Accordingly, the indications for extremity replantations are based on the prediction of sustained satisfactory functional outcome. There are limited reports in the literature regarding replantations of major segments of lower extremities and, particularly, long-term results of those surgeries. However, this analysis is extremely important in refinement of indications for major limb replantations. In this article, evaluation of a patient 23 years after simultaneous replantation of both lower legs is presented.

▶ This is an important anecdotal report of the long-term functional outcome of lower extremity replantation. Despite the initial enthusiasm for lower extremity replantation in the early days of microvascular surgery, many major centers have moved away from aggressively replanting legs and feet. The reasons for this vary, usually include the perception that functional outcomes are terrible and that because of the large mass of the replanted tissue, systemic complications (such as hyperkalemia or acidosis) could threaten the life of the patient. Although this report does not address the question of morbidity and mortality, it does provide a unique window into the functional outcomes that are possible in highly selected cases. It describes follow-up after 23 years of a woman who had both legs amputated (by a farm machine) at the age of 2 years old. Both legs were replanted in a 14-hour operation. The patient did well but required some minor boney work and Ilizarov bone lengthening for leg length discrepancy. At follow-up after 23 years she was able to work as a home attendant, dance, walk, and run with only minor sensory abnormalities. She had no pain or hypersensitivity. This strikingly good result is undoubtedly superior to bilateral lower extremity prostheses. For this reason, this report should make us think twice before judging an injury to be not replantable. This is especially true for the pediatric population, who possess remarkable regenerative capacity.

G. C. Gurtner, MD

Penile Reconstruction: Is the Radial Forearm Flap Really the Standard Technique?

Monstrey S, Hoebeke P, Selvaggi G, et al (Ghent Univ Hosp, Belgium)
Plast Reconstr Surg 124:510-518, 2009

Background.—The ideal goals in penile reconstruction are well described, but the multitude of flaps used for phalloplasty only demonstrates that none of these techniques is considered ideal. Still, the radial forearm flap is the most frequently used flap and universally considered as the standard technique.

Methods.—In this article, the authors describe the largest series to date of 287 radial forearm phalloplasties performed by the same surgical team. Many different outcome parameters have been described separately in previously published articles, but the main purpose of this review is to critically evaluate to what degree this supposed standard technique has been able to meet the ideal goals in penile reconstruction.

Results.—Outcome parameters such as number of procedures, complications, aesthetic outcome, tactile and erogenous sensation, voiding, donor-site morbidity, scrotoplasty, and sexual intercourse are assessed.

Conclusions.—In the absence of prospective randomized studies, it is not possible to prove whether the radial forearm flap truly is the standard technique in penile reconstruction. However, this large study demonstrates that the radial forearm phalloplasty is a very reliable technique for the creation, mostly in two stages, of a normal-appearing penis and scrotum, always allowing the patient to void while standing and in most cases also to experience sexual satisfaction. The relative disadvantages of this technique are the rather high number of initial fistulas, the residual scar on the forearm, and the potential long-term urologic complications. Despite the lack of actual data to support this statement, the authors feel strongly that a multidisciplinary approach with close cooperation between the reconstructive/plastic surgeon and the urologist is an absolute requisite for obtaining the best possible results.

▶ This impressive series of patients (287 reconstructions) provides a number of useful insights into total penile reconstruction. First of all, the authors have been able to develop a logical and staged approach based on careful analysis of their multiple procedures. They conclude that attempting to do everything for a female to male transexual (including mastectomy) at a single stage is really not practical or appropriate. Secondly, they have demonstrated that they can construct a very satisfactory appearing and functioning penis using the radial forearm flap. The examples shown in the article are most likely their best results, but even so, they are impressive. Other, less challenging techniques, including pedicled flap reconstruction, may be easier to do but are likely to yield less consistently successful outcomes. Finally, the reader has to come away from this article with a sense that this is really a complicated operation, probably done best by individuals performing it on a regular basis. The best evidence for this conclusion is the data showing a notably high complication rate in cases done by this group despite their extensive experience. And as is usually the case with complex reconstructive procedures, the participation of multiple cooperating disciplines in the overall effort is likely to result in the highest chance of a successful outcome.

R. L. Ruberg, MD

Sensate Lateral Arm Flap for Defects of the Lower Leg

Kalbermatten DF, Wettstein R, vonkanel O, et al (Univ Hosp of Basel, Switzerland; et al)
Ann Plast Surg 61:40-46, 2008

Ideally, reconstruction of lower extremity soft tissue defects includes not only an esthetically pleasing 3-dimensional shape and solid anchoring to the underlying structures to resist shear forces, but should also address the restoration of sensation. Therefore, we present a prospective study on defect reconstruction of the lower leg and ankle to evaluate the role of sensate free fasciocutaneous lateral arm flap and the impact of sensory nerve reconstruction. Thirty patients were allocated randomly to the study group (n = 15) that obtained end-to-side sensate coaptation using the lower lateral cutaneous brachial nerve to the tibial nerve using the epineural window technique, or to the control group reconstructed without nerve coaptation. At 1-year follow-up the patients were evaluated for pain sensation, thermal sensibility, static and moving 2-point discrimination, and Semmes-Weinstein monofilament tests. Data from both groups were compared and statistically analyzed with the Mann-Whitney U test and the Fisher exact test. Flaps of the study group reached a static and moving 2-point discrimination and Semmes-Weinstein monofilament tests nearly equal to the contralateral leg area and significantly better than flaps of the control group. Donor damage morbidity of the tibial nerve did not occur. To our point of view resensation should be carried out by end-to-side neurorrhaphy to the tibial nerve because of the superior restoration of sensibility.

▶ The authors introduce us to a modification of the lateral arm flap that permits measurably increased sensation of the flap and improved flap integration. Even though they were not able to demonstrate any other benefit of their new approach, they still recommend using their modification. Is this justified? Probably so. The addition of the sensory nerve to the flap probably requires relatively little additional operative time, and is shown to have no detrimental neurological effect at either the donor or recipient site. There are a number of situations in which the improved sensation could have clear clinical benefit. The limitations of the study simply did not permit demonstration of these theoretical benefits. My microsurgical colleagues feel that this is a worthwhile improvement in a very versatile reconstructive technique.

R. L. Ruberg, MD

Outcome of Arterial Reconstruction and Free-Flap Coverage in Diabetic Foot Ulcers: Long-Term Results
Randon C, Vermassen F, Jacobs B, et al (Ghent Univ Hosp, Belgium)
World J Surg 34:177-184, 2010

Background.—Major amputation for advanced soft tissue loss with bone and tendon exposure, can be prevented in diabetes patients with a combined arterial reconstruction and free-flap transfer. We reviewed our 15-year outcome and evaluated the feasibility to save diabetic feet by means of this aggressive strategy.

Methods.—A total of 55 type II diabetes patients (42–80 years of age), hospitalized between January 1992 and December 2006 for a combined arterial reconstruction and free-flap transfer, were followed until December 2007. All would have otherwise required at least a below-knee amputation. Arterial reconstructions, preferentially with autologous vein, were performed in combination with free tissue transfer, simultaneously or staged. The rectus abdominis muscle was the most frequently used muscle graft, although in recent years a growing number of alternative muscle and perforator flaps were used.

Results.—The mean follow-up was 22 months (range: 1–180 months). Major complications occurred in 37% with only one in-hospital death. Major amputations were performed in 15 patients, 5 in the early postoperative period. The 1-year and 3-year limb salvage rates were 75.8 and 64.3%, with a 1-year and 3-year amputation-free survival of 69.5% and 55.8%. The 1-year and 3-year secondary patency for graft and free flap was 78.7% and 60.2%, respectively. Renal insufficiency was a major risk factor for limb loss (Hazard Ratio [HR] 5.581 (95% Confidence Interval [CI] 1.384–22.5)). Independent ambulation was regained in 38 patients.

Conclusions.—Combined arterial reconstruction and free tissue transfer provides an excellent long-term result with regard to amputation-free survival and limb salvage. It should be considered in every diabetes patient with extensive soft tissue deficits before amputation is performed.

▶ This study reaffirms previous reports that show the value of this combined aggressive approach to limb salvage in diabetic patients. Unique to this study are the selection of diabetic patients exclusively and the reporting of long-term results in these patients. The authors don't report a significant complication rate, but also show impressive long-term graft patency and flap viability. The complication rate should be judged acceptable in light of the fact that the alternative treatment is rarely completely successful: return to functional use of an extremity after either below-knee or above-knee amputation in a diabetic patient is very unlikely. However, those patients undergoing this aggressive treatment who don't have, or who survive, complications are likely to have a functional extremity. In this case, the likelihood of a favorable outcome more than justifies the significant risk of the combined vascular reconstruction/free flap approach.

R. L. Ruberg, MD

Long-Term Results of Salvage Surgery in Severely Injured Feet

Ferreira RC, Sakata MA, Costa MT, et al (Santa Casa Med School, São Paulo, Brazil)
Foot Ankle Int 31:113-123, 2010

Background.—The purpose of our study was to analyze the long-term outcome of salvage surgery in severely injured feet.

Material and Methods.—Clinical-functional scores and radiographic findings were used to assess the outcome of 18 patients (19 feet) with severe trauma to the foot treated at a tertiary teaching hospital from January, 1985 to October, 2005. Fourteen males and four females with a mean age of 35 years were studied. The mean followup period was 76 months.

Results.—There was a high incidence of late complications and poor functional results (mean $AOFAS = 68/100$): chronic pain, 15 of 19 (mean analogical pain score 3.4/10); global foot stiffness, 11 of 19 (with radiographic evidence of arthritis of the remaining foot joints in 13 of 19); residual deformity, 13 of 19; arterial-venous insufficiency, 12 of 19; signs of reflex sympathetic dystrophy, seven of 19; chronic ulcers, six of 19; and chronic osteomyelitis, two of 19. Twelve patients had a visible limp and only 8 of 19 returned to work.

Conclusions.—Five years after severe foot injury most patients had painful stiffness and only 40% returned to work. Long-term clinical-functional results of the severely injured foot may be disappointing.

▶ This is a very interesting study. The number of chronic problems in this group is troubling. Years ago a German study showed that salvage of a severely injured lower limb was worth it because even though the initial expenditures are high, the long-term results and costs were better.

While this study does not directly refute that, it does call into question patient selection. Understanding when an amputation is better or not is a real art.

D. J. Smith, Jr, MD

Hand and Finger Replantation After Protracted Ischemia (More Than 24 Hours)

Lin C-H, Aydyn N, Lin Y-T, et al (Chang Gung Univ, Taoyuan, Taiwan)
Ann Plast Surg 64:286-290, 2010

Ischemia tolerance has been a major concern during hand and finger replantation. Because of multiple referrals and damage control resuscitation, ischemia is occasionally prolonged for more than 24 hours. Amputation impairs functional efficiency in amputees; therefore, if there is a favorable indication for replantation, microsurgical replantation can be performed to salvage the function of the affected part to an acceptable extent.

Between 1998 and 2006, 14 patients underwent 25 replantations after prolonged ischemia of more than 24 hours. Of the 14 patients, 12 were referred to our hospital after unsuccessful replantations and admitted to the emergency room. Two of these patients underwent thumb amputations, and 10 patients underwent multiple digit amputations. Two patients underwent wrist amputation with associated polytrauma and profound shock, both hand replantations were performed on the following day after ICU management with damage control resuscitation was performed to control excessive bleeding and stabilize vital signs.

In this study, 16 replantations were successful and 9 failed; thus, the success rate was 64.0%. Several secondary procedures were required for restoring the functional ability of the reconstructed parts.

Ischemia time is critical for limb salvage. Hands and fingers have very little muscle tissue. Hence, replantation of these parts can be performed even in the case of prolonged ischemia to restore the hand function.

▶ Replantation after prolonged ischemic periods is well documented to have higher risk of failure, whether it is due to immediate ischemia-reperfusion injury and no-reflow phenomenon or eventual long-term failure due to poor functional outcomes. Although prolonged ischemia is essentially a clinical determination, periods longer than 6 to 12 hours of warm ischemia or 12 to 24 hours of cold ischemia is generally viewed as contraindications for replantation of digits. In this article, the authors suggest that these periods can be tolerated with a 64% success rate in restoring not only microvascular circulation but also functional outcome. Given that some of their patients had failed a digital replantation attempt at an outside facility and 2 had more proximal amputations at the wrist level, their outcomes are surprisingly good, as these patients undoubtedly had intermittent periods of warm and cold ischemia during their management, and the functional goal of obtaining pinch and opposition are very difficult to match with prostheses. It is difficult to shift paradigms and management strategies in surgery; however, with better than expected success of replantation after prolonged ischemia, this article and previous case reports suggest that it is possible and a worthwhile attempt in the proper clinical setting. Whether mechanical or pharmacologic preconditioning following arterial anastamosis, localized hypothermia, or use of washout solutions on the amputated segment—as in solid organ transplantation—have any additional benefits are questions that should also be addressed in future studies. Also, it raises the question whether replantation centers of excellence should be established. I doubt if any of these referrals would have ever happened in the United States.

D. J. Smith, Jr, MD

Botulinum toxin in preparation of oral cavity for microsurgical reconstruction

Corradino B, Di Lorenzo S, Mossuto C, et al (Università di Palermo, Italy)
Acta Otolaryngol 130:156-160, 2010

Conclusions.—Infiltration of botulinum toxin in the major salivary glands allows a temporary reduction of salivation that begins 8 days afterwards and returns to normal within 2 months. The inhibition of salivary secretion, carried out before the oral cavity reconstructive surgery, could allow a reduction of the incidence of oro-cutaneous fistulas and local complications.

Objectives.—Saliva stagnation is a risk factor for patients who have to undergo reconstructive microsurgery of the oral cavity, because of fistula formation and local complications in the oral cavity. The authors suggest infiltration of botulinum toxin in the major salivary glands to reduce salivation temporarily during the healing stage.

Patients and Methods.—During the preoperative stage, 20 patients with oral cavity carcinoma who were candidates for microsurgical reconstruction underwent sialoscintigraphy and a quantitative measurement of the salivary secretion. Injection of botulinum toxin was carried out in the salivary glands 4 days before surgery. The saliva quantitative measurement was repeated 3 and 8 days after infiltration, sialoscintigraphy after 15 days.

Results.—In all cases, the saliva quantitative measurement revealed a reduction of 50% and 70% of the salivary secretion after 72 h and 8 days, respectively. A lower rate of local complications was observed.

▶ This study is another example of a very innovative use of Botox. Injecting Botox to keep the saliva levels low is an excellent physiologic use in head and neck surgery. It makes sense that this would decrease complications. This is probably worth a try, as there is little downside.

D. J. Smith, Jr, MD

9 Miscellaneous

Assessing the Plastic Surgery Workforce: A Template for the Future of Plastic Surgery

Rohrich RJ, McGrath MH, Lawrence WT, et al (Univ of Texas Southwestern Med Ctr, Dallas; Univ of California San Francisco Med Ctr; Univ of Kansas Med Ctr)

Plast Reconstr Surg 125:736-746, 2010

Background.—The American Society of Plastic Surgeons (ASPS) formed the Plastic Surgery Workforce Task Force to study the size of the plastic surgery workforce and make recommendations about future workforce needs. The ASPS member workforce survey and two supplementary surveys of plastic surgery academic chairs and senior residents were developed to gain insights on current and projected demand for plastic surgery procedures and to find out more about plastic surgeons' current daily practice patterns and plans for the future.

Methods.—The ASPS member workforce survey was mailed to 2500 randomly selected ASPS active members practicing in the United States, and a second mailing was sent to 388 unique members who practice in an academic setting; a total of 1256 surgeons responded (43.5 percent response rate). The survey of academic chairs was distributed to 103 attendees at the annual meeting of the Association of Academic Chairmen of Plastic Surgery, and 74 returned the survey (71.8 percent response rate). The survey of senior residents was e-mailed to 183 graduating residents, of whom 65 responded (35.5 percent response rate).

Results.—Useful demographic information regarding the current plastic surgery workforce was obtained from these surveys. In addition, insight into current trends in practice composition and procedural demand was gained.

Conclusions.—The rapid growth of the U.S. population, combined with a significant number of plastic surgeons approaching retirement and an unchanged number of plastic surgery residency training positions, will lead to a discrepancy between the demand for plastic surgery procedures and the supply of appropriately trained physicians. Without an increase in the number of plastic surgeons trained each year, there will be a significant shortage in the next 10 to 15 years.

▶ Do we need more plastic surgeons? As the authors and many others before them state, it depends on what you mean by plastic surgery and to whom you ask the question. This is an important demographic study from the standpoint of the specialty but fails to answer some very basic questions. One needs to more clearly look at the current and future projected needs and wants of the public for plastic surgical services as defined currently and the types and credentials of the individuals who should and can provide that service in a competent manner. If plastic surgical services and competitors, safe and unsafe, enter the market as they clearly have done in both reconstructive and cosmetic surgeries, will training more plastic surgeons result in a larger market share of reconstructive or cosmetic surgery? As to the former, we have all seen the number of plastic surgeons performing the gamut of noncosmetic procedures (head and neck cancer and reconstruction, hand surgery, facial fractures, pediatric urology, burn surgery, trauma, etc) fall significantly in the last 25 or more years, as other specialists certified by the American Board of Medical Specialties are trained to offer services in these areas and willingly do so. In some instances, this is because of a greater number of those specialists, and in other instances, this is because plastic surgeons have made choices to leave or decrease their involvement in reconstructive procedures. But the bottom line is that patients are being offered these services by professionals conventionally educated and trained to provide them. In practical terms, how will we convince plastic surgeons, as they progress in their professional lives, to voluntarily continue to practice reconstructive surgery? As one moves into the realm of cosmetic surgery, competition is even more keen and the education and training of some providers are less conventional and in some instances are problematic. One of the key issues, from the standpoint of patient safety, is to convince legislatures that their state medical acts need to be amended so that a medical license to practice is not open-ended and must be granted based on accepted national standards of education, training, certification, and maintenance of certification of its licensees.

S. H. Miller, MD, MPH

The World's Experience With Facial Transplantation: What Have We Learned Thus Far?

Gordon CR, Siemionow M, Papay F, et al (Cleveland Clinic, OH; et al)
Ann Plast Surg 63:572-578, 2009

The objective of this review article is to summarize the published details and media citations for all seven face transplants performed to date to point out deficiencies in those reports so as to provide the basis for examining where the field of face transplantation stands, and to act as a stimulus to enhance the quality of future reports and functional outcomes. Overall long-term function of facial alloflaps has been reported satisfactorily in all seven cases. Sensory recovery ranges between 3 and 6 months, and acceptable motor recovery ranges between 9 and 12 months. The risks and benefits of facial composite tissue allotransplantation, which involves mandatory lifelong immunosuppression analogous to kidney transplants, should be deliberated by each institution's multidisciplinary face transplant team. Face transplantation has been shown thus far to be a viable option in some patients suffering severe facial deficits which are not amenable to modern-day reconstructive technique.

▶ In addition to keeping the rest of us informed about the progress of these patients, I believe it is essential for the centers performing this type of surgery to form and maintain a registry for research and to foster information sharing in real time among themselves and other potential centers interested in facial transplantation. Data regarding significant complications and failures needs to be shared quickly.

S. H. Miller, MD, MPH

Quality of life 15 years after sex reassignment surgery for transsexualism
Kuhn A, Bodmer C, Stadlmayr W, et al (Frauenklinik, Univ Hosp and Univ of Bern, Switzerland)
Fertil Steril 92:1685-1689, 2009

Objective.—To evaluate quality of life and patients' satisfaction in transsexual patients (TS) after sex reassignment operation compared with healthy controls.

Design.—A case–control study.

Setting.—A tertiary referral center.

Patient(s).—Patients after sex reassignment operation were compared with a similar group of healthy controls in respect to quality of life and general satisfaction.

Intervention(s).—For quality of life we used the King's Health Questionnaire, which was distributed to the patients and to the control group. Visual analogue scale was used for the determination of satisfaction.

Main Outcome Measure(s).—Main outcome measures were quality of life and satisfaction.

Result(s).—Fifty-five transsexuals participated in this study. Fifty-two were male-to-female and 3 female-to-male. Quality of life as determined by the King's Health Questionnaire was significantly lower in general health, personal, physical and role limitations. Patients' satisfaction was significantly lower compared with controls. Emotions, sleep, and incontinence impact as well as symptom severity is similar to controls. Overall satisfaction was statistically significant lower in TS compared with controls.

Conclusion(s).—Fifteen years after sex reassignment operation quality of life is lower in the domains general health, role limitation, physical limitation, and personal limitation.

▶ Techniques for gender reassignment surgery have continued to improve over time. Aesthetic results are better, and complications appear to be less frequent in both male-to-female and, especially, female-to-male transsexual patients. This study attempts to answer one important question that is not directly related to the technical surgical improvements, but it leaves many other important questions still unanswered. The article clearly shows, using a variety of established measurement tools, that the quality of life for transsexual patients who have undergone gender reassignment surgery is still lower than that of the normal population. Does this mean that the operation is a failure and shouldn't be done? Until there is a study comparing results before surgery and then a number of years after surgery, this question can't be answered. It is certainly possible that the patients actually have substantial improvement in quality of life after this surgery, and therefore the surgery is highly successful. Or the opposite could be true—that their quality of life deteriorates despite the surgery. Without pre- and long-term postoperative quality of life data, the true success (not just the technical success) of gender reassignment surgery can't be determined. This study also should probably be considered valid only for male-to-female patients because the number of female-to-male patients in the series was insufficient to make any reliable conclusion.

R. L. Ruberg, MD

Cutaneous Surgery in Patients on Warfarin Therapy

Nelms JK, Wooten Al, Heckler F (Allegheny General Hosp, Pittsburgh, PA)
Ann Plast Surg 62:275-277, 2009

Warfarin is a commonly used anticoagulant for patients with prosthetic heart valves, atrial fibrillation, stroke, deep vein thrombosis, or pulmonary emboli to prevent thromboembolic events. There is no clear consensus regarding the perioperative management of warfarin therapy for plastic surgery procedures. Our objective is to evaluate the safety and quantify any increased morbidity in patients on warfarin therapy, undergoing soft tissue surgery.

In a retrospective chart review of prospectively collected data, patients undergoing cutaneous surgery on warfarin therapy from 2000 to 2006 were identified. Perioperative complications were evaluated, including major hemorrhage, incisional bleeding, hematoma, wound or flap complications, graft success, and cosmetic surgical outcome. A total of 26 anticoagulated patients who underwent 56 procedures were included. Intraoperative bleeding was controlled in all cases without difficulty. Minor postoperative bleeding was noted in 1 patient, and this was easily controlled with gentle pressure. All wounds healed without complication, including 2 split thickness skin grafts. The cosmesis of all scars was acceptable.

Anticoagulation with warfarin can be safely continued in patients undergoing minor soft tissue procedures, thereby avoiding the risk of potentially devastating thromboembolic events.

▶ This article provides supporting evidence for an approach that myself and many of my colleagues have had for years. For minor procedures done under local anesthesia, it is not necessary to require patients to discontinue warfarin therapy. Of course, it is necessary to define "minor"; but in my experience (and in that of the authors of this article) "minor" includes not just simple excisions, but also local flaps and grafts. We are surgeons capable of achieving hemostasis in complex procedures, so any extra bleeding caused by anticoagulation in a small wound is easily controlled, with a minimum risk for postoperative problems related to bleeding (as documented in this article). I do recommend having some form of cautery device available for these cases, especially because some of these patients are at risk for complications of the administration of epinephrine and must be done without pharmacologic vasoconstriction.

R. L. Ruberg, MD

Cutaneous Surgery in Patients on Warfarin Therapy
Nelms JK, Wooten AI, Heckler F (Allegheny General Hosp, Pittsburgh, PA)
Ann Plast Surg 62:275-277, 2009

Warfarin is a commonly used anticoagulant for patients with prosthetic heart valves, atrial fibrillation, stroke, deep vein thrombosis, or pulmonary emboli to prevent thromboembolic events. There is no clear consensus regarding the perioperative management of warfarin therapy for plastic surgery procedures. Our objective is to evaluate the safety and quantify any increased morbidity in patients on warfarin therapy, undergoing soft tissue surgery.

In a retrospective chart review of prospectively collected data, patients undergoing cutaneous surgery on warfarin therapy from 2000 to 2006 were identified. Perioperative complications were evaluated, including major hemorrhage, incisional bleeding, hematoma, wound or flap complications, graft success, and cosmetic surgical outcome. A total of 26 anticoagulated patients who underwent 56 procedures were included. Intraoperative bleeding was controlled in all cases without difficulty. Minor postoperative bleeding was noted in 1 patient, and this was easily controlled with gentle pressure. All wounds healed without complication, including 2 split thickness skin grafts. The cosmesis of all scars was acceptable.

Anticoagulation with warfarin can be safely continued in patients undergoing minor soft tissue procedures, thereby avoiding the risk of potentially devastating thromboembolic events.

▶ As the population ages, more and more of our patients are being treated with blood thinners, including warfarin, for a variety of thromboembolic conditions. It is critical for us to understand when we must stop such therapy before surgery, and when it can and should be continued to prevent serious subsequent thromboembolic events. The issue has been studied in a variety of different specialties, but not really in plastic surgery. This study is really too small to draw many firm conclusions, but the overwhelming trend suggests that performing minor cutaneous surgery while patients are on warfarin is safe. As the authors suggest, a large prospective, multicenter study defining appropriate management of plastic surgery patients on anticoagulant medication would be extremely worthwhile.

For further reading on this subject I suggest articles by Gallus et al.[1]

S. H. Miller, MD, MPH

Reference

1. Gallus AS, Baker RI, Chong BH, Ockelford PA, Street AM. Consensus guidelines for warfarin therapy. Recommendations from the Australian Society of Thrombosis and Hemostasis. *Med J Aust.* 2000;172:600-605.

Differential judgements about disfigurement: the role of location, age and gender in decisions made by observers
Gardiner MD, Topps A, Richardson G, et al (Royal Free Hosp, London, UK; et al)
J Plast Reconstr Aesthet Surg 63:73-77, 2010

Psychological distress associated with disfiguring facial lesions is common. However, whilst the intrusive behaviour of observers is commonly reported, for example, staring, comments and questions, these factors which may influence the judgements of observers have not been well described. This is important as it may influence a subject's perception of how their appearance is viewed by the external world.

This study is the first to investigate age and gender differences when measuring the importance of location in judgements about facial disfigurement. Observers were asked to rank the impact of simulated lesions in different positions on the face of Caucasian subjects. Age and gender varied in both groups.

Our results show that lesions on the young and female subjects are ranked as having a greater impact than those on the old and male subjects. Lesions on central facial features have a higher impact than those located more peripherally. Both of these findings were not significantly influenced by observer age or gender.

These results are discussed in terms of culturally derived attributions about appearance. It is also suggested that there is a scope to use feedback on how disfigurement is viewed by others as a therapeutic tool in clinical settings.

▶ This is a fascinating study about the role of location, age, and gender in assessing the degree of an artificially contrived disfigurement, a black dot in different locations on the faces of a series of models. The goal, of course, was to assess how observers judge the disfigurements and to potentially use this information to aid those who are disfigured in their social contacts. Findings that central disfigurements in the young and in females had the most impact are not in the least surprising, but it is obvious that these findings need to be explored in greater detail. For example, the study was biased in that Caucasians were the subjects, the observers were predominantly Caucasians, and it was difficult to know what people really thought of the black dot used for disfigurement without asking open-ended questions of the observers. It would also be useful to further delineate the age ranges of the older participants (males or females) over 40 years of age. Finally, it would be very useful to evaluate real subjects to determine how an understanding of what an observer thinks about when he/she sees the disfigurement might affect the social interaction.

S. H. Miller, MD, MPH

Methicillin-Sensitive and Methicillin-Resistant *Staphylococcus aureus*: Preventing Surgical Site Infections Following Plastic Surgery
Elward AM, McAndrews JM, Young VL (Washington Univ School of Medicine, St Louis, MO; St Louis, MO; BodyAesthetic Plastic Surgery & Skin Care Ctr, St Louis, MO)
Aesthet Surg J 29:232-244, 2009

Learning Objectives.—The reader is presumed to have a broad understanding of aesthetic surgical procedures. After studying this article, the participant should be able to:

1. Explain the microbiology of *Staphylococcus* species and discuss antibiotic resistance development in *Staphylococcus* species and assess how clinical outcomes are affected.
2. Identify the epidemiology of *Staphylococcus* carriers and the impact on the clinical practice and regulation. Practice effective measures that prevent surgical site infections.
3. Practice screening for and decolonizing of patients with methicillin-resistant *Staphylococcus aureus* (MRSA).

Physicians may earn 2.5 AMA PRA Category 1 Credit™ by successfully completing the examination based on material covered in this article. The examination begins on page 245. As a meaure of the success of the education we hope you will receive from this article, **we encourage you to log on to the Aesthetic Society website and take the preexamination before reading this article.** Once you have completed the article, you may then take the examination again for CME credit. The Aesthetic Society will be able to compare your answers and use this data for future reference as we attempt to continually improve the CME articles we offer. ASAPS members can complete this CME examination online by logging on to the ASAPS Members-Only Website (http://www.surgery.org/members) and clicking on "Clinical Education" in the menu bar.

Staphylococcus aureus is the most common cause of surgical site infections (SSI), with both methicillin-sensitive and methicillin-resistant strains causing these infections. The incidence of methicillin-resistant *S aureus* (MRSA) has increased in the US over the past decade, largely due to the emergence of community-acquired MRSA (CA-MRSA). This article reviews the microbiology and epidemiology of methicillin-sensitive *S aureus* (MSSA) and MRSA, risk factors for surgical site infections among plastic surgery patients, the evidence supporting preoperative screening and decolonization measures to prevent surgical site infections caused by MRSA, recommendations for anti-microbial prophylaxis, and treatment recommendations for surgical site infections. Other proven methods of reducing SSI, including maintenance of normothermia during surgery, glucose control, cessation of nicotine use, and not shaving the surgical site preoperatively are discussed.

▶ Given the morbidity, potential mortality, medical-legal implications, and economic costs of methicillin-resistant *Staphylococcus aureus* (MRSA) infections, all surgeons should be familiar with the most current thoughts and recommendations for preventing infections and treating infected patients. Although plastic surgery specific guidelines are not available, we can draw upon experience from other surgical specialties. The spread of MRSA from the community to health care facilities has resulted in a new classification of health care-acquired MRSA (HA-MRSA) and community-acquired MRSA (CA-MRSA). Still to be determined is the role of preoperative screening and active surveillance, need for MRSA decolonization, and risk factors specific to plastic surgery patients. Recent state legislation and public reporting of nosocomial infections reinforces the need to take active measures in addressing this problem. This article provides an excellent update on MRSA infections and should be read.

K. A. Gutowski, MD

20-Year Experience With the Conrad Modification of the Freer Elevator as a Pull-in Suture Introducer
Torgerson C, Conrad K (Univ of Toronto, Ontario, Canada)
Arch Facial Plast Surg 11:267-269, 2009

A modified Freer elevator was created to aid the safe placement of alloplasts in a subcutaneous dissection pocket. We believe that this innovation represents a better way to insert nonrigid facial alloplasts and grafts and that it contributes to the reduced technique-related complications of migration, kinking, and asymmetry; it also minimizes tissue trauma and unnecessary surgical explorations.

▶ This article describes a very simple but clever modification of the standard freer elevator that expands its capabilities. Essentially a groove is fashioned into the side of the elevator that can contain a Keith needle. The elevator is used to create the pocket, and then the Keith needle can be released into the most distal portion of the pocket and passed through the skin. The suture is passed through the implant and is then used to pull the implant into the proper position. For anyone who has tried to pass a needle precisely down a tunneled path without engaging the sides (and thus preventing the graft of the implant from following the suture) this is a very appealing concept. The pulling of implants or cartilage grafts in this manner is more predictable than the pushing of these materials down very constrained passageways. Although it is not clear that this will result in a decreased number of malposition complications (as is stated in the article) it will certainly facilitate the operative conduct of these maneuvers.

G. C. Gurtner, MD

The osmotic tissue expander: a three-year clinical experience
Obdeijn MC, Nicolai J-PA, Werker PMN (Univ of Groningen, The Netherlands)
J Plast Reconstr Aesthet Surg 62:1219-1222, 2009

Closure of defects after trauma or excision of neoplasms is a basic skill in plastic surgery. Local, regional and distant flaps lead to additional scars. Skin recruitment by serial excision or skin expansion is a less damaging option for defects that must be closed. Advantages of tissue expansion include good colour and texture match. Disadvantages are the need for a second operation, use of an implant with the attendant risk of infection, time needed for inflation of the device, repeat visits to the clinic, and punctures to inflate the expander. To overcome the last disadvantage, an osmotic expander was developed in Germany in 1999 by OSMED GmbH (Ilmenau).

▶ A refreshing study from the Netherlands outlining a less than stellar experience with the Holy Grail of tissue expansion, the self-inflating expander, OSMED. The device was manufactured in Germany and approved for use in Europe for a wide variety of conditions, but only for anophthalmia in the United States. The expanders used are all quite small and the end volume of fluid as measured, when possible and only in a few cases, upon removal did not exceed 100 cc, and in many instances was considerably less. The authors report a complication rate of 77% and a premature removal rate of 55%. They conclude that their experience was not as positive as the experience described by Ronert in 2004.[1] Evidently the new era of osmotic tissue expanders is not yet here.

S. H. Miller, MD, MPH

Reference

1. Ronert MA, Hofheinz H, Manassa E, Asgarouladi H, Olbrisch RR. The beginning of a new era in tissue expansion: self-filling osmotic tissue expander–four-year clinical experience. *Plast Reconstr Surg*. 2004;114:1025-1031.

Article Index

Chapter 1: Congenital

Chapter 2: Neoplastic, Inflammatory and Degenerative Conditions

Chapter 3: Trauma

Chapter 4: Hand and Upper Extremity

Chapter 5: Aesthetic

Chapter 6: Breast

Chapter 7: Scars and Wound Healing

Chapter 8: Grafts, Flaps, and Microsurgery

Chapter 9: Miscellaneous

Author Index

Printed and bound by CPI Group (UK) Ltd, Croydon, CR0 4YY

08/05/2025

01864677-0006